Cancer Drug Discovery and Development

Series Editor

Beverly A. Teicher
Genzyme Corporation, Framington, MA, USA

For further volumes:
http://www.springer.com/series/7625

Derek LeRoith
Editor

Insulin-like Growth Factors and Cancer

From Basic Biology to Therapeutics

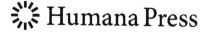

Editor
Derek LeRoith MD PhD
Chief of the Division of Endocrinology
Diabetes & Bone Diseases
Mt. Sinai School of Medicine
1 Gustave Levy Place
New York, NY 10029, USA
derek.leroith@mssm.edu

ISBN 978-1-4614-0597-9   e-ISBN 978-1-4614-0598-6
DOI 10.1007/978-1-4614-0598-6
Springer New York Dordrecht Heidelberg London

Library of Congress Control Number: 2011935731

© Springer Science+Business Media, LLC 2012
All rights reserved. This work may not be translated or copied in whole or in part without the written permission of the publisher (Springer Science+Business Media, LLC, 233 Spring Street, New York, NY 10013, USA), except for brief excerpts in connection with reviews or scholarly analysis. Use in connection with any form of information storage and retrieval, electronic adaptation, computer software, or by similar or dissimilar methodology now known or hereafter developed is forbidden.
The use in this publication of trade names, trademarks, service marks, and similar terms, even if they are not identified as such, is not to be taken as an expression of opinion as to whether or not they are subject to proprietary rights.
While the advice and information in this book are believed to be true and accurate at the date of going to press, neither the authors nor the editors nor the publisher can accept any legal responsibility for any errors or omissions that may be made. The publisher makes no warranty, express or implied, with respect to the material contained herein.

Printed on acid-free paper

Humana Press is part of Springer Science+Business Media (www.springer.com)

Preface

The insulin-like growth factor (IGF) system has long been known from cell culture systems to be involved in cancer cell biology. Most varieties of cancer cells express components of the IGF system; ligands, receptors, or IGF-binding proteins (IGFBPs). Furthermore, proliferation and cell survival are affected by manipulations of this system. Only recently has this important relationship become clinically relevant; both from a diagnostic and a therapeutic point of view. In this compilation of chapters by world-authorities on the topic, we have aimed at presenting this concept from the epidemiological, basic biology, and therapeutic aspects.

Epidemiologically, studies have demonstrated that the relative risk for various epithelial cancers, such as prostate, breast, and colon, are associated with circulating IGF-1 levels that are in the upper quartiles of the normal range. Both aging and obesity are associated with increased cancer risk and its relationship with these normal physiological processes maybe explained by varying IGF-1 levels. On the other hand, obesity and Type 2 diabetes are conditions that commonly cause endogenous hyperinsulinemia secondary to the insulin resistance, and the elevated circulating insulin levels have recently been shown to be related to increased cancer risk.

Basic biological studies have given further insights into the connection between cancer and the IGF system. Most cancer cells and indeed tumor samples demonstrate increased expression of the IGF-1 receptor (IGF-1R). The levels of IGF-1Rs are the result, in many cases, of mutations in tumor suppressor gene products, such as p53, WT1, PTEN, and BRAC1/2 genes. These proteins normally inhibit the IGF-1R promoter, but when mutated cause increased gene expression. Activation of the receptor by the ligands, insulin, IGF-1, or IGF-2 results in increased proliferation of the cells, with IGF-2 demonstrating the most powerful mitogenic effects of the three. While the insulin receptor (IR) was generally considered a purely metabolic receptor, studies have identified a mitogenic subtype of the receptor (IR-A) that is also expressed in some common cancers, such as breast cancer. Since insulin and IGF-2 both activate this receptor equally, it may play an important role in the cancer biology.

Inhibition of these effects has become a potentially important therapeutic tool in oncology; from antibodies to the receptor or the ligands to tyrosine kinase inhibitors.

Indeed, many potential drugs have been developed and are being tested in preclinical and phase 1–3 clinical trials.

Thus, the IGF system and cancer is a prime example of translational research, where epidemiology has driven to some degree the basic science, and the basic science is now driving clinical therapeutics. Bringing these concepts and information to the reader has required enormous efforts by the most outstanding investigators in this field and we are all extremely grateful for their devotion and hard work.

New York, NY, USA   Derek LeRoith

Contents

1 Epidemiology of IGF-1 and Cancer 1
Katharina Nimptsch and Edward Giovannucci

2 Aging and Cancer: The IGF-I Connection 25
Kalina Biernacka, Claire Perks, and Jeff Holly

3 Obesity, Type 2 Diabetes and Cancer 37
Rosalyn D. Ferguson and Derek LeRoith

4 IGF System and Breast Cancer 73
Marc A. Becker and Douglas Yee

**5 The Role of Insulin-Like Growth Factor Signaling in Prostate
Cancer Development and Progression** 85
Bruce Montgomery, James Dean, and Stephen Plymate

**6 IGF-1 Cellular Action and its Relationship to Cancer:
Evidence from in Vitro and in Vivo Studies** 105
Rosalyn D. Ferguson, Nyosha Alikhani, Archana Vijayakumar,
Yvonne Fierz, Dara Cannata, and Shoshana Yakar

7 Insulin-Like Growth Factor Signaling in Pediatric Sarcomas 147
Xiaolin Wan, Su Young Kim, and Lee J. Helman

**8 Cancer Genes, Tumor Suppressors, and Regulation
of IGF1-R Gene Expression in Cancer** 159
Haim Werner, Zohar Attias-Geva, Itay Bentov, Rive Sarfstein,
Hagit Schayek, Doron Weinstein, and Ilan Bruchim

9 Mouse Models of IGF-1R and Cancer 179
Craig I. Campbell, James J. Petrik, and Roger A. Moorehead

**10 Targeting the Insulin-Like Growth Factor-I Receptor
in Cancer Therapy** 193
David R. Clemmons

vii

11 Targeting Insulin-Like Growth Factor Receptor 1 (IGF-1R) and Insulin Receptor Signaling by Tyrosine Kinase Inhibitors in Cancer ... 215

Joan M. Carboni, Mark Wittman, and Fei Huang

12 Calories and Cancer: The Role of Insulin-Like Growth Factor-1 ... 231

Stephen D. Hursting, Sarah D. Smith, Alison E. Harvey, and Laura M. Lashinger

13 Cancer Cell Metabolism ... 245

Akash Patnaik, Jason W. Locasale, and Lewis C. Cantley

14 Overlaps Between the Insulin and IGF-I Receptor and Cancer ... 263

Antonino Belfiore and Roberta Malaguarnera

Index ... 279

Contributors

Nyosha Alikhani Division of Endocrinology, Diabetes and Bone Diseases, The Samuel Bronfman Department of Medicine, Mount Sinai School of Medicine, New York, NY, USA

Zohar Attias-Geva Department of Human Molecular Genetics and Biochemistry, Sackler School of Medicine, Tel Aviv University, Tel Aviv, Israel

Marc A. Becker Department of Pharmacology, University of Minnesota, Minneapolis, MN, USA

Antonino Belfiore Endocrinology, Department of Clinical and Experimental Medicine, University of Catanzaro, Catanzaro, Italy

Itay Bentov Department of Human Molecular Genetics and Biochemistry, Sackler School of Medicine, Tel Aviv University, Tel Aviv, Israel

Kalina Biernacka IGFs & Metabolic Endocrinology Group, School of Clinical Sciences, University of Bristol, Learning and Research Building, Southmead Hospital, Bristol, UK

Ilan Bruchim Department of Human Molecular Genetics and Biochemistry, Sackler School of Medicine, Tel Aviv University, Tel Aviv, Israel

Craig I. Campbell Department of Biomedical Sciences, Ontario Veterinary College, University of Guelph, Guelph, ON, Canada,

Dara Cannata Division of Endocrinology, Diabetes and Bone Diseases, The Samuel Bronfman Department of Medicine, Mount Sinai School of Medicine, New York, NY, USA

Lewis C. Cantley Division of Signal Transduction, Department of Medicine, Beth Israel Deaconess Medical Center, Boston, MA, USA

Department of Systems Biology, Harvard Medical School, Boston, MA, USA

Joan M. Carboni Oncology Drug Discovery, Bristol Myers Squibb Company, Princeton, NJ, USA

David R. Clemmons Division of Endocrinology, University of North Carolina, School of Medicine, Burnett-Womack, Chapel Hill, NC, USA

James Dean Division of Oncology, Department of Medicine, University of Washington, Seattle Cancer Care Alliance, Seattle, WA, USA

Rosalyn D. Ferguson Division of Endocrinology, Diabetes and Bone Diseases, The Samuel Bronfman Department of Medicine, Mount Sinai School of Medicine, New York, NY, USA

Yvonne Fierz Division of Endocrinology, Diabetes and Bone Diseases, The Samuel Bronfman Department of Medicine, Mount Sinai School of Medicine, New York, NY, USA

Edward Giovannucci Department of Nutrition, Harvard School of Public Health, Boston, MA, USA

Department of Epidemiology, Harvard School of Public Health, Boston, MA, USA

Alison E. Harvey Department of Nutritional Sciences, The University of Texas at Austin, Austin, TX, USA

Lee J. Helman Pediatric Oncology Branch, Center for Cancer Research, National Cancer Institute, National Institute of Health, Bethesda, MD, USA

Jeff Holly IGFs & Metabolic Endocrinology Group, School of Clinical Sciences, University of Bristol, Learning and Research Building, Southmead Hospital, Bristol, UK

Fei Huang Clinical Biomarkers-Oncology/DMCP, Princeton, NJ, USA

Stephen D. Hursting Department of Nutritional Sciences, The University of Texas at Austin, Austin, TX, USA

Department of Carcinogenesis, The University of Texas MD Anderson Cancer Center, Smithville, TX, USA

Su Young Kim Pediatric Oncology Branch, Center for Cancer Research, National Cancer Institute, National Institute of Health, Bethesda, MD, USA

Laura M. Lashinger Department of Nutritional Sciences, The University of Texas at Austin, Austin, TX, USA

Derek LeRoith Division of Endocrinology, Diabetes and Bone Diseases, The Samuel Bronfman Department of Medicine, Mount Sinai School of Medicine, New York, NY, USA

Jason W. Locasale Division of Signal Transduction, Department of Medicine, Beth Israel Deaconess Medical Center, Boston, MA, USA

Department of Systems Biology, Harvard Medical School, Boston, MA, USA

Roberta Malaguarnera Endocrinology, Department of Clinical and Experimental Medicine, University of Catanzaro, Catanzaro, Italy

Bruce Montgomery Division of Oncology, Department of Medicine, University of Washington, Seattle Cancer Care Alliance, Seattle, WA, USA

VA Puget Sound Health Care System, Seattle, WA, USA

Roger A. Moorehead Department of Biomedical Sciences, Ontario Veterinary College, University of Guelph, Guelph, ON, Canada

Katharina Nimptsch Department of Nutrition, Harvard School of Public Health, Boston, MA, USA

Akash Patnaik Division of Hematology/Oncology, Department of Medicine, Beth Israel Deaconess Medical Center, Boston, MA, USA

Division of Signal Transduction, Department of Medicine, Beth Israel Deaconess Medical Center, Boston, MA, USA

Department of Systems Biology, Harvard Medical School, Boston, MA, USA

Claire Perks IGFs & Metabolic Endocrinology Group, School of Clinical Sciences, University of Bristol, Learning and Research Building, Southmead Hospital, Bristol, UK

James J. Petrik Department of Biomedical Sciences, Ontario Veterinary College, University of Guelph, Guelph, ON, Canada

Stephen Plymate VA Puget Sound Health Care System, Seattle, WA, USA

Division of Geriatrics and Gerontology, Department of Medicine, University of Washington School of Medicine, Seattle, WA, USA

Rive Sarfstein Department of Human Molecular Genetics and Biochemistry, Sackler School of Medicine, Tel Aviv University, Tel Aviv, Israel

Hagit Schayek Department of Human Molecular Genetics and Biochemistry, Sackler School of Medicine, Tel Aviv University, Tel Aviv, Israel

Sarah D. Smith Department of Nutritional Sciences, The University of Texas at Austin, Austin, TX, USA

Archana Vijayakumar Division of Endocrinology, Diabetes and Bone Diseases, The Samuel Bronfman Department of Medicine, Mount Sinai School of Medicine, New York, NY, USA

Xiaolin Wan Pediatric Oncology Branch, Center for Cancer Research, National Cancer Institute, National Institute of Health, Bethesda, MD, USA

Doron Weinstein Department of Human Molecular Genetics and Biochemistry, Sackler School of Medicine, Tel Aviv University, Tel Aviv, Israel

Haim Werner Department of Human Molecular Genetics and Biochemistry, Sackler School of Medicine, Tel Aviv University, Tel Aviv, Israel

Mark Wittman Oncology Chemistry, Wallingford, CT, USA

Shoshana Yakar Division of Endocrinology, Diabetes and Bone Diseases, The Samuel Bronfman Department of Medicine, Mount Sinai School of Medicine, New York, NY, USA

Douglas Yee Masonic Cancer Center, University of Minnesota, Minneapolis, MN, USA

Department of Pharmacology, University of Minnesota, Minneapolis, MN, USA

Department of Medicine, University of Minnesota, Minneapolis, MN, USA

Chapter 1
Epidemiology of IGF-1 and Cancer

Katharina Nimptsch and Edward Giovannucci

Introduction

The incidence rates of cancer have been increasing steadily during the last 20 years in industrially developed parts of the world, notably Western Europe and North America (IARC 2008). The wide variation in cancer rates across the world as well as the observed increase in cancer risk among migrants moving from low-risk to high-risk countries convincingly suggest that environmental factors associated with a Western lifestyle may be major determinants of cancer risk. Western lifestyle is characterized by a diet high in total and saturated fat, refined sugars, and animal protein accompanied by physical inactivity. These lifestyle factors and overweight, which is most commonly related to Western diet and lifestyle, have been associated with insulin resistance and postprandial hyperinsulinemia, and many of them have been positively associated with different types of cancer in epidemiological studies. Both insulin and IGF-1 can enhance tumor development by stimulating cell proliferation and by inhibiting apoptosis. It has been hypothesized that variations in the insulin and insulin-like growth factor (IGF) pathways could account for the nutritional and lifestyle risk factors and the high cancer incidence in Western countries.

In this chapter, we first provide background information on the physiology of IGF-1 and its possible mechanistic links to cancer risk followed by a review of the literature of epidemiologic studies relating IGF-1 directly or indirectly to cancer risk.

E. Giovannucci (✉)
Department of Nutrition, Harvard School of Public Health,
Boston, MA, USA

Department of Epidemiology, Harvard School of Public Health,
Boston, MA, USA
e-mail: egiovann@hsph.harvard.edu

D. LeRoith (ed.), *Insulin-like Growth Factors and Cancer: From Basic Biology to Therapeutics*, Cancer Drug Discovery and Development,
DOI 10.1007/978-1-4614-0598-6_1, © Springer Science+Business Media, LLC 2012

Physiology of IGF-1 and Mechanism by Which IGF-1 May Influence Cancer Risk

The IGF System

The IGF family is formed by the two IGFs (IGF-1, IGF-2), two cell-membrane receptors (IGF-1R and IGF-2R) and six IGF binding proteins (IGFBP-1 to IGFBP-6). IGFs and IGFBPs are synthesized in most major tissue types, although the liver is the primary origin of these proteins that can be measured in the blood (Giovannucci 2001). IGF-1 and certain IGFBPs are upregulated by growth hormone. The two forms of IGF are structurally similar to insulin, sharing 40% homology in the amino-acid sequence with proinsulin (Furstenberger and Senn 2002).

IGFBPs are modulators of the action of IGFs regulating their bioavailability. In general, IGFs bound to IGFBPs have less affinity to IGF receptors (Pollak 2008). However, under certain circumstances some IGFBPs (-1, -2, -3, -5) may increase the IGF-1 binding to its receptor (Kaaks and Lukanova 2001; Pollak 2008). The major binding protein of IGF-1 is IGFBP-3, which forms a ternary complex with more than 90% of circulating IGF-1 and an acid-labile subunit.

Interrelation of IGF-1 and Insulin

The metabolism of IGF-1 is tightly linked to insulin. Both insulin and IGF act as tissue growth factors but also as hormones regulating energy metabolism and stimulating cell proliferation and anabolic processes (Pollak 2008). While the immediate effects of insulin on metabolism are mainly of short term (i.e., postprandial), the IGF-axis exerts longer-term growth-stimulating effects. Circulating insulin increases the bioactivity of IGF-1 by two mechanisms (Kaaks and Lukanova 2001; Pollak 2008), as summarized in Fig. 1.1. First, insulin enhances the hepatic IGF-1 synthesis through actions on growth hormone. Second, insulin reduces the hepatic secretion of two of their binding proteins (IGFBP-1 and IGFBP-2), resulting in higher free or bioactive IGF-1 levels (Fig. 1.1). Thus, although insulin has tumor growth-promoting properties itself, many of the mitogenic and antiapoptotic effects of insulin are believed to operate through the IGF-1 axis.

Receptor Signaling

The responses of insulin and IGFs are mediated by insulin and IGF receptors that are widely expressed on normal tissues. Cells that coexpress insulin and IGF-receptors have been shown to express an additional type of receptor which shows

1 Epidemiology of IGF-1 and Cancer

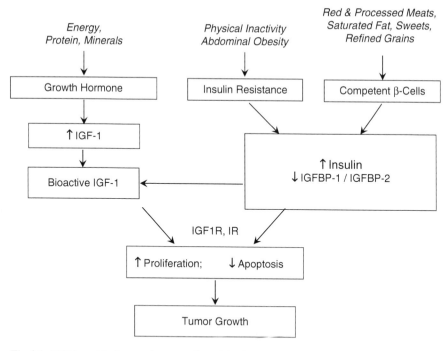

Fig. 1.1 IGF-1 metabolism and proposed model whereby Western lifestyle and dietary factors may affect tumor growth through alterations in the insulin/IGF axis

features of both types of receptors and is referred to as hybrid receptors (Pollak 2008). Besides normal tissues, insulin receptors (IR) and IGF-1 receptors (IGF1R) are expressed by most neoplastic cell lines. There are two types of insulin receptors. While one of them, the B isoform, primarily mediates metabolic effects of insulin in normal tissue, the A isoform is expressed on cancer cells and stimulates insulin-mediated mitogenesis (Pollak 2008). On the tumor level, insulin and IGF-1 act similar: binding to their receptors is followed by downstream signaling which may stimulate cell proliferation and inhibit apoptosis. These features are of crucial importance in the growth and development of cancer and also cancer-specific phenotypes such as invasion and metastasis are stimulated by binding of insulin or IGF-1 to their receptors (Pollak 2008). Both premalignant and cancerous stages can be influenced by insulin and IGF-1 (Giovannucci 2001). There is abundant evidence from in vitro as well as in vivo studies that IGF-1 may directly influence growth of various neoplasms (Pollak et al. 1998). Among others, growth stimulating effects of IGF-1 have been demonstrated in the mammary gland, endometrium, colorectum, and prostate (Kaaks and Lukanova 2001; Monti et al. 2007). Insulin may affect cancer development by both exerting mitogenic effects itself and by decreasing IGFBPs, thereby increasing the bioactivity of IGF-1, which is a generally stronger mitogen than insulin.

Determinants of IGF-1 Levels

Relatively few determinants of normal variation of IGF-1 levels are known. Prolonged energy and protein restriction leads to substantial decreases in plasma IGF-1 levels (Kaaks 2004). In well-fed populations, genetic factors may be dominant determinants of IGF-1 levels (Harrela et al. 1996). Between 38% and 80% of variance in IGF-1 levels can be explained by inherited genetic variation (Schumacher et al. 2010). Age is another determinant of IGF-1 concentrations, since with aging, production of growth-hormone decreases, leading to a decrease in circulating IGF-1 (Brabant and Wallaschofski 2007). Two cross-sectional studies in generally well-nourished male and female populations have shown that habitual dietary intake of protein is the major dietary determinant of circulating IGF-1 levels. The protein sources milk and cheese, as well as minerals such as potassium, zinc, and magnesium, were also positively associated with IGF-1 levels (Holmes et al. 2002; Giovannucci et al. 2003). Energy intake, however, was only weakly associated with IGF-1 levels. This weak association, which was mainly restricted to lean individuals (BMI <25 kg/m^2), is not surprising, since energy restriction was not present in these populations, and assessment of energy intake might have been imprecise, especially among overweight participants.

Insulin resistance is characterized by reduced response of tissues to the physiological actions of insulin. Common Western lifestyle associated risk factors for cancer such as obesity, physical inactivity and Western dietary pattern characterized by high consumption of red and processed meats, saturated fat, sweets, and refined grains are not associated with circulating IGF-1 levels but are determinants of insulin resistance (Giovannucci et al. 2004). Factors that increase insulin resistance will produce a compensatory fasting and postprandial hyperinsulinemia, which, in turn, may increase the bioactivity of IGF-1 by reducing hepatic IGFBP secretion. Thus, we can distinguish between direct determinants of IGF-1 levels, such as high protein intake, and factors that may indirectly increase IGF-1 exposure via actions on insulin levels (Fig. 1.1).

Epidemiologic Evidence that IGF-1 Is Associated with Cancer Risk

While experimental and laboratory studies strongly suggest that IGF-1 may affect the growth and progression of cancer cells in various tissues, they cannot give information on whether these observations at the cellular level are also relevant on the population level. Epidemiological studies measuring concentrations of IGF-1 and its major binding protein IGFBP-3 in blood samples of study participants have been conducted to answer this question since the early 1990s. In case–control studies where blood samples from case participants were drawn after diagnosis, it cannot be excluded that circulating IGF-1 levels are influenced by the existence of the tumor.

Thus, etiological inference from these studies is limited. In case–control studies nested within prospective cohort studies blood samples are drawn before diagnosis, which reduces the possibility of the existence of the tumor influencing the results. However, especially in studies with short follow-up times the tumor could have been present undiagnosed at the time of blood collection in later case participants, and thus have influenced hormone levels.

Studying the association between circulating IGFBP-3 and cancer risk is challenging, since IGFBP-3 may influence cancer risk by modulating the bioavailability of IGF-1, but can also have direct antiproliferative and proapoptotic effects, independent of its IGF-1 binding properties (Baxter 2001). Moreover, IGFBP-3 level is typically highly correlated with IGF-1 level, reflecting the fact that synthesis of both is controlled by growth hormone and that IGF-1 is typically bound to IGFBP-3.

Whether IGF-1 alone or IGF-1 and IGFBP-3 are entered simultaneously to the statistical models has different interpretation. While a model with IGF-1 only represents the effect of total circulating IGF-1 in relation to cancer risk, a risk estimate for IGF-1 mutually adjusted for IGFBP-3 might be a better estimate for the effect of bioavailable IGF-1 in relation to cancer risk.

A common limitation of epidemiologic studies relating IGF-1 or IGFBP-3 levels to risk of cancer is that most studies have only one blood sample collected and thus, rely on a single measurement to reflect long-term exposure. However, both IGF-1 and IGFBP-3 seem to be relatively stable over time. In a male cohort where blood samples were collected at two time points (3 ± 0.5 years apart) correlation coefficients between two measurements of IGF-1 and IGFBP-3 were 0.70 and 0.68, respectively (Platz et al. 1999).

In addition to measuring IGF-1 exposure directly in blood, epidemiological studies relating factors associated with IGF-1 levels or bioavailability to cancer risk may indirectly provide evidence for a potential role of IGF-1 in cancer development. Since high circulating insulin levels increase the bioactivity of IGF-1 by various mechanisms, determinants of hyperinsulinemia such as obesity, physical inactivity and Western diet may indirectly influence IGF-1 exposure.

Colorectal Cancer

Among the most common cancer types, colorectal cancer incidence is most strongly associated with Western lifestyle factors such as being overweight, physically inactive and consuming an energy-dense diet high in total and saturated fat and rapidly digestible carbohydrates (World Cancer Research Fund/American Institute for Cancer 2007). In addition, many studies have found that individuals with adult type II diabetes mellitus are at increased risk of colon cancer (Larsson et al. 2005). Since all of these factors are related to hyperinsulinemia, the hypothesis that alterations in the insulin/IGF-axis play a role in the association between Western lifestyle and colorectal cancer risk seems plausible and is supported by experimental studies (Giovannucci 2001).

Indirect Evidence

Acromegaly is a disease of somatic growth caused by excessive production of growth hormone. Patients with this condition typically have hyperinsulinemia and extraordinarily high IGF-1 concentrations are found in their blood. It has been shown that the colonic epithelial cell proliferation is increased among patients with acromegaly (Cats et al. 1996). Despite the rarity of the disease, a few epidemiologic studies were able to show that the incidence of colorectal adenomas (which are a precursor of colorectal cancer) and colorectal cancer is increased among people with acromegaly (Brunner et al. 1990; Ron et al. 1991; Jenkins et al. 1997, 2000). Jenkins et al. (2000) showed that the increased adenoma risk among patients with acromegaly is associated with increased IGF-1 concentrations. Also, fasting insulin concentrations and hyperinsulinemia have been positively associated with colorectal adenoma risk among patients with acromegaly (Colao et al. 2007; Foltyn et al. 2008).

IGF-1 levels during childhood and adolescence influence linear growth (Juul et al. 1994). While adult attained height correlates weakly with adult IGF-1 levels, height may be an indirect marker for IGF-1 exposure during childhood and adolescence. Several studies have shown that adult tallness is positively associated with risk of colorectal cancer (Wei et al. 2004; Engeland et al. 2005; Pischon et al. 2006), which might be explained by the IGF-hypothesis.

Other risk factors of colorectal cancer such as type 2 diabetes, BMI, waist circumference, Western diet as well as physical inactivity are probably primarily related to alterations in insulin metabolism but may indirectly support a role of IGF-1 in colorectal carcinogenesis through the aforementioned effects of insulin on the IGF-1 bioactivity.

Serologic Evidence

A number of epidemiological studies have been conducted to elucidate the association between circulating IGF-1 and risk of colorectal cancer. A small case–control study found significantly higher serum IGF-1 concentrations among 29 colorectal cancer cases compared with 159 tumor-free controls (Glass et al. 1994). A second case–control study comprising 41 colorectal cancer patients and 50 control subjects suggested that high IGF-1 concentrations and low IGFBP-3 concentrations are associated with increased risk of colorectal cancer (Manousos et al. 1999). In both studies, blood samples of cases were drawn post diagnosis, and thus, levels in cases may have been influenced by the existence of the tumor, limiting the causal inference from these studies.

The first prospective evidence came in 1999 from a case–control study nested within the Physicians' Health Study, showing that high prediagnostic IGF-1 concentrations were associated with increased risk of colorectal cancer (Ma et al. 1999). Comparing the highest with the lowest quintile, the relative risk (RR) for colorectal cancer was 1.36. The association became stronger and statistically significant after mutual adjustment for IGFBP-3 (RR, 2.51). Two subsequent prospective studies among female US populations [Nurses' Health Study (Giovannucci et al. 2000) and the New York University Women's Health Study (Kaaks et al. 2000)] showed positive associations of similar magnitude, which, however, did not reach statistical significance.

Epidemiological research in colorectal cancer has suggested that there may be etiological differences according to location, i.e., risk factors may differ between colon and rectal cancer (Wei et al. 2004). A prospective study from Sweden found no distinct association with colorectal cancer (Palmqvist et al. 2002), but a significant positive association was observed between IGF-1 and colon cancer, while a nonsignificant inverse association was observed with rectal cancer. Similarly, a study among Japanese-American men showed increased ORs for IGF-1 concentrations with colon and decreased ORs with rectal cancer (Nomura et al. 2003). An update from the Nurses' Health study with 6 years more follow-up time and more than twice the number of cases (Wei et al. 2005) compared to the first analysis (Giovannucci et al. 2000) found a positive association between IGF-1 concentrations and colon cancer, which was of similar magnitude as the earlier observed association with colorectal cancer. It has been proposed that the different associations for colon and rectal cancer might be related to differential tissue-specific expression of insulin and IGF receptors (Wei et al. 2004).

While until 2005 studies from Western populations consistently showed moderate positive associations between prediagnostic IGF-1 concentrations and risk of colorectal, or at least colon cancer, two studies from Asia found no associations between IGF-1 and colorectal cancer, even when studying colon and rectal cancer separately (Probst-Hensch et al. 2001; Otani et al. 2007). This discrepancy is somewhat surprising and raises the question whether the impact of IGF-1 concentrations on colorectal cancer may differ in different target populations. Since the means and distributions of IGF-1 levels in the Asian studies were comparable to those in the studies among Western populations, less variability in IGF-1 levels among Asians cannot serve as an explanation. It is noteworthy that a positive association between adult height (as a proxy for energy balance related to insulin and IGF-1 levels during childhood and adolescence) has been observed in Western populations (Wei et al. 2004; Engeland et al. 2005; Pischon et al. 2006) but not in a large prospective study among Japanese men and women (Otani et al. 2005). However, a study among Japanese-Americans living in Hawaii showed a positive association between IGF-1 and colon cancer comparable to the results from other Western studies (Nomura et al. 2003). Thus, the apparent discrepancy in results might not point to different associations in Asian as compared to Western populations but rather be explainable by different study designs, or by geographical location or type of diet (e.g., Western or traditional Asian).

The four most recent studies relating prediagnostic IGF-1 concentrations to incidence of colorectal cancer found no associations (Morris et al. 2006; Gunter et al. 2008; Max et al. 2008; Rinaldi et al. 2010). The multicenter European Prospective Investigation into Cancer and Nutrition (EPIC) cohort study is the largest study on the topic so far comprising 1,121 colorectal cancer cases and 1,121 controls (Rinaldi et al. 2010).

Comparing the highest with the lowest quintile in IGF-1 concentrations, RR for colorectal cancer was 1.07, which was attenuated by mutual adjustment for IGFBP-3 (RR, 1.01). No association was observed with colon or rectal cancer. However, the authors of this study investigated the association between IGF-1 and colorectal cancer stratified by dietary intake and found significant positive associations among subjects with low intake of milk and dairy calcium.

The most recent meta-analysis published in 2010 by the authors of the EPIC analysis shows a moderately significantly increased risk of colorectal cancer (RR per SD increase in IGF-1 1.07), even when including the null-finding from the large EPIC study (Rinaldi et al. 2010). This meta-analysis included only studies that published RRs for IGF-1 that were not adjusted for IGFBP-3, and thus did not include the study among 282 male Japanese-American case–control pairs, which observed a nonsignificant positive association between IGF-1 and colon cancer risk (Nomura et al. 2003).

The association between prediagnostic concentrations of IGFBP-3 and risk of colorectal cancer has been inconclusive so far. While the two earliest prospective studies relating IGF to colorectal cancer observed significant inverse associations with IGFBP-3 (Ma et al. 1999; Giovannucci et al. 2000), other studies observed nonsignificantly increased associations (Kaaks et al. 2000; Probst-Hensch et al. 2001; Palmqvist et al. 2002) or no association (Morris et al. 2006; Gunter et al. 2008; Max et al. 2008; Rinaldi et al. 2010). The updated analysis from the Nurses' Health Study (Wei et al. 2005) did not confirm the inverse association for IGFBP-3 observed in the first analysis (Giovannucci et al. 2000). With more follow-up time, the authors found no association between IGFBP-3 and risk of colon cancer, with or without mutual adjustment for IGF-1 (Wei et al. 2005). It has been suggested that the inconsistent results for the association between IGFBP-3 and colorectal cancer may be due to differences in assays, i.e., depend on whether intact or total IGFBP-3 is measured (Rinaldi et al. 2005). The analysis from the EPIC study applied two IGFBP-3 assays, one of them measuring total IGFBP-3 (which is most commonly measured in other studies) and one measuring intact IGFBP-3 only (Rinaldi et al. 2010). Neither total nor intact IGFBP-3 was associated with risk of colorectal cancer in EPIC. A meta-analysis from 2006 including seven prospective studies showed a pooled RR for colorectal cancer of 0.98 comparing the highest versus lowest quartile of IGFP-3 (Morris et al. 2006).

Considering the differential associations of IGFBP-3 with colorectal cancer risk observed in the various studies, it is not surprising that adding IGFBP-3 to the models changed RRs for IGF-1 in various directions. While adjustment for IGFBP-3 strengthened the association between IGF-1 and colorectal cancer in some studies (Ma et al. 1999; Giovannucci et al. 2000), essentially those which observed inverse associations for IGFBP-3 and colorectal cancer, in most other studies adjustment for IGFBP-3 slightly attenuated the positive association between IGF-1 and colorectal cancer (Kaaks et al. 2000; Probst-Hensch et al. 2001; Wei et al. 2005; Allen et al. 2007; Rinaldi et al. 2010).

In addition to measuring IGF-1, a number of epidemiologic studies have examined markers of hyperinsulinemia such as fasting or nonfasting insulin levels or C-peptide, which is an indicator of insulin secretion. In the New York University Women's Health Study, a threefold higher risk of colorectal cancer was observed comparing the top and bottom quartiles of C-peptide (Kaaks et al. 2000). In a cohort study from Northern Sweden, while no association was observed between fasting and nonfasting insulin and colorectal cancer, a nonsignificant positive association was observed when considering only fasting (>4 h) blood samples (Palmqvist et al. 2003). In the Physicians' Health Study, plasma C-peptide was significantly positively associated with risk of colorectal cancer, adjusting for BMI and exercise (Ma et al. 2004). A recent meta-analysis found significant excess risks of colorectal cancer associated with higher circulating insulin or C-peptide (Pisani 2008). Very few studies investigated the joint or interactive association between insulin and IGF-1 concentrations. In the Nurses' Health study, the positive association between total IGF-1 and IGF-1/IGFBP-3 ratio and colon cancer risk was primarily observed in women with low insulin exposure represented by low C-peptide or high IGFBP-1 (Wei et al. 2005). The joint analysis revealed that being high in either IGF-1 or insulin exposure was sufficient to substantially elevate colon cancer risk, while being high in both did not additionally increase risk beyond being high in either one. This result requires confirmation by further studies, but suggests that in people who are at high risk for colorectal cancer because of hyperinsulinemia, high total IGF-1 does not further increase risk. Consequently, IGF-1 exposure may be more relevant in individuals without hyperinsulinemia. More studies investigating the joint association between IGF-1 and insulin are required to investigate whether the established positive association between hyperinsulinemia and colorectal cancer is due to direct effects of insulin on tumor growth or due to the metabolic effects of insulin on IGF-1 bioactivity.

Taken together, the majority of prospective studies show a positive but mostly nonsignificant association between prediagnostic IGF-1 concentrations and colorectal cancer. With respect to the individual association of IGFBP-3 and risk of colorectal cancer, the inconsistent results from the prospective studies suggest that there is no major association. Several studies have observed positive associations of hyperinsulinemia represented by high plasma C-peptide or fasting insulin in relation to colorectal cancer and one study investigating IGF-1 and insulin exposure jointly showed that either high IGF-1 or insulin exposure are sufficient to increase risk.

Prostate Cancer

The rise in prostate cancer incidence in Western countries during the twentieth century and the increase in incidence rates among migrants moving from countries with low rates to those countries with high rates strongly suggest an association between Western lifestyle and prostate cancer risk. However, individual Western lifestyle factors such as obesity, physical inactivity and Western diet have been less clearly associated with prostate as compared to colorectal cancer (World Cancer Research

Fund/American Institute for Cancer 2007). The evidence that physical activity or body fatness are associated with the risk of prostate cancer is limited, although there is suggestion of associations with more aggressive disease (Giovannucci et al. 2007; Hsing et al. 2007). The epidemiological prostate cancer research has been challenged by the fact that in many industrialized countries since the mid-nineties the majority of prostate cancer cases are initially detected by PSA-screening. Screening patterns resulted in a change in the case-mix in studies, i.e., a growing number of early, localized cancer, part of which never become clinically significant during the lifetime (Savage et al. 2010), and a decreasing proportion of advanced cancers. Results from numerous epidemiological studies suggest that risk factors for prostate cancer may differ according to stage of disease (advanced versus nonadvanced), or Gleason grade. The heterogeneous nature of prostate cancer leads to difficulties in interpretation of studies and may have contributed to the inconsistent results in terms of body weight, physical activity and Western diet in relation to prostate cancer. However, laboratory studies clearly suggest that the insulin and IGF-1 axes play a role in prostate cancer (Pollak et al. 1998).

Indirect Evidence

Compared to colorectal cancer, only limited evidence exists for an association between higher levels of IGF-1 and prostate cancer risk in acromegalics (Jenkins 2004). However, due to the rarity of the disease and possible confounding by treatment an association cannot be excluded (Pollak 2008). In addition, hypogonadism is common in patients with acromegaly, and androgens seem to play a role in prostate cancer development (Monti et al. 2007). More consistently, adult attained height reflecting early-life exposure to IGF-1 as well as birthweight, which reflects early-life exposure to IGF-1, IGF-2, and insulin, has been associated with increased risk of prostate cancer. In the Health Professionals Follow-up Study, adult height was not associated with overall prostate cancer, but a significant positive association was observed with advanced or fatal prostate cancer (Giovannucci et al. 2007). A meta-analysis estimated a significantly increased RR per 10 cm increment in adult height of 1.06 for total prostate cancer, which was stronger for advanced/aggressive prostate cancer (RR, 1.12) (Zuccolo et al. 2008).

Apart from age one of the best established risk factors for prostate cancer is African-American descent (Giovannucci et al. 2007). It has been suggested that the increased risk of prostate cancer among African-Americans might at least partly be explained by IGF-1 levels. However, a cross-sectional study observed higher concentrations of both IGF-1 and IGFBP-3 in Whites than in African Americans (Platz et al. 1999). Similarly, higher IGF-1 and IGFBP-3 concentrations were observed in the cord blood from White as compared to African-American male neonates (Rohrmann, CEBP 2009). These results seem to contradict the hypothesis of IGF as possible explanation for the higher prostate cancer risk among African-Americans. Nevertheless, the observed lower IGFBP-3 concentrations in African-American neonates and adults, may contribute to the increased risk via more bioavailable IGF-1.

Serologic Evidence

Since 1993, numerous retrospective and prospective epidemiological studies have been conducted to investigate whether higher levels of circulating IGF-1 are associated with increased risks of prostate cancer. Two case–control studies published in 1993 (Cohen et al. 1993; Kanety et al. 1993), however, failed to demonstrate an association between IGF-1 and risk of prostate cancer. The first significant positive association between IGF-1 and prostate cancer was observed in a small case–control study in 1997 (Mantzoros et al. 1997). Comparing 52 subjects with prostate cancer to age- and weight-matched controls, the RR per 60 ng/ml increment in IGF-1 was 1.91. A meta-analysis identified 31 retrospective studies on the association between IGF-1 and prostate cancer and found a significantly increased pooled RR per standard deviation increase in IGF-1 of 1.26 (Rowlands et al. 2009).

In 1998, the first prospective analysis on circulating IGF-1 in relation to risk of prostate cancer was published by Chan et al. using data from the Physicians' Health Study (1998) with blood samples collected on average 7 years before diagnosis. The authors observed in a nested case–control setting including 152 prostate cancer cases and an equal number of age-matched controls a strong positive association between IGF-1 and total prostate cancer. A twofold higher risk of prostate cancer was observed in those in the top quartile of IGF-1, and a fourfold higher risk was seen after adjustment for IGFBP-3. Similarly, in an analysis from the Baltimore Longitudinal Study on Aging published in 2000 including 72 cases with an average time between blood collection and diagnosis of 9 years, circulating IGF-1 concentrations were nonsignificantly positively associated with prostate cancer and stronger positively associated in a model adjusting for IGFBP-3 (Harman et al. 2000). Several subsequent prospective studies relating circulating IGF-1 to prostate cancer showed increased, but mostly not significant RRs with increasing IGF-1 for total prostate cancer (Stattin et al. 2000; Meyer et al. 2005; Platz et al. 2005; Morris et al. 2006; Allen et al. 2007). Other prospective studies, however, did not observe an association between IGF-1 and total prostate cancer (Lacey et al. 2001; Woodson et al. 2003; Severi et al. 2006; Weiss et al. 2007; Johansson et al. 2009). Possible reasons for this heterogeneity include study characteristics such as age at recruitment, lag time between blood collection and diagnosis as well as differences in biochemical assay methods. In addition, different results might be related to whether a study was conducted in a setting where PSA-screening was common, i.e., whether the majority of cases were PSA-detected or not, which results in differences in case-mix.

The two most recent meta-analyses consistently suggest that risk of prostate cancer is moderately increased with increasing IGF-1 concentrations (Roddam et al. 2008; Rowlands et al. 2009). In one of them, analyzing individual patient data from 12 prospective studies including 3,700 cases and 5,200 controls a significantly increased pooled RR of 1.38 for total prostate cancer was estimated comparing the highest versus lowest quintile of IGF-1. In a meta-analysis including 31 retrospective and 16 prospective studies the overall pooled RR was 1.21 per standard deviation increase in IGF-1 (prospective studies only, RR, 1.07).

IGF-1 might act differently according to tumor stage or grade. The question whether IGF-1 is related to advanced rather than overall prostate cancer implies information on the time when IGF-1 is relevant for cancer development. If IGF-1 was equally associated with advanced and nonadvanced prostate cancer, this would favor the hypothesis that IGF-1 acts during early steps of prostate carcinogenesis. By contrast, stronger associations between IGF-1 and advanced as opposed to nonadvanced prostate cancer would support a role of IGF-1 during progression from indolent to clinically symptomatic disease. Some of the prospective studies report risk estimates stratified by cancer stage or some study-specific definition of aggressiveness of disease (Chan et al. 2002; Stattin et al. 2004; Meyer et al. 2005; Severi et al. 2006; Allen et al. 2007; Weiss et al. 2007; Nimptsch et al. 2010). In the follow-up publication of the Physicians' Health Study in 2002, including 530 cases, no association between IGF-1 and total prostate cancer was observed (Chan et al. 2002). However, men with IGF-1 levels in the top versus bottom quartile had a 5-fold significantly increased risk of advanced prostate cancer, while no association was seen for nonadvanced prostate cancer (RR, 1.2). Similarly, in a Swedish nested case–control study significantly increased RRs were observed for advanced (RR highest versus lowest quartile 2.87), but not nonadvanced (RR, 1.69) prostate cancer (Stattin et al. 2004). Other prospective studies did not observe substantial differences according to the stage of prostate cancer (Severi et al. 2006; Weiss et al. 2007; Nimptsch et al. 2010).

Few prospective studies investigated whether the association between IGF-1 and prostate cancer differs by Gleason grade (Chan et al. 2002; Meyer et al. 2005; Allen et al. 2007; Nimptsch et al. 2010). Three of these observed stronger associations for low-grade (Gleason score <7) than for high-grade prostate cancer (Chan et al. 2002; Allen et al. 2007; Nimptsch et al. 2010), although no significant heterogeneity was observed in any of these studies. Stronger associations between IGF-1 and low-grade versus high-grade prostate cancer might reflect that high-grade tumors are more autonomous in their growth, possibly due to constitutively activated IGF-1 signaling (McMenamin et al. 1999), and are thus less sensitive to variations in circulating IGF-1 levels (Chan et al. 2002; Nimptsch et al. 2010).

The two most recent meta-analyses differ in their conclusions in terms of potential heterogeneity by stage or grade of disease. The pooled analysis by Roddam et al. (2008) observed higher RRs for low-grade than for high-grade prostate cancer (2010 low-grade and 954 high-grade cases, p-heterogeneity, 0.027), while no heterogeneity was seen by stage of disease (514 advanced, 1949 localized cases, p-heterogeneity, 0.78) (Rowlands et al. 2009). By contrast, using data from four prospective studies, the meta-analysis by Rowlands et al. (2008, 2009) shows higher pooled RRs for advanced than for localized prostate cancer (p-heterogeneity, 0.06), but did not observe any heterogeneity by grade of disease (p-heterogeneity, 0.50).

Since prostate cancer can be present for many years but asymptomatic, it is questionable whether the observed positive associations between IGF-1 and prostate cancer in prospective studies reflect an etiologic relationship or whether IGF-1 is rather a tumor marker, i.e., the observed associations might be due to IGF-1 secretion by extant cancers of the prostate. The common approach to elucidate this question is to exclude cases that were diagnosed early after blood collection. Three prospective studies report unchanged or even stronger associations between IGF-1 and prostate cancer when excluding cases diagnosed within 2 (Nimptsch et al. 2010), 5 (Stattin et al. 2004) or 9 (Chan et al. 2002) years after blood collection. These observations argue against the possibility that the observed associations were the result of IGF-1 production by prevalent tumors. However, after the first studies showing an association between IGF-1 and prostate cancer risk were published, there was substantial hope that IGF-1 could serve as a diagnostic marker in addition to PSA. In particular, it was suggested the IGF-1 could help reducing the number of false-positive PSA tests and prevent unnecessary biopsy examinations. Three prospective studies investigated whether IGF-1 improves the sensitivity or specificity of PSA as a diagnostic marker (Chan et al. 1998; Harman et al. 2000; Stattin et al. 2004), but all of them concluded that IGF-1 in addition to PSA does not improve sensitivity or specificity substantially. A study among men with elevated serum PSA concluded that serum IGF-1 is not a useful diagnostic test for prostate cancer (Finne et al. 2000). The failure of IGF-1 as a potential diagnostic marker is not surprising considering the moderate association between IGF-1 and prostate cancer risk.

The association between concentrations of IGFBP-3 and prostate cancer has been studied extensively, with, however, inconsistent results. Several studies show significant (Stattin et al. 2004; Severi et al. 2006; Johansson et al. 2009; Nimptsch et al. 2010) or nonsignificant (Morris et al. 2006; Allen et al. 2007; Weiss et al. 2007) positive associations between IGFBP-3 and overall prostate cancer, while other studies observed nonsignificant inverse (Harman et al. 2000; Chen et al. 2005; Meyer et al. 2005) or no association (Lacey et al. 2001). As in the studies on colorectal cancer this heterogeneity may be due to differences in assay specificity and the stage of proteolytic cleavage of the measured form of IGFBP-3 (Rinaldi et al. 2005). In addition, studies differ with respect to study design, age of included participants, sample size, and case mix, which could all contribute to heterogeneity of results.

The meta-analysis using individual patient data shows a significantly increased RR for IGFBP-3 (RR highest versus lowest quintile 1.23), which, however, is substantially attenuated after adjustment for IGF-1, suggesting that that the association of IGFBP-3 with prostate cancer is secondary to IGF-1 (Roddam et al. 2008). The meta-analysis by Rowlands et al. shows no association between IGFBP-3 and prostate cancer when pooling 13 prospective studies (RR per standard deviation increase in IGFBP-3, 1.00), but a significant inverse pooled RR among 16 retrospective studies (RR, 0.78).

Insulin and C-peptide levels have been investigated in relation to prostate cancer in several studies. In a Chinese case–control study, a 2.6-fold higher risk of prostate cancer was observed when comparing top and bottom tertiles of fasting plasma insulin (Hsing et al. 2003). In the Northern Sweden Health and Disease Cohort Study, no association between insulin levels and risk of prostate cancer was observed (Stattin et al. 2000). Another Swedish study found a significant inverse association between C-peptide and overall prostate cancer, but with aggressive prostate cancer there was tendency of a positive association (Stocks et al. 2007). In the Physicians'

Health Study, among men with prostate cancer, those with high prediagnostic C-peptide had twofold risk of dying from prostate cancer and this association was stronger among overweight individuals (Ma et al. 2008). In a cohort of Finnish men, elevated fasting levels of serum insulin were positively associated with risk of prostate cancer (Albanes et al. 2009). Although not entirely consistent, these results suggest that high insulin may increase risk of prostate cancer or at least prostate cancer progression. The pattern of an association with aggressive prostate cancer or prostate cancer mortality, but inconsistent results with incident prostate cancer is consistent with studies investigating obesity and physical inactivity, the main determinants of hyperinsulinemia, in relation to prostate cancer. No study so far has investigated the joint or interactive effects of IGF-1 and insulin exposure with respect to prostate cancer incidence or progression.

To summarize, a large body of epidemiological evidence is in favor of a moderate positive association between circulating IGF-1 and risk of prostate cancer, which is supported by two recent meta-analyses. The possibility of reverse causation due to IGF-1 production by extant cancers is rather unlikely as several studies show that exclusion of cases diagnosed within the first years after blood collection did not change the results. The association between IGFBP-3 and prostate cancer is inconclusive so far. There is some evidence that IGF-1 might be more important for low-grade than for high-grade prostate cancer and for advanced versus nonadvanced prostate cancer. Insulin exposure may be relevant for the progression of prostate cancer.

Breast Cancer

Estrogens are an important factor in the etiology of breast cancer. Besides risk factors directly related to hormone status, such as early menarche, late menopause, nulliparity, or late first pregnancy, obesity is an established risk factor for postmenopausal breast cancer (World Cancer Research Fund/American Institute for Cancer 2007). It has been widely assumed that the association between obesity and breast cancer risk is due to the higher circulating estrogen levels present in the blood of obese women. However, due to the hyperinsulinemia often accompanied by obesity, it is plausible that the insulin and IGF-1 axes play a role in this association, too. IGF-1 may directly affect breast carcinogenesis by exhibiting mitogenic and antiapoptotic effects, and hyperinsulinemic states may increase risks of breast cancer by enhancing the bioavailability of IGF-1. In addition, there is evidence for cross talk occurring between the IGF and estrogen signaling pathways in breast tissue (Dupont and Le Roith 2001).

Breast tissue, hormones, and hormone-receptors status vary at different stages in life and factors that modify the risk of breast cancer may act differently depending on the menopausal status or age. Thus, menopausal status is a potential effect modifier, which is why most epidemiological studies present results separately for premenopausal and postmenopausal populations.

Indirect Evidence

Besides obesity as an established risk factor for breast cancer possibly related in part to the insulin/IGF-1 axis, birth weight and adult attained height, both of which reflect early-life exposure to IGF-1 and, in the case of birthweight, also to IGF-2 and insulin, are positively associated with the risk of breast cancer (World Cancer Research Fund/American Institute for Cancer 2007).

In a large pooled cross-sectional analysis, IGF-1 concentrations were associated with established risk factors for breast cancer including height, age at menarche, and age at first full-term pregnancy, suggesting that these factors may affect breast cancer risk at least partly through their relationships with IGF-1 (Key et al. 2010).

In addition, IGF-1 concentrations as well as genetic variation in IGF-related genes have been related – although not entirely consistently – to mammographic density, a strong risk factor for breast cancer (Becker and Kaaks 2009).

Serologic Evidence

Several case–control studies conducted between 1993 and 1998 showed positive associations between circulating IGF-1 and risk of breast cancer in young premenopausal women (Peyrat et al. 1993; Bruning et al. 1995; Bohlke et al. 1998). In line with these results, the early prospective studies suggested that prediagnostic circulating IGF-1 might be positively associated with risk of breast cancer in premenopausal women. Four nested case–control studies published between 1998 and 2002 observed positive associations between IGF-1 and breast cancer among premenopausal but not postmenopausal women (Hankinson et al. 1998; Toniolo et al. 2000; Krajcik et al. 2002; Muti et al. 2002). In all of these studies, risk estimates for women who had high premenopausal IGF-1 levels were two- to threefold higher. In the Nurses' Health Study, a nested case–control study including 305 premenopausal and 76 postmenopausal breast cancer cases (menopausal status was defined at the time of blood collection), showed that circulating IGF-1 was significantly positively associated with breast cancer in premenopausal women (Hankinson et al. 1998). Comparing the highest versus lowest tertile, RR for premenopausal breast cancer was twofold increased. This association became stronger after adjustment for IGFBP-3 (RR, 2.88). No association between IGF-1 and breast cancer among postmenopausal women was observed in the same study, although the number of postmenopausal breast cancer cases was very limited. However, an updated analysis within the Nurses' Health Study confirmed a positive association among women who were premenopausal at blood collection (447 cases) and no association among postmenopausal women (237 cases) (Schernhammer et al. 2005).

The second published prospective study on the topic used data from the New York University Women's Health Study and observed a nonsignificant positive association between IGF-1 and breast cancer among premenopausal women (172 cases), but no association among postmenopausal women (115 cases) (Toniolo et al. 2000). Similarly to the Nurses' Health Study, these results were confirmed at a later update analysis with more follow-up and more cases (Rinaldi et al. 2005). Three further nested case–control studies showed consistently increased risks for premenopausal women, and nonsignificantly decreased risks for postmenopausal women (Krajcik et al. 2002; Muti et al. 2002; Allen et al. 2005). One of them (Krajcik et al. 2002) defined menopausal status at the time of diagnosis, while all other previously mentioned nested case–control studies stratified by menopausal status at the time of blood collection. In contrast to these studies, a large study nested within two Swedish cohorts observed no noteworthy association between plasma IGF-1 and breast cancer risk regardless of menopausal status or age (Kaaks et al. 2002).

Using data from the prospective cohorts Clue I and II, Rollison et al. (2006) aimed to specifically investigate whether circulating IGF-1 levels prior to menopause are related to breast cancer diagnosed after menopause. They observed no association between postmenopausal breast cancer and high circulating IGF-1 levels measured before (175 cases) or after (91 cases) menopause. However, stratification by age at blood draw revealed significantly increased risks in the youngest (25–35 years, 37 cases) premenopausal age group and the oldest (61–74 years, 40 cases) postmenopausal age group. Since the power for age-specific associations was very limited, these results should be interpreted cautiously.

The largest study to date was conducted within the European Prospective Investigation into Cancer and Nutrition (EPIC) comprising 1,081 breast cancer cases and 2,098 controls (Rinaldi et al. 2006). The authors observed a significant moderate positive association between IGF-1 and overall breast cancer (RR, 1.34). The EPIC study was the first study that had sufficient power to show heterogeneity in the association between IGF-1 levels and breast cancer depending on the time between blood donation and breast cancer diagnosis. The association between serum IGF-1 levels and risk of breast cancer was stronger in subjects in whom breast cancer was diagnosed two or more years after blood donation (RR, 1.51), than in subjects with a breast cancer diagnosis within the first 2 years of follow-up (RR, 0.76; p-heterogeneity 0.0004). The authors showed that the observed heterogeneity by follow-up time could not be attributed to time-dependent differences in the distribution of other breast cancer risk factors such as BMI, reproductive or menstrual history, previous HRT use, or tumor characteristics. The results from the EPIC study contrast with those from previous prospective studies, as no obvious differences were observed in the association between IGF-1 levels and breast cancer risk when stratifying by menopausal status at blood collection. Circulating IGF-1 levels were nonsignificantly positively associated with breast cancer among both premenopausal and postmenopausal women. One important difference that might contribute to this heterogeneity is that the median follow-up time in the EPIC study (2.8 years) was substantially lower than in the previously published nested case–control studies [between 4.8 (Toniolo et al. 2000) and 10.5 years (Krajcik et al. 2002)]. Unexpectedly, results from the Nurses' Health Study II did not confirm an association between IGF-1 and breast cancer among women who were premenopausal at baseline (Schernhammer et al. 2006), which contrasts results from most previous studies, including the first Nurses' Health Study. An Australian case–cohort analysis found no association of IGF-1 for women who were premenopausal at baseline, but significant positive associations were observed for postmenopausal women (Baglietto et al. 2007). By contrast, four prospective studies including only women who were postmenopausal at the time of blood collection did not observe a positive association between IGF-1 and breast cancer (Keinan-Boker et al. 2003; Gronbaek et al. 2004; Gunter et al. 2009; Schairer et al. 2010).

Four systematic reviews and meta-analyses published before 2005 indicated a positive association between IGF-1 and risk of breast cancer in premenopausal women, while no association was observed for postmenopausal women (Renehan 2004; Shi 2004; Sugumar 2004; Fletcher 2005). An updated meta-analysis published by Renehan et al. in 2006 recognized an attenuation of the positive association between IGF-1 and premenopausal breast cancer risk in more recent publications, but still observed an overall significant positive association (RR, 1.69) between IGF-1 and risk of breast cancer in women who were premenopausal at baseline. In contrast to these meta-analyses, a pooled analysis including all prospective studies on IGF-1 and breast cancer risk published to date observed significant positive associations for both premenopausal and postmenopausal women (Key et al. 2010). The overall pooled risk estimate comparing the highest versus lowest study-specific quintiles was 1.21 for premenopausal and 1.33 for postmenopausal women at baseline.

Given the strong association between estrogen levels and breast cancer and the cross talk in cells between IGF-1 and estrogen signaling pathways, it was hypothesized that the association between IGF-1 and risk of breast cancer might depend on estrogen levels or estrogen receptor (ER) status of the tumor. Few of the prospective studies explicitly stratify by estrogen receptor status, and none of them had observed significant associations before stratification (Gronbaek et al. 2004; Schernhammer et al. 2006; Gunter et al. 2009). Of these studies, one study among postmenopausal women reported a significant positive association between IGF-1 and ER positive but not ER negative breast cancer (Gronbaek et al. 2004), while none of the other studies observed differences by estrogen receptor status. The pooled analysis, however, was able to use information on estrogen receptor status also from studies that had not explicitly investigated this association in their publications (Key et al. 2010). Investigating 1414 ER positive and 479 ER negative breast cancer cases, the authors found IGF-1 to be associated with significantly increased RRs for ER positive, but not ER negative breast cancer (p-heterogeneity 0.007). Only one of the prospective studies on IGF-1 and breast cancer simultaneously measured endogenous estradiol to assess independent associations between IGF-1 levels and the risk of breast cancer (Gunter et al. 2009). In this study, no association between IGF-1 and postmenopausal breast cancer was observed with or without adjustment for endogenous estradiol levels, while estradiol was independently positively associated with breast cancer risk.

Most studies investigating the association between IGF-1 and risk of breast cancer also studied IGFBP-3. The first prospective study including IGFBP-3 (Toniolo et al. 2000) did not observe an association among either premenopausal or postmenopausal women. Further prospective studies mostly consistently found no substantial evidence for an association between IGFBP-3 and breast cancer risk.

While most studies in premenopausal women observed no association between circulating IGFBP-3 and risk of breast cancer (Allen et al. 2005; Schernhammer et al. 2005, 2006; Rinaldi et al. 2006; Rollison et al. 2006; Baglietto et al. 2007), three studies observed significant positive associations (Krajcik et al. 2002; Muti et al. 2002; Allen et al. 2007). In terms of postmenopausal breast cancer, no association for IGFBP-3 was seen in seven prospective studies (Gronbaek et al. 2004; Allen et al. 2005; Schernhammer et al. 2005, 2006; Vatten et al. 2008; Gunter et al. 2009), while four studies observed significant (Rinaldi et al. 2006) or nonsignificant (Keinan-Boker et al. 2003; Rollison et al. 2006; Baglietto et al. 2007) positive associations and two studies observed nonsignificant inverse associations (Krajcik et al. 2002; Muti et al. 2002). The pooled estimates from prospective studies indicate no association for premenopausal women, but a significant positive association for postmenopausal breast cancer (RR highest versus lowest study-specific quintile 1.23) (Key et al. 2010).

As seen in the studies for colorectal and prostate cancer, mutual adjustment for IGFBP-3 did in some studies (Hankinson et al. 1998; Allen et al. 2005) potentiate associations between IGF-1 and breast cancer, and in others attenuate associations (Krajcik et al. 2002; Rinaldi et al. 2006; Allen et al. 2007).

Four prospective studies have investigated plasma insulin or C-peptide in relation to risk of breast cancer, and no association was observed with overall (Toniolo et al. 2000; Muti et al. 2002; Verheus et al. 2006; Eliassen et al. 2007) or premenopausal or postmenopausal (Toniolo et al. 2000; Muti et al. 2002) breast cancer. A meta-analysis observed excess risk of breast cancer with high circulating C-peptide or insulin, which was, however, entirely driven by case–control studies (Pisani 2008).

In summary, the body of epidemiological studies suggests that IGF-1 plays a role for breast cancer development although as to date it remains unclear whether the association varies by menopausal status or age. While the early prospective studies clearly suggested a positive association between IGF-1 and premenopausal breast cancer, this association was less obvious in more recent publications. The pooled estimates of the most recent meta-analysis are driven by the findings from the EPIC study, which by far is the largest study conducted so far and found positive association between IGF-1 and risk of breast cancer regardless of menopausal status. There is suggestion that the association between IGF-1 and breast cancer is confined to estrogen receptor positive breast tumors. In prospective studies, plasma levels of C-peptide or insulin were not associated with breast cancer and the joint or interactive effects of insulin and IGF-1 have not been studied so far.

Conclusion

In the past 20 years, considerable evidence has accumulated from both experimental and epidemiological studies suggesting that the IGF axis is involved in the development of cancer. Mechanistically, experimental data provide strong rationale for IGF-1 influencing carcinogenesis by promoting proliferation and inhibiting apoptosis. Epidemiologic evidence suggests positive associations between circulating IGF-1 and risk of colorectal, prostate, and breast cancer, albeit the strength of the associations are moderate. By showing positive associations even after exclusion of several years of follow-up after blood draw, many epidemiological studies support the hypothesis that IGF-1 might be an etiological factor rather than a tumor marker. Circumstantial evidence of markers of high IGF-1 levels, such as adult attained height with respect to cancer at different sites adds indirectly evidence for an association between IGF-1 and cancer risk.

Together, these data support the hypothesis that IGF-1 is a link between obesity and hyperinsulinemia associated with Western lifestyle and the high cancer rates in industrialized countries. However, further studies with slightly different study designs are warranted to further elucidate the association between insulin and IGF-1 axis with respect to cancer risk and cancer progression. To better understand the interactions between insulin and IGF-1 future studies need to consider carefully the independent and joint roles of these two hormones with respect to cancer development. Furthermore, in the case of breast cancer, more studies investigating IGF-1 and estrogen levels simultaneously are required to attain a better understanding of their joint effects on breast carcinogenesis. The comparability of future studies could be improved by standardization of the assay methods used. With multiple blood collections in different years of follow-up, the time-line of the effect of IGF-1 on cancer incidence and progression could be better elucidated. These studies should be complemented by studies based on tumor tissue factors, such as insulin and IGF-1 receptors, that may mediate the action of circulating IGF-1 levels.

References

Albanes, D., S. J. Weinstein, et al. (2009). "Serum insulin, glucose, indices of insulin resistance, and risk of prostate cancer." J Natl Cancer Inst **101**(18): 1272–9.

Allen, N. E., T. J. Key, et al. (2007). "Serum insulin-like growth factor (IGF)-I and IGF-binding protein-3 concentrations and prostate cancer risk: results from the European Prospective Investigation into Cancer and Nutrition." Cancer Epidemiol.Biomarkers Prev **16**(6): 1121–1127.

Allen, N. E., A. W. Roddam, et al. (2005). "A prospective study of serum insulin-like growth factor-I (IGF-I), IGF-II, IGF-binding protein-3 and breast cancer risk." Br J Cancer **92**(7): 1283–7.

Baglietto, L., D. R. English, et al. (2007). "Circulating insulin-like growth factor-I and binding protein-3 and the risk of breast cancer." Cancer Epidemiol Biomarkers Prev **16**(4): 763–8.

Baxter, R. C. (2001). "Signalling pathways involved in antiproliferative effects of IGFBP-3: a review." Mol Pathol **54**(3): 145–8.

Becker, S. and R. Kaaks (2009). "Exogenous and endogenous hormones, mammographic density and breast cancer risk: can mammographic density be considered an intermediate marker of risk?" Recent Results Cancer Res **181**: 135–57.

Bohlke, K., D. W. Cramer, et al. (1998). "Insulin-like growth factor-I in relation to premenopausal ductal carcinoma in situ of the breast." Epidemiology **9**(5): 570–3.

Brabant, G. and H. Wallaschofski (2007). "Normal levels of serum IGF-I: determinants and validity of current reference ranges." Pituitary **10**(2): 129–33.

Bruning, P. F., J. Van Doorn, et al. (1995). "Insulin-like growth-factor-binding protein 3 is decreased in early-stage operable pre-menopausal breast cancer." Int J Cancer **62**(3): 266–70.

Brunner, J. E., C. C. Johnson, et al. (1990). "Colon cancer and polyps in acromegaly: increased risk associated with family history of colon cancer." Clin Endocrinol (Oxf) **32**(1): 65–71.

Cats, A., R. P. Dullaart, et al. (1996). "Increased epithelial cell proliferation in the colon of patients with acromegaly." Cancer Res **56**(3): 523–6.

Chan, J. M., M. J. Stampfer, et al. (1998). "Plasma insulin-like growth factor-I and prostate cancer risk: a prospective study." Science **279**(5350): 563–6.

Chan, J. M., M. J. Stampfer, et al. (2002). "Insulin-like growth factor-I (IGF-I) and IGF binding protein-3 as predictors of advanced-stage prostate cancer." J Natl Cancer Inst **94**(14): 1099–106.

Chen, C., S. K. Lewis, et al. (2005). "Prostate carcinoma incidence in relation to prediagnostic circulating levels of insulin-like growth factor I, insulin-like growth factor binding protein 3, and insulin." Cancer **103**(1): 76–84.

Cohen, P., D. M. Peehl, et al. (1993). "Elevated levels of insulin-like growth factor-binding protein-2 in the serum of prostate cancer patients." J Clin Endocrinol Metab **76**(4): 1031–5.

Colao, A., R. Pivonello, et al. (2007). "The association of fasting insulin concentrations and colonic neoplasms in acromegaly: a colonoscopy-based study in 210 patients." J Clin Endocrinol Metab **92**(10): 3854–60.

Dupont, J. and D. Le Roith (2001). "Insulin-like growth factor 1 and oestradiol promote cell proliferation of MCF-7 breast cancer cells: new insights into their synergistic effects." Mol Pathol **54**(3): 149–54.

Eliassen, A. H., S. S. Tworoger, et al. (2007). "Circulating insulin and c-peptide levels and risk of breast cancer among predominately premenopausal women." Cancer Epidemiol Biomarkers Prev **16**(1): 161–4.

Engeland, A., S. Tretli, et al. (2005). "Height and body mass index in relation to colorectal and gallbladder cancer in two million Norwegian men and women." Cancer Causes Control **16**(8): 987–96.

Finne, P., A. Auvinen, et al. (2000). "Insulin-like growth factor I is not a useful marker of prostate cancer in men with elevated levels of prostate-specific antigen." J Clin Endocrinol Metab **85**(8): 2744–7.

Fletcher O., L. Gibson, et al. (2005). "Polymorphisms and circulating levels in the insulin-like growth factor system and risk of breast cancer: a systematic review." Cancer Epidemiol Biomarkers Prev **14**(1):2–19.

Foltyn, W., B. Kos-Kudla, et al. (2008). "Is there any relation between hyperinsulinemia, insulin resistance and colorectal lesions in patients with acromegaly?" Neuro Endocrinol Lett **29**(1): 107–12.

Furstenberger, G. and H. J. Senn (2002). "Insulin-like growth factors and cancer." Lancet Oncol **3**(5): 298–302.

Giovannucci, E. (2001). "Insulin, insulin-like growth factors and colon cancer: a review of the evidence." J Nutr **131**(11 Suppl): 3109S–20S.

Giovannucci, E., Y. Liu, et al. (2007). "Risk factors for prostate cancer incidence and progression in the health professionals follow-up study." Int J Cancer.

Giovannucci, E., M. Pollak, et al. (2003). "Nutritional predictors of insulin-like growth factor I and their relationships to cancer in men." Cancer Epidemiol Biomarkers Prev **12**(2): 84–9.

Giovannucci, E., M. N. Pollak, et al. (2000). "A prospective study of plasma insulin-like growth factor-1 and binding protein-3 and risk of colorectal neoplasia in women." Cancer Epidemiol Biomarkers Prev **9**(4): 345–9.

Giovannucci, E., E. B. Rimm, et al. (2004). "Height, predictors of C-peptide and cancer risk in men." Int J Epidemiol **33**(1): 217–25.

Glass, A. R., J. W. Kikendall, et al. (1994). "Serum concentrations of insulin-like growth factor 1 in colonic neoplasia." Acta Oncol **33**(1): 70–1.

1 Epidemiology of IGF-1 and Cancer

Gronbaek, H., A. Flyvbjerg, et al. (2004). "Serum insulin-like growth factors, insulin-like growth factor binding proteins, and breast cancer risk in postmenopausal women." Cancer Epidemiol Biomarkers Prev **13**(11 Pt 1): 1759–64.

Gunter, M. J., D. R. Hoover, et al. (2008). "Insulin, insulin-like growth factor-I, endogenous estradiol, and risk of colorectal cancer in postmenopausal women." Cancer Res **68**(1): 329–37.

Gunter, M. J., D. R. Hoover, et al. (2009). "Insulin, insulin-like growth factor-I, and risk of breast cancer in postmenopausal women." J Natl Cancer Inst **101**(1): 48–60.

Hankinson, S. E., W. C. Willett, et al. (1998). "Circulating concentrations of insulin-like growth factor-I and risk of breast cancer." Lancet **351**(9113): 1393–6.

Harman, S. M., E. J. Metter, et al. (2000). "Serum levels of insulin-like growth factor I (IGF-I), IGF-II, IGF-binding protein-3, and prostate-specific antigen as predictors of clinical prostate cancer." J Clin Endocrinol Metab **85**(11): 4258–65.

Harrela, M., H. Koistinen, et al. (1996). "Genetic and environmental components of interindividual variation in circulating levels of IGF-I, IGF-II, IGFBP-1, and IGFBP-3." J Clin Invest **98**(11): 2612–5.

Holmes, M. D., M. N. Pollak, et al. (2002). "Dietary correlates of plasma insulin-like growth factor I and insulin-like growth factor binding protein 3 concentrations." Cancer Epidemiol Biomarkers Prev **11**(9): 852–61.

Hsing, A. W., Y. T. Gao, et al. (2003). "Insulin resistance and prostate cancer risk." J Natl Cancer Inst **95**(1): 67–71.

Hsing, A. W., L. C. Sakoda, et al. (2007). "Obesity, metabolic syndrome, and prostate cancer." Am J Clin Nutr **86**(3): s843-57.

IARC (2008). World Cancer Report 2008. Lyon, World Health Organization, International Agency for Research on Cancer.

Jenkins, P. J. (2004). "Acromegaly and cancer." Horm Res **62 Suppl 1**: 108–15.

Jenkins, P. J., P. D. Fairclough, et al. (1997). "Acromegaly, colonic polyps and carcinoma." Clin Endocrinol (Oxf) **47**(1): 17–22.

Jenkins, P. J., V. Frajese, et al. (2000). "Insulin-like growth factor I and the development of colorectal neoplasia in acromegaly." J Clin Endocrinol Metab **85**(9): 3218–21.

Johansson, M., J. D. McKay, et al. (2009). "Genetic and plasma variation of insulin-like growth factor binding proteins in relation to prostate cancer incidence and survival." Prostate **69**(12): 1281–91.

Juul, A., P. Bang, et al. (1994). "Serum insulin-like growth factor-I in 1030 healthy children, adolescents, and adults: relation to age, sex, stage of puberty, testicular size, and body mass index." J Clin Endocrinol Metab **78**(3): 744–52.

Kaaks, R. (2004). "Nutrition, insulin, IGF-1 metabolism and cancer risk: a summary of epidemiological evidence." Novartis Found Symp **262**: 247–60; discussion 260–68.

Kaaks, R. and A. Lukanova (2001). "Energy balance and cancer: the role of insulin and insulin-like growth factor-I." Proc Nutr Soc **60**(1): 91–106.

Kaaks, R., E. Lundin, et al. (2002). "Prospective study of IGF-I, IGF-binding proteins, and breast cancer risk, in northern and southern Sweden." Cancer Causes Control **13**(4): 307–16.

Kaaks, R., P. Toniolo, et al. (2000). "Serum C-peptide, insulin-like growth factor (IGF)-I, IGF-binding proteins, and colorectal cancer risk in women." J Natl Cancer Inst **92**(19): 1592–600.

Kanety, H., Y. Madjar, et al. (1993). "Serum insulin-like growth factor-binding protein-2 (IGFBP-2) is increased and IGFBP-3 is decreased in patients with prostate cancer: correlation with serum prostate-specific antigen." J Clin Endocrinol Metab **77**(1): 229–33.

Keinan-Boker, L., H. B. Bueno De Mesquita, et al. (2003). "Circulating levels of insulin-like growth factor I, its binding proteins −1,-2, -3, C-peptide and risk of postmenopausal breast cancer." Int J Cancer **106**(1): 90–5.

Key, T. J., P. N. Appleby, et al. (2010) "Insulin-like growth factor 1 (IGF1), IGF binding protein 3 (IGFBP3), and breast cancer risk: pooled individual data analysis of 17 prospective studies." Lancet Oncol **11**(6): 530–42.

Krajcik, R. A., N. D. Borofsky, et al. (2002). "Insulin-like growth factor I (IGF-I), IGF-binding proteins, and breast cancer." Cancer Epidemiol Biomarkers Prev **11**(12): 1566–73.

Lacey, J. V., Jr., A. W. Hsing, et al. (2001). "Null association between insulin-like growth factors, insulin-like growth factor-binding proteins, and prostate cancer in a prospective study." Cancer Epidemiol Biomarkers Prev **10**(10): 1101–2.

Larsson, S. C., N. Orsini, et al. (2005). "Diabetes mellitus and risk of colorectal cancer: a meta-analysis." J Natl Cancer Inst **97**(22): 1679–87.

Ma, J., E. Giovannucci, et al. (2004). "A prospective study of plasma C-peptide and colorectal cancer risk in men." J Natl Cancer Inst **96**(7): 546–53.

Ma, J., H. Li, et al. (2008). "Prediagnostic body-mass index, plasma C-peptide concentration, and prostate cancer-specific mortality in men with prostate cancer: a long-term survival analysis." Lancet Oncol **9**(11): 1039–47.

Ma, J., M. N. Pollak, et al. (1999). "Prospective study of colorectal cancer risk in men and plasma levels of insulin-like growth factor (IGF)-I and IGF-binding protein-3." J Natl Cancer Inst **91**(7): 620–5.

Manousos, O., J. Souglakos, et al. (1999). "IGF-I and IGF-II in relation to colorectal cancer." Int J Cancer **83**(1): 15–7.

Mantzoros, C. S., A. Tzonou, et al. (1997). "Insulin-like growth factor 1 in relation to prostate cancer and benign prostatic hyperplasia." Br J Cancer **76**(9): 1115–8.

Max, J. B., P. J. Limburg, et al. (2008). "IGF-I, IGFBP-3, and IGF-I/IGFBP-3 ratio: no association with incident colorectal cancer in the Alpha-Tocopherol, Beta-Carotene Cancer Prevention Study." Cancer Epidemiol Biomarkers Prev **17**(7): 1832–4.

McMenamin, M. E., P. Soung, et al. (1999). "Loss of PTEN expression in paraffin-embedded primary prostate cancer correlates with high Gleason score and advanced stage." Cancer Res **59**(17): 4291–6.

Meyer, F., P. Galan, et al. (2005). "A prospective study of the insulin-like growth factor axis in relation with prostate cancer in the SU.VI.MAX trial." Cancer Epidemiol Biomarkers Prev **14**(9): 2269–72.

Monti, S., L. Proietti-Pannunzi, et al. (2007). "The IGF axis in prostate cancer." Curr Pharm Des **13**(7): 719–27.

Morris, J. K., L. M. George, et al. (2006). "Insulin-like growth factors and cancer: no role in screening. Evidence from the BUPA study and meta-analysis of prospective epidemiological studies." Br J Cancer **95**(1): 112–7.

Muti, P., T. Quattrin, et al. (2002). "Fasting glucose is a risk factor for breast cancer: a prospective study." Cancer Epidemiol Biomarkers Prev **11**(11): 1361–8.

Nimptsch, K., E. A. Platz, et al. (2010). "Plasma insulin-like growth factor 1 is positively associated with low-grade prostate cancer in the Health Professionals Follow-up Study 1993–2004." Int J Cancer.

Nomura, A. M., G. N. Stemmermann, et al. (2003). "Serum insulin-like growth factor I and subsequent risk of colorectal cancer among Japanese-American men." Am J Epidemiol **158**(5): 424–31.

Otani, T., M. Iwasaki, et al. (2005). "Body mass index, body height, and subsequent risk of colorectal cancer in middle-aged and elderly Japanese men and women: Japan public health center-based prospective study." Cancer Causes Control **16**(7): 839–50.

Otani, T., M. Iwasaki, et al. (2007). "Plasma C-peptide, insulin-like growth factor-I, insulin-like growth factor binding proteins and risk of colorectal cancer in a nested case-control study: the Japan public health center-based prospective study." Int J Cancer **120**(9): 2007–12.

Palmqvist, R., G. Hallmans, et al. (2002). "Plasma insulin-like growth factor 1, insulin-like growth factor binding protein 3, and risk of colorectal cancer: a prospective study in northern Sweden." Gut **50**(5): 642–6.

Palmqvist, R., P. Stattin, et al. (2003). "Plasma insulin, IGF-binding proteins-1 and −2 and risk of colorectal cancer: a prospective study in northern Sweden." Int J Cancer **107**(1): 89–93.

Peyrat, J. P., J. Bonneterre, et al. (1993). "Plasma insulin-like growth factor-1 (IGF-1) concentrations in human breast cancer." Eur J Cancer **29A**(4): 492–7.

Pisani, P. (2008). "Hyper-insulinaemia and cancer, meta-analyses of epidemiological studies." Arch Physiol Biochem **114**(1): 63–70.

Pischon, T., P. H. Lahmann, et al. (2006). "Body size and risk of colon and rectal cancer in the European Prospective Investigation Into Cancer and Nutrition (EPIC)." J Natl Cancer Inst **98**(13): 920–31.

Platz E. A., M. N. Pollak, et al. (1999). "Racial variation in insulin-like growth factor-1 and binding protein-3 concentrations in middle-aged men." Cancer Epidemiol Biomarkers Prev **8**(12):1107–10.

Platz, E. A., M. N. Pollak, et al. (2005). "Plasma insulin-like growth factor-1 and binding protein-3 and subsequent risk of prostate cancer in the PSA era." Cancer Causes Control **16**(3): 255–62.

Pollak, M. (2008). "Insulin and insulin-like growth factor signalling in neoplasia." Nat Rev Cancer **8**(12): 915–28.

Pollak, M., W. Beamer, et al. (1998). "Insulin-like growth factors and prostate cancer." Cancer Metastasis Rev **17**(4): 383–90.

Probst-Hensch, N. M., J. M. Yuan, et al. (2001). "IGF-1, IGF-2 and IGFBP-3 in prediagnostic serum: association with colorectal cancer in a cohort of Chinese men in Shanghai." Br J Cancer **85**(11): 1695–9.

Renehan A. G., M. Zwahlen, et al. (2004). "Insulin-like growth factor (IGF)-I, IGF binding protein-3, and cancer risk: systematic review and meta-regression analysis." Lancet **363**(9418): 1346–53.

Renehan, A. G., M. Harvie, et al. (2006). "Insulin-like growth factor (IGF)-I, IGF binding protein-3, and breast cancer risk: eight years on." Endocr Relat Cancer **13**(2): 273–8.

Rinaldi, S., R. Cleveland, et al. (2010). "Serum levels of IGF-I, IGFBP-3 and colorectal cancer risk: results from the EPIC cohort, plus a meta-analysis of prospective studies." Int J Cancer **126**(7): 1702–15.

Rinaldi, S., R. Kaaks, et al. (2005). "Insulin-like growth factor-I, IGF binding protein-3, and breast cancer in young women: a comparison of risk estimates using different peptide assays." Cancer Epidemiol Biomarkers Prev **14**(1): 48–52.

Rinaldi, S., P. H. Peeters, et al. (2006). "IGF-I, IGFBP-3 and breast cancer risk in women: The European Prospective Investigation into Cancer and Nutrition (EPIC)." Endocr Relat Cancer **13**(2): 593–605.

Roddam, A. W., N. E. Allen, et al. (2008). "Insulin-like growth factors, their binding proteins, and prostate cancer risk: analysis of individual patient data from 12 prospective studies." Ann Intern Med **149**(7): 461–71, W83-8.

Rollison, D. E., C. J. Newschaffer, et al. (2006). "Premenopausal levels of circulating insulin-like growth factor I and the risk of postmenopausal breast cancer." Int J Cancer **118**(5): 1279–84.

Ron, E., G. Gridley, et al. (1991). "Acromegaly and gastrointestinal cancer." Cancer **68**(8): 1673–7.

Rowlands, M. A., D. Gunnell, et al. (2009). "Circulating insulin-like growth factor peptides and prostate cancer risk: a systematic review and meta-analysis." Int J Cancer **124**(10): 2416–29.

Savage, C. J., H. Lilja, et al. (2010) "Empirical estimates of the lead time distribution for prostate cancer based on two independent representative cohorts of men not subject to prostate-specific antigen screening." Cancer Epidemiol Biomarkers Prev **19**(5): 1201–7.

Schairer, C., McCarty, C.A., Isaacs, C., Sue, L.Y., Pollak, M.N., Berg, C.D., Ziegler, R.G. (2010). "Circulating insulin-like growth factor (IGF)-1 and IGF binding protein (IGFBP)-3 levels and postmenopausal breast cancer risk in the Prostate, Lung, Colorectal and Ovarian Cancer Screening Trial (PLCO) Cohort." Hormones and Cancer(1): 100–111.

Schernhammer, E. S., J. M. Holly, et al. (2006). "Insulin-like growth factor-I, its binding proteins (IGFBP-1 and IGFBP-3), and growth hormone and breast cancer risk in The Nurses Health Study II." Endocr Relat Cancer **13**(2): 583–92.

Schernhammer, E. S., J. M. Holly, et al. (2005). "Circulating levels of insulin-like growth factors, their binding proteins, and breast cancer risk." Cancer Epidemiol Biomarkers Prev **14**(3): 699–704.

Schumacher, F. R., I. Cheng, et al. (2010). "A comprehensive analysis of common IGF1, IGFBP1 and IGFBP3 genetic variation with prospective IGF-I and IGFBP-3 blood levels and prostate cancer risk among Caucasians." Hum Mol Genet.

Severi, G., H. A. Morris, et al. (2006). "Circulating insulin-like growth factor-I and binding protein-3 and risk of prostate cancer." Cancer Epidemiol Biomarkers Prev **15**(6): 1137–41.

Shi R., H. Yu, et al. (2004). "IGF-I and breast cancer: a meta-analysis." Int J Cancer **111**(3):418–23.

Stattin, P., A. Bylund, et al. (2000). "Plasma insulin-like growth factor-I, insulin-like growth factor-binding proteins, and prostate cancer risk: a prospective study." J Natl Cancer Inst **92**(23): 1910–7.

Stattin, P., S. Rinaldi, et al. (2004). "High levels of circulating insulin-like growth factor-I increase prostate cancer risk: a prospective study in a population-based nonscreened cohort." J Clin Oncol **22**(15): 3104–12.

Stocks, T., A. Lukanova, et al. (2007). "Insulin resistance is inversely related to prostate cancer: a prospective study in Northern Sweden." Int J Cancer **120**(12): 2678–86.

Sugumar A., Y. C. Liu, et al. (2004). " Insulin-like growth factor (IGF)-I and IGF-binding protein 3 and the risk of premenopausal breast cancer: a meta-analysis of literature." Int J Cancer **111**(2): 293–7.

Toniolo, P., P. F. Bruning, et al. (2000). "Serum insulin-like growth factor-I and breast cancer." Int J Cancer **88**(5): 828–32.

Vatten, L. J., J. M. Holly, et al. (2008). "Nested case-control study of the association of circulating levels of serum insulin-like growth factor I and insulin-like growth factor binding protein 3 with breast cancer in young women in Norway." Cancer Epidemiol Biomarkers Prev **17**(8): 2097–100.

Verheus, M., P. H. Peeters, et al. (2006). "Serum C-peptide levels and breast cancer risk: results from the European Prospective Investigation into Cancer and Nutrition (EPIC)." Int J Cancer **119**(3): 659–67.

Wei, E. K., E. Giovannucci, et al. (2004). "Comparison of risk factors for colon and rectal cancer." Int J Cancer **108**(3): 433–42.

Wei, E. K., J. Ma, et al. (2005). "A prospective study of C-peptide, insulin-like growth factor-I, insulin-like growth factor binding protein-1, and the risk of colorectal cancer in women." Cancer Epidemiol Biomarkers Prev **14**(4): 850–5.

Weiss, J. M., W. Y. Huang, et al. (2007). "IGF-1 and IGFBP-3: Risk of prostate cancer among men in the Prostate, Lung, Colorectal and Ovarian Cancer Screening Trial." Int J Cancer **121**(10): 2267–73.

Woodson, K., J. A. Tangrea, et al. (2003). "Serum insulin-like growth factor I: tumor marker or etiologic factor? A prospective study of prostate cancer among Finnish men." Cancer Res **63**(14): 3991–4.

World Cancer Research Fund/American Institute for Cancer, R. (2007). Food, Nutrition, Physical Activity, and the Prevention of Cancer: a Global Perspective. . Washington DC AICR.

Zuccolo, L., R. Harris, et al. (2008). "Height and prostate cancer risk: a large nested case-control study (ProtecT) and meta-analysis." Cancer Epidemiol Biomarkers Prev **17**(9): 2325–36.

Chapter 2
Aging and Cancer: The IGF-I Connection

Kalina Biernacka, Claire Perks, and Jeff Holly

Introduction

Over the last decade there has been an explosion of interest in IGFs in two fields: that of cancer, culminating in the development of many new cancer therapies targeting the IGF-system, and that of aging, where experimental manipulations of the IGF-system have consistently been found to alter lifespan. In order to understand the role that IGFs may play in cancer and its relationship with aging this has to be considered within the context of the evolving concepts of cancer aetiology.

Molecular Aetiology of Cancer

Cancer is caused by gene mutations: either from gain of function of oncogenes or from loss of function of tumour suppressor genes. Cells that are actively dividing are at much greater risk for acquiring such mutations than non-dividing cells, and tumours generally originate from rapidly proliferating tissues. Cell proliferation is most active during early development and childhood but despite this human cancer is generally a disease of aging and the majority of cancers are not inherited. The replication of DNA does not occur with 100% fidelity, and mutations in all genes including neoplastic mutations are a frequent natural occurrence, but these only very rarely result in clinical cancers. Estimations of the rate of natural damage to DNA indicate a very high burden of mutations (Singer and Grunberger 1983). There are, however, many inbuilt safeguards: the integrity of the genome is tightly guarded

---

J.P. Holly (✉)
IGFs & Metabolic Endocrinology Group, School of Clinical Sciences,
University of Bristol, Learning and Research Building,
Southmead Hospital, Bristol, UK
e-mail: jeff.holly@bristol.ac.uk

D. LeRoith (ed.), *Insulin-like Growth Factors and Cancer: From Basic Biology to Therapeutics*, Cancer Drug Discovery and Development,
DOI 10.1007/978-1-4614-0598-6_2, © Springer Science+Business Media, LLC 2012

with a complex array of monitoring and repair mechanisms. Even with this potential for repair it has been reported that in normal skin epithelium mutations in the oncogenic gene p53 occur in around 50 clones within every square centimetre of skin, each clone containing between 60 and 30,000 cells (Jonason et al. 1996). Despite this huge number of cells with p53 mutations, they only very rarely result in cancers. This is because although neoplasias are initiated by oncogenic mutations, cells with potential transforming mutations then still have to evade controls such as contact-inhibition of growth, cell senescence and damage-induced apoptosis in order to progress to initiate cancers. For a cancer to develop there has to be background deregulation of cell proliferation together with a reduction in apoptosis and evasion of cell senescence: indeed it has been proposed that there are six essential controls that have to be overcome for a cancer to progress (Hanahan and Weinberg 2000). It is now clear that many of these safeguards are regulated processes and hence open to influence by environmental cues.

There are several other observations which indicate that the initiating mutations are not sufficient to generate a clinical cancer. The incidence of lung cancer increases rapidly in smokers, but then in individuals who cease to smoke the incidence remains roughly constant, and does not fall for many years despite the cessation of exposure to carcinogen (Halpern et al. 1993). This implies that other factors independent of smoking are responsible for the progression from mutated cell to clinical cancer. The importance of the local tissue environment for a transformed cell to become a cancer is also indicated by genetic cancer syndromes caused by highly penetrant mutations, such as Bloom syndrome, neurofibromatosis and BRCA1/2 mutations (Vineis 2003). Even in such syndromes where there is a clearly identified heritable risk, despite these mutations occurring throughout the whole body, they only result in cancers within specific tissues where presumably the milieu provides the favourable setting. In all other tissues, these mutations do not result in tumours and therefore by themselves these are not alone sufficient to cause cancer. Thus, while cancers are initiated by oncogenic mutations, some selective advantage for the cell within its environment is also required for the cancer to develop to clinical disease.

By the early 1990s, it was realised that cancers arise due to not one but a series of mutations (Vogelstein and Kinzler 1993) and since then many have attempted to define the actual number of mutations that are responsible for cancers. It soon became apparent that most tumours harbour many mutations and estimates ranged up to many tens of thousands although it was appreciated that many of these may be passenger mutations that provide no advantage to the tumour rather than driver mutations. Recent advances in technology made it possible to assess the mutations in the vast majority of genes that actually encode for proteins in two of the most common human cancers, colorectal and breast (Wood et al. 2007; Sjoblom 2008). These studies conclude that there were around 80 mutations that alter amino acid sequences in proteins that may contribute to the development of these cancers. In this newly mapped cancer genome landscape there were mountains, which comprised a small number of commonly mutated, well known cancer-related genes such as p53, but the landscape was really dominated by a much larger number of infrequently mutated genes referred to as gene "hills." These gene hills were surprisingly not hopelessly complex, but many were genes that could be mapped to a limited number of cell signalling pathways and it was concluded that it was these pathways rather than individual genes which appeared to govern the course of tumorigenesis (Vogelstein and Kinzler 2004; Wood et al. 2007). One signalling pathway prominent for both breast and colorectal cancers was the PI3k–Akt/PKB pathway. This signalling pathway is obviously one of the canonical signalling pathways activated by the IGF-I receptor. These new findings added to the wealth of existing evidence implying an important role for the IGFs in many different cancers. As reviewed in many of the other contributions to this issue evidence has amassed from cell and animal models demonstrating that IGFs have multiple actions that could support and promote carcinogenesis and evidence from clinical studies have also demonstrated that there were alterations to the IGF-system in many human cancers.

Cancer and Aging

The one clear common risk factor for many human cancers is age; the prevalence in human populations of most clinical cancers increases exponentially with advancing age, and as longevity increases in most developed countries the incidence of cancer also inevitably increases. In respect to the age-distribution of its prevalence, cancer is no different in its trajectory and relationship to lifespan from many age-related degenerative diseases. Aging is generally considered as an overall decline of the integrity and functions of many systems; decrease in lean muscle mass, accumulation of body fat, loss of bone mineral density, decreased reproductive capacity, reduced cognitive function and ultimately increased mortality. In humans, more than 80% of neoplastic diseases are diagnosed after the age of 50 years. Nearly 1.5 million cancer cases were diagnosed in 2009 in US study (US Census Bureau) and an estimated 60% of cancer incidences and 70% of cancer-related mortality occurred in subjects older than 65 years. There are some marked site-specific variations in the age-related incidence of different cancers (Rubin et al. 2010) but the most prevalent cancers all occur after the age of 50.

Carcinogenesis is a multistage, multifactor process and the mechanisms involved parallel to those involved in normal tissue development, maintenance, and senescence but in cancers these processes occur inappropriately. Many of the molecular, cellular and physiological events that are associated with aging are also implicated in carcinogenesis and subsequent tumour growth (Dix et al. 1980). Aging and cancer both may result from accumulated cellular damage and both may be related to the control of specific genes in the damage/repair response. While the association between cancer prevalence and aging is clear, there remains some uncertainty in relation to the underlying mechanisms. There are several mechanisms that may contribute to the effect of age on cancer prevalence. The first relates to the duration of exposure and to the length of time for accumulation of genetic aberrations. There is considerable evidence indicating that the number of genetic alterations in cells and tissues increases with age in experimental animals and in humans (Vijg 2007). Consistent with this there is evidence indicating that spontaneous neoplasias increase with age across a broad range of species from invertebrates through to humans (Anisimov et al. 2009). As discussed above, however, there is evidence that the actual burden of mutations is very high throughout the lifespan and the accumulation of defects may not just reflect duration of exposure to damaging agents but could also be due to an age-related deterioration in DNA repair mechanisms (Gorbunova et al. 2007). The second consideration is that progressive changes in the internal milieu with age may provide a more favourable environment for the induction and development of neoplastic lesions and also for the growth of latent malignant cells. For example, age-related alterations in the immune and endocrine systems may contribute to establishing this more favourable internal environment. There is experimental evidence which clearly shows that changes in the internal milieu with age does influence tumour development. When neoplastically transformed liver epithelial cells were transplanted into rats of different ages their tumorigenic potential increased with advancing age of the recipient rats (McCullough et al. 1994). In contrast, when rhabdomyosarcoma cells were inoculated into rats of different ages the number of resulting lung tumours was greatest in the youngest rats and correlated positively with the IGF-I-activity in the lung (Anisimov et al. 1988). There is also some clinical evidence that age-related changes in the internal milieu affect tumour growth. For example, the local recurrence of breast cancer 4 years after partial mastectomy was reported to be 18% in women younger than 55 years but only 3% in women older than 55 (Veronesi et al. 2001). Another mechanism that may contribute to the age-dependency of cancers relates to age-related cellular changes that may predispose to neoplasia including epigenetic gene silencing, telomere shortening and altered stromal derived factors.

Over the last decade it has become increasingly clear that the IGF-system plays a pivotal role in both aging and in the development of many cancers. Reports that various manipulations of the IGF-system can dramatically alter lifespan have generated considerable interest in the role that IGFs may play in aging. Avoiding cancer is clearly one route to a long lifespan but the links go beyond this obvious truism and it has become clear from work in many experimental models that the IGFs have a fundamental role in aging which has been conserved throughout evolution (Kenyon 2010). Genetic studies have established that many genes that affect lifespan are stress-response genes or nutrient sensors which in periods when harsh conditions are encountered enhance the ability of the organism to survive. These genes appear to enable the organism to shift its physiology from its normal program for growth and reproduction to one in which cell protection and maintenance are prioritised. Although this shift does not favour selection for longevity per se, however, the evolution of such mechanisms would enable organisms to survive better through harsh, life-threatening environments and as a secondary consequence would have naturally prolonged lifespan by the enhanced cell-protection pathways also reducing the wear and tear that contribute to aging. The most well-studied environmental stress is that of nutrient deprivation. In the last great depression in the 1930s, there was concern that hunger may shorten the lives of those affected but studies at the time addressing

2 Aging and Cancer: The IGF-I Connection

this in rats established that in fact it had the opposite effect. This has subsequently been confirmed in many experimental models and including recently in primates (Colman et al. 2009). It was initially thought that nutritional deprivation prolonged lifespan merely due to decreased nutrient metabolism resulting in a reduced rate of cellular damage but it gradually became clear that the effect was mediated by nutrient sensing pathways which engage a switch from cell growth to cell maintenance. Dietary restriction in most experimental animals decreases the activity of the insulin/IGF axis and this mediates the increase in lifespan in many circumstances. The two pathways overlap is confirmed by the lack of effect of dietary restriction in mice that already have an extended lifespan due to deficiencies in activity of the IGF-system (Bartke 2008; Arum et al. 2009). For almost as long as it has been known to extend lifespan it has been recognised that the most robust strategy for reducing cancer is also by dietary restriction. Dietary restriction is known to lower IGF-I levels and mice with reduced IGF-I-activity not only have increased lifespan but they also have reduced susceptibility to cancer (Ikeno et al. 2003) as reviewed by Shoshana Yakar in Chap. 6. Replacing the reduced IGF-I in calorie-restricted mice negates the benefits in terms of preventing tumour promotion (Dunn et al. 1997) indicating that IGF-I mediates this beneficial effect of dietary restriction. That reduced IGF-I activity and reduced nutritional intake act via a common pathway is also indicated by the observation that dietary restriction fails to inhibit cancers induced by constitutive activation of signalling pathways downstream of the IGF-I receptor (Kalaany and Sabatini 2009).

Occult Tumours and Clinical Cancers in Human Populations

From the very high rates of oncogenic mutations it should be expected that neoplastic lesions would also be common. Many different sources of evidence relating to the prevalence of latent neoplastic lesions indicate that they are indeed very common in the general population and in many tissues these lesions increase with age. A very high prevalence of latent, clinically asymptomatic cancers has been universally discovered incidentally in both screening and autopsy studies of normal populations. Both autopsy studies and colonoscopy screening studies indicate an increasing presence of colonic adenomas with age such that the incidence reached around 50% by the age of 80 years (Renehan et al. 2000). Even more extensive data are available for latent prostate neoplasias in men; again, autopsy studies reveal very prevalent rates of latent cancers in the general population (Delongchamps et al. 2006). All studies indicate a steady increase with age, with prevalence estimates of 50% of all men by the age of 70 years (Sakr et al. 1994) and up to 80% of men aged over 90 years (Sheldon et al. 1980). Further evidence for the high prevalence of latent cancers comes from data from biopsies taken from men with normal prostate-specific antigen (PSA) and digital rectal examinations in the Prostate Cancer Prevention Trial. The prevalence of latent cancers detected from biopsies (15.2%) was lower than in comparable autopsy series (18.5–38.8%) (Thompson et al. 2004;

Gosselaar et al. 2005), but this difference would be expected because of the under-detection rate when comparing small biopsies with whole-mount prostate analysis that is possible at autopsy. Although data are only available for a limited number of specific tissues in the body, it is clear that all individuals are probably harbouring one or more subclinical latent neoplastic lesions by the age of 70, and a large proportion of the population have such lesions present by the age of 50.

Despite the recognition that oncogenic transforming mutations occur at an extremely high rate and the observations that neoplastic lesions are very prevalent and increase with age, it is clear that the incidence of clinical cancers is very much lower which indicates that few of the neoplastic lesions actually progress to clinical disease. The explanation for this discrepancy is that for a clinical cancer to develop, in addition to the initiating mutations there has also to be a permissive internal environment. This internal milieu may initially determine whether a mutated cell survives and avoids cell senescence, but then may also determine its subsequent rate of proliferation and hence its propensity to progress to become a clinical cancer.

There is some evidence for variations in the prevalence of latent neoplasias according to geographical location around the world. For example, there are up to twofold differences in the prevalence of latent prostate neoplasias in different regions; but this is very small compared to the global variations in incidence of clinical prostate cancer which vary by up to 100-fold (Haas et al. 2008). This indicates that even in regions where the incidence of clinical prostate cancer is very low, such as Japan and China, the prevalence of clinically undetected occult cancers are very high but obviously less progress to clinical disease. The clear conclusion from this evidence is that there is a relatively small variation in the high rates of initiation of cancers between different regions, consistent with the high inherent rate of oncogenic mutations; but in contrast there is a relatively large variation in the rates of progression to clinical disease. This variation in progression to clinical disease appears to be mostly due to differences in lifestyle and/or environmental exposures. This is clearly indicated by studies of migrants who have moved between regions of the world with different rates of clinical cancers; such studies demonstrate that cancer rates in migrants soon converge to that of their new locale (Peto 2001; Iwasaki et al. 2004; Lee et al. 2007; Rastogi et al. 2008). This excludes simple genetic explanations for the large geographical variations as clearly somatic genes do not change within just a few generations. For example, the incidence of breast, colon and prostate cancers is considerably lower in Japan than in America, but in Japanese migrants who have relocated to Hawaii the incidence of these cancers becomes similar to that of indigenous Hawaiian Caucasians within one generation (Peto 2001). This clearly indicates that environmental exposures are a strong determinant of the rate of progression to clinical disease. Similar implications can be made from studies within countries where environmental exposures have rapidly changed due to changes in lifestyle. Japan was virtually closed to Western influences until the 1950s, since then there has been a remarkable Westernisation of dietary habits (Tominaga and Kuroishi 1997). This change in exposure has been accompanied by a rapid increase in the height of Japanese girls, followed – with a

2 Aging and Cancer: The IGF-I Connection

30-year lag-period – by a parallel increase in the incidence of breast cancer (Michels and Willett 2004). This indicates that changing environmental exposures which resulted in increased childhood growth may also have influenced the subsequent risk of this cancer. These large changes throughout the society in Japan have also been accompanied by an increase in the observed prevalence of latent prostate cancers; the age-adjusted rate was estimated as 22.5% from an autopsy series between 1965 and 1979 and had increased to 34.6% from a similar series between 1982 and 1986 (Yatani et al. 1988). This was then comparable to the rate of 34.6% in white men in the USA (Yatani et al. 1982) despite the incidence of clinical prostate cancers being at least tenfold higher in the USA than in Japan (Watanabe et al. 2000). If the effect of environmental exposures was an effect of initiating carcinogens, then the rates of latent cancers would be expected to increase in migrants who move from regions of the world with low incidence of cancers to regions with high incidence. The limited available data, however, indicate that the prevalence of latent prostate cancers were similar in Japanese migrants to Hawaii as in indigenous Japanese (Shiraishi et al. 1994), despite the large increase in clinical cancers.

The relatively small genetic contribution to the risk of most common cancers has also been indicated in studies of very large cohorts of twins comparing incidence of sporadic cancers in monozygotic twins (who share all of their genes) with dizygotic twins (who share 50% of their segregated genes) (Lichtenstein et al. 2000). From this comparison, it was estimated that the risk of breast cancer was 27% due to heritable factors and 73% due to environmental factors. The importance of environmental exposures is even apparent when there is a clearly identified strong heritable risk such as BRCA1/2 mutations. Within a community of over 1,000 Ashkenazi Jewish women with inherited mutations in BRCA1/2, the risk of developing clinical breast cancer by the age of 50 was 24% in those born before 1940 but increased to 67% in those born after 1940, with physical exercise and obesity being factors determining cancer onset (King et al. 2003). Similarly, for women in Iceland with BRCA2 mutations the risk of developing breast cancer by the age of 70 was 18.6% in 1920 and had risen to 71.9% by 2002; over the same time period in the general population the increased risk was from 1.8 to 7.5% (Tryggvadottir et al. 2006). The relative temporal increase in cancer risk due to environmental changes was therefore approximately the same in women with a clearly identified heritable risk as it was for women with sporadic cancers. A recent study of French Canadian families with inherited BRCA1/2 mutations found that diet was a strong determinant of cancer risk (Nkondjock et al. 2006). These studies indicate that exposures that determine progression to clinical disease have a large effect and operate independently of the initiating factors. Taken together these different lines of evidence indicate that although cancers are initiated by gene defects, genetic susceptibility makes a relatively small contribution towards the risk of these common cancers developing into clinical disease compared to a major role played by environmental exposures. In addition, it also importantly suggests that most cancers are in principle avoidable, even when there is a high genetic risk. This makes it important to characterise the environmental exposures that affect this risk; with the important question relating not to the risk of initiating neoplastic lesions but to the risk of progression to clinical disease. These common cancers are prevalent in all developed "Westernised" societies in which industrialisation and advances in technology have dramatically changed both the pattern and amount of physical activity and also completely changed the composition and quantity of dietary intake (Cordain et al. 2005). A "Westernised" lifestyle is characterised by the consumption of large volumes of energy-dense processed foods combined with very sedentary lifestyles. This causes a large energy imbalance which has resulted in an epidemic of obesity with associated metabolic and hormonal imbalances (Mistry et al. 2007). The geographic distribution of Westernised industrialisation and urban development mirrors closely the variations in incidence of these common clinical cancers, such as prostate cancer (Mistry et al. 2007). When considering the exposures that may be responsible for the promotion of latent neoplastic lesions into clinical cancers the metabolic and hormonal imbalance are prime suspects as factors like IGFs are nutritionally dependent and have many actions that could promote cancer progression.

IGFs, Aging and Cancer

There is a gradual decline in circulating IGF-I levels throughout adult life. This has been termed the "somatopause," in analogy with the menopause, and there has been a long debate about whether hormone replacement therapy should be used to prevent the decline in GH and IGF-I analogous to estrogen replacement therapy in post-menopausal women (Lieberman and Hoffman 1997). However, unlike the menopause which is triggered by an abrupt life-event: the switch-off of ovarian function signalling the end of a woman's reproductive life, the decline in IGF-I is a gradual process starting in early adult life soon after puberty. The debate in relation to replacement therapy for the somatopause is controversial with many sides of the risk/benefit balance unclear. In respect to cancer there are important points that should be considered in this debate. There is very limited evidence to indicate that variations in IGF-I may initiate the oncogenic process. Studies in experimental animals which examine whether raised GH/IGF-I levels cause cancer are therefore not relevant to the elderly human population in which most individuals will already harbour latent occult neoplasias. The relevant question in elderly human populations is whether altering the level of IGF-I will affect the development of the neoplastic lesions that are already present. There is now much evidence from experimental animals that lower IGF-I levels reduce the progression of induced cancers as reviewed by Shoshana Yakar in Chap. 6 and there is also considerable epidemiology indicating that in human populations individuals with lower levels of IGF-I are relatively protected from the common cancers (Roddam et al. 2008; Key et al. 2010). These observations could imply that the age-related decline in IGF-I levels is a protective mechanism. As reviewed above the evidence from research

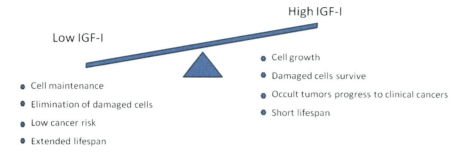

Fig. 2.1 Balancing factors that affect the links between IGF, aging and cancer

into aging in a variety of experimental models suggests that lower IGF-I levels are part of a mechanism that enables a shift from growth and development to cell protection and maintenance. This mechanism for protection against stress also appears to apply to genotoxic stress; reducing levels of IGF-I protects against carcinogens by permitting more effective elimination of damaged cells by apoptosis (Dunn et al. 1997; Longo et al. 2008). These studies imply that the age-related decline in IGF-I may have a function in facilitating the removal of damaged cells that increasingly occur with age and therefore reducing the risk of cancers developing. At least in some tissues the apoptosis that is induced by genotoxic stress however declines with age, as observed in the liver of rats (Suh et al. 2002). This reduced ability to eliminate mutated cells could contribute to the increase in cancers with age and suggests that at least in this tissue reduced levels of IGF-I with age do not over-ride and provide protection. The levels of IGF-I receptors are however very low in hepatocytes which may therefore be relatively insensitive to changes in IGF-I and the situation may be very different in tissues where IGF-I receptors are prevalent such as in glandular epithelial cells.

Conclusions

As humans age the prevalence of occult tumours increases such that most elderly individuals harbour latent cancers. Whether these neoplastic lesions progress to clinical disease is then dependent on environmental exposures; in particular, a Western lifestyle with its associated metabolic and endocrine imbalances promotes the development of clinical cancers. From early adult life IGF-I levels gradually decline. With age cellular damage increases, at least partly due to deterioration in DNA repair mechanisms. Lower IGF-I levels may promote an extended lifespan by enabling a switch from cell growth to cell protection and maintenance; and they may also facilitate the elimination of damage cells which occur with increasing frequency with age (Fig. 2.1).

References

Anisimov, V. N., E. Sikora, et al. (2009). "Relationships between cancer and aging: a multilevel approach." Biogerontology **10**(4): 323–338.

Anisimov, V. N., N. V. Zhukovskaya, et al. (1988). "Influence of host age on lung colony forming capacity of injected rat rhabdomyosarcoma cells." Cancer Lett **40**(1): 77–82.

Arum, O., M. S. Bonkowski, et al. (2009). "The growth hormone receptor gene-disrupted mouse fails to respond to an intermittent fasting diet." Aging Cell **8**(6): 756–760.

Bartke, A. (2008). "Insulin and aging." Cell Cycle **7**(21): 3338–3343.

Colman, R. J., R. M. Anderson, et al. (2009). "Caloric restriction delays disease onset and mortality in rhesus monkeys." Science **325**(5937): 201–204.

Cordain, L., S. B. Eaton, et al. (2005). "Origins and evolution of the Western diet: health implications for the 21st century." Am J Clin Nutr **81**(2): 341–354.

Delongchamps, N. B., A. Singh, et al. (2006). "The role of prevalence in the diagnosis of prostate cancer." Cancer Control **13**(3): 158–168.

Dix, D., P. Cohen, et al. (1980). "On the role of aging in cancer incidence." J Theor Biol **83**(1): 163–173.

Dunn, S. E., F. W. Kari, et al. (1997). "Dietary restriction reduces insulin-like growth factor I levels, which modulates apoptosis, cell proliferation, and tumor progression in p53-deficient mice." Cancer Res **57**(21): 4667–4672.

Gorbunova, V., A. Seluanov, et al. (2007). "Changes in DNA repair during aging." Nucleic Acids Res **35**(22): 7466–7474.

Gosselaar, C., M. J. Roobol, et al. (2005). "Prevalence and characteristics of screen-detected prostate carcinomas at low prostate-specific antigen levels: aggressive or insignificant?" BJU Int **95**(2): 231–237.

Haas, G. P., N. Delongchamps, et al. (2008). "The worldwide epidemiology of prostate cancer: perspectives from autopsy studies." Can J Urol **15**(1): 3866–3871.

Halpern, M. T., B. W. Gillespie, et al. (1993). "Patterns of absolute risk of lung cancer mortality in former smokers." J Natl Cancer Inst **85**(6): 457–464.

Hanahan, D. and R. A. Weinberg (2000). "The hallmarks of cancer." Cell **100**(1): 57–70.

Ikeno, Y., R. T. Bronson, et al. (2003). "Delayed occurrence of fatal neoplastic diseases in ames dwarf mice: correlation to extended longevity." J Gerontol A Biol Sci Med Sci **58**(4): 291–296.

Iwasaki, M., C. P. Mameri, et al. (2004). "Cancer mortality among Japanese immigrants and their descendants in the state of Sao Paulo, Brazil, 1999–2001." Jpn J Clin Oncol **34**(11): 673–680.

Jonason, A. S., S. Kunala, et al. (1996). "Frequent clones of p53-mutated keratinocytes in normal human skin." Proc Natl Acad Sci U S A **93**(24): 14025–14029.

Kalaany, N. Y. and D. M. Sabatini (2009). "Tumours with PI3K activation are resistant to dietary restriction." Nature **458**(7239): 725–731.

Kenyon, C. J. (2010). "The genetics of ageing." Nature **464**(7288): 504–512.

Key, T. J., P. N. Appleby, et al. (2010). "Insulin-like growth factor 1 (IGF1), IGF binding protein 3 (IGFBP3), and breast cancer risk: pooled individual data analysis of 17 prospective studies." Lancet Oncol **11**(6): 530–542.

King, M. C., J. H. Marks, et al. (2003). "Breast and ovarian cancer risks due to inherited mutations in BRCA1 and BRCA2." Science **302**(5645): 643–646.

Lee, J., K. Demissie, et al. (2007). "Cancer incidence among Korean-American immigrants in the United States and native Koreans in South Korea." Cancer Control **14**(1): 78–85.

Lichtenstein, P., N. V. Holm, et al. (2000). "Environmental and heritable factors in the causation of cancer--analyses of cohorts of twins from Sweden, Denmark, and Finland." N Engl J Med **343**(2): 78–85.

Lieberman, S. A. and A. R. Hoffman (1997). "The somatopause: should growth hormone deficiency in older people Be treated?" Clin Geriatr Med **13**(4): 671–684.

2 Aging and Cancer: The IGF-I Connection

Longo, V. D., M. R. Lieber, et al. (2008). "Turning anti-ageing genes against cancer." Nat Rev Mol Cell Biol **9**(11): 903–910.

McCullough, K. D., W. B. Coleman, et al. (1994). "Age-dependent regulation of the tumorigenic potential of neoplastically transformed rat liver epithelial cells by the liver microenvironment." Cancer Res **54**(14): 3668–3671.

Michels, K. B. and W. C. Willett (2004). "Breast cancer--early life matters." N Engl J Med **351**(16): 1679–1681.

Mistry, T., J. E. Digby, et al. (2007). "Obesity and prostate cancer: a role for adipokines." Eur Urol **52**(1): 46–53.

Nkondjock, A., A. Robidoux, et al. (2006). "Diet, lifestyle and BRCA-related breast cancer risk among French-Canadians." Breast Cancer Res Treat **98**(3): 285–294.

Peto, J. (2001). "Cancer epidemiology in the last century and the next decade." Nature **411**(6835): 390–395.

Rastogi, T., S. Devesa, et al. (2008). "Cancer incidence rates among South Asians in four geographic regions: India, Singapore, UK and US." Int J Epidemiol **37**(1): 147–160.

Renehan, A. G., P. Bhaskar, et al. (2000). "The prevalence and characteristics of colorectal neoplasia in acromegaly." J Clin Endocrinol Metab **85**(9): 3417–3424.

Roddam, A. W., N. E. Allen, et al. (2008). "Insulin-like growth factors, their binding proteins, and prostate cancer risk: analysis of individual patient data from 12 prospective studies." Ann Intern Med **149**(7): 461–471, W483–468.

Rubin, P., J. P. Williams, et al. (2010). "Cancer genesis across the age spectrum: associations with tissue development, maintenance, and senescence." Semin Radiat Oncol **20**(1): 3–11.

Sakr, W. A., D. J. Grignon, et al. (1994). "High grade prostatic intraepithelial neoplasia (HGPIN) and prostatic adenocarcinoma between the ages of 20–69: an autopsy study of 249 cases." In Vivo **8**(3): 439–443.

Sheldon, C. A., R. D. Williams, et al. (1980). "Incidental carcinoma of the prostate: a review of the literature and critical reappraisal of classification." J Urol **124**(5): 626–631.

Shiraishi, T., M. Watanabe, et al. (1994). "The frequency of latent prostatic carcinoma in young males: the Japanese experience." In Vivo **8**(3): 445–447.

Singer, B. and D. Grunberger (1983). Molecular biology of mutagens and carcinogens. New York; London, Plenum.

Sjoblom, T. (2008). "Systematic analyses of the cancer genome: lessons learned from sequencing most of the annotated human protein-coding genes." Curr Opin Oncol **20**(1): 66–71.

Suh, Y., K. A. Lee, et al. (2002). "Aging alters the apoptotic response to genotoxic stress." Nat Med **8**(1): 3–4.

Thompson, I. M., D. K. Pauler, et al. (2004). "Prevalence of prostate cancer among men with a prostate-specific antigen level < or =4.0 ng per milliliter." N Engl J Med **350**(22): 2239–2246.

Tominaga, S. and T. Kuroishi (1997). "An ecological study on diet/nutrition and cancer in Japan." Int J Cancer **Suppl 10**: 2–6.

Tryggvadottir, L., H. Sigvaldason, et al. (2006). "Population-based study of changing breast cancer risk in Icelandic BRCA2 mutation carriers, 1920–2000." J Natl Cancer Inst **98**(2): 116–122.

Veronesi, U., E. Marubini, et al. (2001). "Radiotherapy after breast-conserving surgery in small breast carcinoma: long-term results of a randomized trial." Ann Oncol **12**(7): 997–1003.

Vijg, J. (2007). Aging of the genome : the dual role of the DNA in life and death. Oxford, Oxford University Press.

Vineis, P. (2003). "Cancer as an evolutionary process at the cell level: an epidemiological perspective." Carcinogenesis **24**(1): 1–6.

Vogelstein, B. and K. W. Kinzler (1993). "The multistep nature of cancer." Trends Genet **9**(4): 138–141.

Vogelstein, B. and K. W. Kinzler (2004). "Cancer genes and the pathways they control." Nat Med **10**(8): 789–799.

Watanabe, M., T. Nakayama, et al. (2000). "Comparative studies of prostate cancer in Japan versus the United States. A review." Urol Oncol **5**(6): 274–283.

Wood, L. D., D. W. Parsons, et al. (2007). "The genomic landscapes of human breast and colorectal cancers." Science **318**(5853): 1108–1113.

Yatani, R., I. Chigusa, et al. (1982). "Geographic pathology of latent prostatic carcinoma." Int J Cancer **29**(6): 611–616.

Yatani, R., T. Shiraishi, et al. (1988). "Trends in frequency of latent prostate carcinoma in Japan from 1965–1979 to 1982–1986." J Natl Cancer Inst **80**(9): 683–687.

Chapter 3
Obesity, Type 2 Diabetes and Cancer

Rosalyn D. Ferguson and Derek LeRoith

Introduction

A large percentage of the developed world's population is now either officially overweight or obese; meanwhile, cancer rates have been rising steadily. Cases of type 2 diabetes have also become alarmingly common. In this chapter, we discuss the epidemiological evidence which suggests that obesity, type 2 diabetes and cancer are linked. Possible mechanisms for obesity leading to type 2 diabetes and cancer are discussed, as well as the recent studies which potentially uncover therapies to treat aspects and reduce the rates of cancer associated with obesity and type 2 diabetes.

Obesity

The World Health Organization classifies body mass index (BMI) into four broad groups: underweight (BMI < 18.5 kg/m^2), normal weight (BMI 18.5–24.9 kg/m^2), overweight (BMI 25–29.9 kg/m^2), and obese ($\geq$30 kg/m^2) (WHO 1995). Statistics show that globally, in 2005, around 23% of the world's population was overweight and 9.8% were obese and, from now to 2030, these figures are predicted to increase (Kelly et al. 2005). Reports for specific countries show substantial variations on these figures, with the most recent NHANES data from 2007 to 2008 showing the rates of overweight and obese individuals in the USA to be standing at 68 and

---

D. LeRoith (✉)
Division of Endocrinology, Diabetes and Bone Diseases,
The Samuel Bronfman Department of Medicine, Mount Sinai
School of Medicine, New York, NY, USA
e-mail: Derek.leroith@mssm.edu

D. LeRoith (ed.), *Insulin-like Growth Factors and Cancer: From Basic Biology
to Therapeutics*, Cancer Drug Discovery and Development,
DOI 10.1007/978-1-4614-0598-6_3, © Springer Science+Business Media, LLC 2012

33.8% respectively (Flegal et al. 1999). From this data, a climb to 86.3% overweight and 51.1% obese US individuals is forecast by 2030 (Wang et al. 2008). The most recent Health Survey for England reveals that 61% of adults there are overweight, and of these, 24.5% are classified as obese (NHS 2008). In Australia, 48.2% of men and 29.9% of women were classed as overweight in 2000; of these, 19.3% of men and 22.2% of women were officially obese. In China, Japan, and India, although the percentage of obese individuals (all <5%) is lower than in those countries mentioned above, the average BMI has been rising steadily between 1997 and 2002 and is predicted to continue doing so over the next two decades (McMichael 2008).

With the rise in easily affordable, high-calorie processed food and a decline in physical activity, obesity trends may not reverse in the near future. The cost of the obesity epidemic is increasing yearly. Associated with obesity are a host of other health issues, which at present have an annual medical cost of $147 billion (Finkelstein et al. 2009), while in the UK the direct cost of obesity and related illness to the National Health Service is currently £4.3 billion annually – 5% of the total budget. Worldwide, on average, countries spend between 0.7 and 2.8% of the total health budget on the treatment of obesity-related disorders (Withrow and Alter 2010).

Obesity and Type 2 Diabetes

Diabetes mellitus is a disease characterized by a collection of serious dysfunctions including impaired insulin action, inadequate insulin secretion (or both of these), chronically elevated circulating glucose levels and impaired carbohydrate, fat and protein metabolism. Diabetes mellitus was the seventh leading cause of death in the USA in 2006 and, at present, 23.6 million people or 7.8% of the population have diabetes, consisting of 17.9 million diagnosed and a further 5.7 million undiagnosed cases (Diabetes Research and Statistics 2007). In the UK in 2009, 2.6 million cases of diabetes mellitus were diagnosed and an estimated 0.5 million cases remain undiagnosed (Diabetes UK 2010). Although cases of diabetes mellitus may be classified as type 1, type 2, or gestational diabetes mellitus (Alberti and Zimmet 1998), the huge rise in numbers of diabetics is largely attributable to an increase in type 2 diabetes. At present, 85–95% of diabetics suffer this form of the disease.

Although type 2 diabetes is associated with older age, family history of diabetes, history of gestational diabetes, physical inactivity and race/ethnicity (African Americans, Hispanic/Latino Americans and American Indians are at particularly high risk for type 2 diabetes and its complications) the most critical risk factor for developing type 2 diabetes is obesity. Almost 70–80 % of type 2 diabetics are obese; moreover, several long-term prospective studies have shown a higher risk of diabetes with increasing body weight. An NHANES survey 25 years ago highlighted an association between being overweight and suffering from diabetes (Van Itallie 1985). A 13.5-year prospective metabolic study on a group of 54-year-old Swedish men showed a clear correlation between increased BMI and type 2 diabetes (Ohlson et al. 1988). A 12-year long prospective study on a group of 50-year-old Swedish women also associated increased BMI with type 2 diabetes (Lundgren et al. 1989). A study on British men aged 40–59 reported that an increased BMI was the dominant risk factor for diabetes (Perry et al. 1995). In the USA, a study of 30- to 55-year-old women demonstrated that BMI and type 2 diabetes were positively associated (Colditz et al. 1995). Recently, it has been discovered that even apparently metabolically healthy overweight or obese men are still at significantly higher risk of developing type 2 diabetes (Arnlov 2009).

Obesity and Cancer

As well as type 2 diabetes, other complications including coronary heart disease (Willett et al. 1995; Rimm et al. 1995; Krauss et al. 1998; Rexrode et al. 1997; Kato et al. 1992; Anderson and Felson 1988), and numerous cancers (WHO 2002) are all now included as risks associated with obesity. Cancer is one of the leading causes of death worldwide, accounting for around 7.4 million deaths in 2004 (ACS 2010). In the USA, cancer is the second most common cause of death after heart disease, and The American Cancer Society predicts that this year alone, 1.5 million Americans will die from cancer (ACS 2010). In 2002 it was officially recognized by the International Agency for Research into Cancer (WHO 2002) that an increased risk of cancer of the colon, breast (postmenopausal), endometrium, kidney, and esophagus was associated with obesity (Vainio et al. 2002). A large, US-based Cancer Prevention Study II (CPSII) reported that for men with a BMI of 35–40 kg/m^2 or above 40 kg/m^2 the relative risk of dying from any cancer was 1.20 and 1.52 times that of the normal weight individual, respectively. Similarly, for women with BMI values of 30–35 kg/m^2 or greater than 40 kg/m^2, the relative risk for dying from any cancer rose from that of the normal weight individual to 1.32 and 1.62, respectively (Calle et al. 2003). This study specifically stated that cancer of the colon, rectum, liver, gallbladder, pancreas, and kidney as well as esophageal adenocarcinoma, non-Hodgkin's lymphoma, and multiple myeloma were all associated with overweight or obesity. Furthermore, significant trends of increasing risk with higher BMI values were reported for cancers of the stomach and prostate in men and of the breast (postmenopausal), uterus, cervix, and ovary in women (Calle et al. 2003). Obesity has continued to be linked to cancer of the breast (postmenopausally) (Lahmann et al. 2004; Berclaz et al. 2004; Dossus et al. 2010; Moore et al. 2004; Larsson and Wolk 2007a; Moghaddam et al. 2007; Larsson et al. 2007), pancreas (Larsson et al. 2007) and also adenocarcinoma of the esophagus (Corley et al. 2008), and remains associated with an increase in the risk of B-cell lymphoma (Larsson and Wolk 2007b) and multiple myeloma (Birmann et al. 2007). Gastric cardia cancer (Kubo and Corley 2006) and intrahepatic cholangiocarcinoma (Welzel et al. 2007) have additionally been reported to be associated with obesity. In 2007, the World

Cancer Research Fund reported that increased body adiposity is related to pancreatic, colorectal, breast (postmenopausal), endometrial and kidney cancer (McMichael 2008). A study of British men recently showed that being overweight or obese raised the risk of mortality from carcinoma of the rectum, bladder, colon and liver, and from lymphoma (Batty et al. 2008). Similar studies in Canada, Japan and other areas of Europe yielded similar results (Bergstrom et al. 2001; Pan et al. 2004; Kuriyama et al. 2005). In 2008, a large meta-analysis of 221 datasets showed that obesity significantly increased the risk of colon, renal and thyroid cancer, esophageal adenocarcinoma and malignant and multiple myeloma and furthermore, for the first time, highlighted that Asia-Pacific populations have rates of obesity-related cancers similar to the USA, Europe, and Australia (Renehan et al. 2008). In 2010, the European Prospective Investigation into Cancer and Nutrition (EPIC) reported a significant association between increased BMI and postmenopausal breast and colorectal cancers (Gonzalez and Riboli 2010). Meanwhile, being overweight appears to have a protective effect on breast cancer in premenopausal women (Ursin et al. 1995; van den Brandt et al. 2000) and is in fact inversely associated with lung cancer, although results have been confounded somewhat by smoking and body weight issues (Renehan et al. 2008). Data on ovarian cancer are inconsistent (Olsen et al. 2007); likewise, a clear relationship between obesity and prostate cancer has yet to be defined (Ma et al. 2008; Wallstrom et al. 2009; Khan et al. 2010).

Type 2 Diabetes and Cancer

Evidence is now emerging for a direct association between type 2 diabetes and cancer, independent of the effects of obesity. In the CPSII, it was reported that type 2 diabetes was associated with a higher risk of cancer mortality (Calle et al. 2003). Consistent with this finding, a study of around one million US adults has demonstrated that diabetes is an independent predictor of mortality from several cancers (Coughlin et al. 2004) and an analysis of 1.3 million Koreans showed that elevated fasting serum glucose and a diagnosis of diabetes are independent risk factors for several major cancers (Jee et al. 2005). A smaller study of around 100,000 Japanese adults also reported significantly higher total cancer rates for diabetics, although these were greater for men than for women (Inoue et al. 2006). Recently, a large meta-analysis of five Japanese studies suggested that, independent of all other factors, the relative risk of type 2 diabetic patients developing cancer was higher than in nondiabetics, although this risk was higher for men than women (1.7 vs. 1.23) (Noto et al. 2010).

Regarding specific cancers, the relationship between type 2 diabetes and breast cancer has been studied extensively. In a case–control study of 700 women aged 38–75, it was found that hyperinsulinemia and insulin resistance were significant risk factors for breast cancer independent of general adiposity or body fat distribution as shown by raised circulating C-peptide levels, a commonly used biomarker for insulin secretion in type 2 diabetics (Bruning et al. 1992). A prospective study in Sweden of 80,000 women (average age 64.2 years) found that individuals with type 2 diabetes had an increased incidence of breast cancer (Weiderpass et al. 1997) and in another prospective study in 2003, an increased risk of estrogen positive breast cancer, postmenopausally, was found to be associated with type 2 diabetes (Michels et al. 2003). A recent meta-analysis cautions that the positive associations between C-peptide and insulin levels in breast cancer case–control studies are more reliable than those found in prospective studies (Pisani 2008); however, two very recent and large prospective studies demonstrate a significant positive association between raised circulating nonfasting C-peptide levels and postmenopausal breast cancer (Verheus et al. 2006; Gunter et al. 2009). An increase in overall mortality from breast cancer has also been reported, independent of obesity (Coughlin et al. 2004; Yancik et al. 2001; Verlato et al. 2003).

The relationship between type 2 diabetes and pancreatic cancer is complex and has been the subject of numerous studies. Although type 2 diabetics are known to be at high risk of developing pancreatic cancer (Coughlin et al. 2004; Pisani 2008; Rousseau et al. 2006; Kuriki et al. 2007; Michaud et al. 2007), it has also been discovered that pancreatic cancer can cause diabetes, through islet cell death and also insulin resistance (Permert et al. 1994; Isaksson et al. 2003). Colorectal cancer is associated positively with type 2 diabetes. A prospective study on women aged 30–55 years demonstrated that type 2 diabetics had an increased relative risk for colorectal or fatal colorectal cancer of 1.43 and 2.39, respectively (Hu et al. 1999). A case–control study of around 10,000 adults in the UK showed that the risk of both colonic and rectal cancers is increased in both male and female diabetic patients (odds ratio = 1.42) (Yang et al. 2005; Sturmer et al. 2006) and the Physician's Health Study, during a 19-year follow-up, showed that in a group of 22,000 male physicians, the relative risk of colorectal cancer in sufferers of type 2 diabetes was 1.5 (Sturmer et al. 2006). Endometrial cancer risk has also been shown to be directly related to high circulating insulin or C-peptide levels and mortality risk is relatively high in diabetes compared to some other cancers (relative risk ≥ 2) (Folsom et al. 2004).

Type 2 diabetes has been found to be inversely associated with prostate cancer, at least for nonaggressive tumors. In several prospective studies, no association was found between elevated C-peptide or insulin levels and prostate cancer risk. One of these was on a study of around 800 men from the USA and Canada (Borugian et al. 2007). Another on around 350 American men also showed no association between serum insulin and prostate cancer (Chen et al. 2005). Fasting insulin and glucose levels were also unrelated to prostate cancer risk in an analysis of around 800 subjects (Hubbard et al. 2004). Several meta-analyses have also shown a negative association between type 2 diabetes and prostate cancer (Coughlin et al. 2004; Bonovas et al. 2004; Kasper and Giovannucci 2006). Obese patients, however, who do develop prostate cancer and have high circulating C-peptide levels, are at higher risk of dying from the disease, suggesting an risk between insulin and aggressive, high-grade prostatic tumors specifically (Ma et al. 2008).

Obesity, Type 2 Diabetes and Mechanisms of Cancer Development

Both obesity and type 2 diabetes are known to increase incidence, progression and sometimes mortality of specific cancers, as shown by epidemiological evidence. In terms of finding possible treatments for cancers related to these conditions, it is necessary to dissect out the various metabolic disruptions that typify the setting of both obesity and diabetes and identify which of these could be risks for cancer development. In the following sections, the major metabolic changes related to obesity and type 2 diabetes are discussed in light of how they may affect cancer outcome.

Adipose Tissue and Cancer

Far from being inert, adipose tissue is a highly metabolically active mass of cells which can affect metabolism, immune function, neuroendocrine function, and sex-steroid production. Indeed, adipose tissue is often classed as an endocrine organ (Kershaw and Flier 2004). Adipose tissue contains adipocytes (around 80% of total), macrophages, fibroblasts, and epithelial cells, as well as blood vessels, nerve tissue, and extracellular matrix. Cells in adipose tissue secrete many different proteins with endocrine functions, including resistin, adiponectin, leptin, interleukin-6 (IL-6), tumor necrosis factor (TNF)-α, aromatase, complement and complement-related proteins, and proteins involved in lipid transport. Collectively, these peptides are termed adipocytokines. During obesity, excess adipose tissue causes significant and prolonged fluctuations in adipocytokine output, resulting in a surprisingly wide range of disorders such as insulin resistance, hypertension, proinflammatory and prothrombotic conditions, and cardiovascular disease (Grundy 2004). In terms of cancer development, the most important of these adiposity-related disorders is insulin resistance. Here, the mechanisms responsible for adipose tissue-mediated insulin resistance are discussed, as well as how the characteristic conditions of insulin resistance, principally hyperinsulinemia, hyperglycemia, and hyperlipidemia, are potential mediators of cancer development.

Insulin Signaling and Insulin Resistance

Insulin Signaling

Biologically active insulin is released postprandially from pancreatic beta cells as a 5.8-kDa monomer composed of two polypeptide chains tethered by two disulfide bridges (Chang et al. 1997). The heterotetrameric insulin receptor (IR) exists as two isoforms known as IR-A and IR-B, which are formed by alternative splicing of the IR transcript; exon 11 is present in IR-B but not in IR-A (Mosthaf et al. 1990). IR-B is generally expressed in muscle, liver, and adipose tissues, while IR-A is expressed mainly in fetal tissues and several cancer cell types but is also coexpressed with IR-B on some adult cells. The minor structural variation between IR-A and IR-B leads to significant modifications in signaling pathways, which then define the roles of the two receptors. IR-B mediates insulin's essential metabolic effects: glucose uptake, glycogen synthesis, and gluconeogenic inhibition. Insulin binding to IR-B causes autophosphorylation of tyrosine residues present in the β-subunit (Van Obberghen et al. 1993). Phosphotyrosine-binding (PTB) domains of the insulin receptor substrate (IRS) family adaptor proteins recognize and bind these residues, causing phosphorylation of key tyrosine residues on IRS proteins (Lizcano and Alessi 2002) some of which are then recognized by the Src homology 2 (SH2) domain of the p85 regulatory subunit of PI 3-kinase. PI 3-kinase contains a catalytic subunit, p110, which phosphorylates phosphatidylinositol (4,5) bisphosphate [PtdIns (4,5) P_2], leading to the formation of PtdIns (3,4,5) P_3, which effects the recruitment of Akt (protein kinase B) to the plasma membrane. After complete activation by protein kinase 3-phosphoinositide-dependent protein kinase-1 (PDK1) serine phosphorylation, Akt enters the cytoplasm and causes the translocation of a glucose transporter (GLUT)-4 to the plasma membrane to initiate glucose uptake. Akt phosphorylates, and thus deactivates, glycogen synthase kinase 3 (GSK-3), which releases its inhibition of glycogen synthase, thereby allowing glycogen synthesis to proceed (Lizcano and Alessi 2002). In hepatocytes, insulin signaling inhibits gluconeogenesis and glycogenolysis, mainly by suppressing the expression of the genes for the key gluconeogenic enzymes PEPCK and G-6-Pase (Puigserver et al. 2003). In adipose tissue, insulin signaling increases lipoprotein lipase activity, thereby promoting triglyceride clearance in plasma. Insulin also inhibits the release of free fatty acids from adipose tissue by inhibiting lipolysis (Castan et al. 1999).

Signaling through IR-A, differently, executes antiapoptotic and mitogenic signaling pathways (Sciacca et al. 1999). The mechanism for the differential signaling of IR-A and IR-B is still under investigation; one study has proposed that the differential activation of IR-A or IR-B is due to the spatial arrangement in the plasma membrane, which controls the availability of specific adapter proteins, which can act as key switches in initiating different signal transduction pathways (Uhles et al. 2003). Differences also exist in the ligand specificities of the two receptors. IR-B has a high affinity for insulin only, whereas IR-A binds insulin with high affinity, insulin-like growth factor-II (IGF-II) with moderate affinity and IGF-I with low affinity (Frasca et al. 1999). Binding of both insulin and IGF-II to IR-A have been shown to initiate the classic mitogenic pathway involving MAP kinase as well as a mitogenic signaling cascade through activation of the mammalian target of rapamycin (mTOR) complex (Sacco et al. 2009). Furthermore, IGF-I can also activate ERK1/2 and mTOR pathways through IR-A activation (Sacco et al. 2009). mTOR is a potent stimulator of protein translation by its phosphorylation of 4E-BP1 and the subsequent release of eIF-4E, which then allows mRNA to engage in a ribosomal initiation complex for protein translation (Galbaugh et al. 2006). Active mTOR, in concert with phosphoinositide-dependent kinase-1 PDK1, phosphorylates and activates p70S6 kinase (p70S6K) (Isotani et al. 1999). Active p70S6K then stimulates protein synthesis through activation of p70S6 ribosomal protein and components of translational machinery (Flynn et al. 1996). p70S6K can also engage in a positive feedback loop with mTOR by phosphorylating its negative regulatory domain at two sites, which causes further activation of mTOR (Holz et al. 2005).

Insulin Resistance

The efficacy of IR signaling is sensitive to many external factors, and may be compromised in several ways, such as through loss of receptor concentration or kinase activity, concentration or phosphorylation of the IRS proteins, PI-3-kinase activity, GLUT-4 translocation, and the concentration of different intracellular enzymes (Le Marchand-Brustel et al. 1985; Pessin and Saltiel 2000). Furthermore, insulin resistance in the different target tissues results in different metabolic effects. In adipose tissue, insulin resistance primarily results in abnormalities in triglyceride (TG) and free fatty acid (FFA) levels due to the lack of lipolytic inhibition normally bestowed by insulin signaling (Brassard et al. 2008). In the liver, insulin resistance results in excessive rates of hepatic gluconeogenesis (Boden et al. 2002), while in skeletal muscle, insulin resistance results in inhibited glucose uptake and reduced mitochondrial oxidation capacity (Patti et al. 2003; Peterson et al. 2004). A severe lack of insulin sensitivity may have a wholly genetic basis, such as in the rare cases of leprechaunism, Rabson Mendenhall Syndrome, or type A syndrome of insulin resistance (Taylor and Arioglu 1998). The milieu of dysfunctions found in type 2 diabetes is also caused largely by a reduction in insulin sensitivity, which can be polygenically inherited and may involve polymorphisms in genes associated with insulin signaling, pancreatic insulin secretion, or the formation of intermediary signaling metabolites (Stern 2000). Evidence for the genetic predisposition to type 2 diabetes comes from studies which show that both adipose and muscle insulin resistance are present in lean, nondiabetic subjects with a family history of diabetes long before the development of hyperglycemia or obesity (Gulli et al. 1992; Kashyap et al. 2003).

The huge rise in cases of type 2 diabetes that has been observed over the last two decades, however, is difficult to explain by genetics. Rather, the increase in obesity and proven epidemiological links between obesity and type 2 diabetes suggests than an increase in adiposity may antagonize insulin signaling and cause insulin resistance, in adipose tissue itself, as well as in muscle and liver. A lipocentric view of type 2 diabetes was proposed almost 20 years ago (McGarry 1992) and since then evidence has been growing that increased adiposity is central to the cause of total insulin resistance. Studies have shown that the various adipokines released from adipose tissue may initiate insulin resistance locally, leading to reduced insulin sensitivity in adipose tissue, followed by an increase in circulating FFA.

An increase of systemic adipocytokines from adipose tissue, coupled with elevated circulating FFA, then are proposed to mediate further insulin resistance in both liver and muscle tissues.

Adipose Tissue and Insulin Resistance

Tumor Necrosis Factor Alpha

TNF-α was originally described as an endotoxin-induced factor which caused tumor necrosis in septic animals and was then found to be identical to cachexin, a factor responsible for mediating cachexia in body-wasting diseases such as cancer (Coppack 2001). TNF-α, produced as active 17-kDa monomers, is now recognized as a multifunctional, regulatory cytokine involved in insulin resistance, inflammation, apoptosis, survival and cytotoxicity. TNF-α was first implicated in the pathogenesis of obesity and insulin resistance when it was found to be upregulated in obese mice and then humans (Hotamisligil 2003, 2005). Adipocytes were discovered to be a major source of TNF-α and TNF-α receptors, revealing both a paracrine and autocrine role for TNF-α in adipose tissue. TNF-α promotes insulin resistance through the serine kinase inhibitor of nuclear factor κB (IKK-beta), which serine phosphorylates IRS-1 and IRS-2, making them unavailable as substrates for the IR, and also promoting their degradation (Hotamisligil 2003). Total levels of the key IR downstream signaling protein Akt have also been shown to be negatively correlated with TNF-α levels (Levinger et al. 2010). TNF-α also stimulates lipolysis in adipose tissue, thus triggering FFA release from adipose tissue into the circulation (Zhang et al. 2002). In vivo, TNF-α infused into adult rats caused rapid and significant changes in adipocyte gene expression and caused downregulation of IRS-1, GLUT-4, PPAR-γ, and adiponectin (Ruan et al. 2002). Fewer and less rapid changes occur in hepatic gene expression, suggesting that adipose tissue is an immediate local target of TNF-α (Ruan et al. 2002). NFkB is an essential mediator of most TNF-α responses and has been shown to antagonize gene expression regulated by peroxisome proliferator-activated receptor (PPAR)-α, which may also contribute to insulin resistance in adipose tissue (Ye 2008). In a mouse model of nonalcoholic steatohepatitis where insulin resistance is typically advanced, TNF has recently been shown to be reduced after treatment with the insulin sensitizing PPAR agonist rosiglitazone (Liu et al. 2010).

Interleukin-6

IL-6 is both a pro- and anti-inflammatory cytokine which is secreted by T cells and macrophages as part of an immune response to tissue trauma. IL-6 is also secreted from adipocytes and adipose matrix (Fain et al. 2004), and its proinflammatory properties make this cytokine one of the most common mediators of insulin resistance in obesity. IL-6 is secreted as a glycosylated protein ranging in size from 22 to 27 kDa and binds either a soluble or membrane bound receptor. Unlike TNF-α, IL-6 circulates systemically, and circulating levels of IL-6 positively correlate with obesity, impaired glucose tolerance, and insulin resistance (Vozarova et al. 2001). Weight loss reduces IL-6 levels (Esposito et al. 2003), while healthy human or rodent subjects administered IL-6 demonstrate hyperglycemia, hyperlipidemia, and insulin resistance (Stith and Luo 1994; Tsigos and Chrousos 1994). The proposed mechanism of IL-6-mediated insulin resistance involves suppressor of cytokine signaling (SOCS)-3, which is increased in adipocyte cell lines in vitro following IL-6 stimulation (Lagathu et al. 2003) and also in the adipose tissue of obese, insulin-resistant, nondiabetic individuals (Rieusset et al. 2004). SOCS-3 targets and ubiquitinates IRS-1 and IRS-2, thereby causing the proteasomal degradation of these important IR adaptor molecules (Emanuelli et al. 2000). Insulin resistance caused by IL-6 preferentially occurs in hepatic and adipose tissue; minimal effects have been observed on insulin sensitivity in muscle as a result of elevated IL-6 (Klover et al. 2003).

Resistin

Resistin is a 12.5-kDa protein belonging to the family of proteins called resistin-like molecules, which are identical to the proteins of the inflammatory zone family known as the FIZZ proteins (Banerjee and Lazar 2003). Resistin was first identified during a screening for genes induced during differentiation of mouse adipocytes. Resistin was found to be downregulated by the insulin-sensitizing thiazolidinediones (TDZ) and was thus suggested as a factor involved in adipocyte-mediated insulin resistance. In the same study, it was found that mice fed a high fat diet for 8 weeks demonstrated increased resistin levels that correlated with the onset of obesity and insulin resistance. An infusion of recombinant resistin promoted hyperglycemia and hyperinsulinemia in mice while an infusion of antiresistin antibodies reversed these effects (Steppan et al. 2001). In other murine studies, resistin gene expression was shown to be upregulated at the onset of high fat diet-induced obesity in rats (Li et al. 2002). Conversely, several studies have also reported that insulin resistance and obesity are actually associated with decreased resistin expression (Juan et al. 2001; Le Lay et al. 2001; Haugen et al. 2001) suggesting that the role of resistin may not be as clear as first proposed. In humans, the role of resistin is also uncertain. The human protein shares only 64% homology with the murine form and is expressed poorly in adipocytes (Banerjee and Lazar 2003). Furthermore, several epidemiological studies failed to prove a definite link between circulating resistin levels and adiposity or insulin resistance (Banerjee and Lazar 2003). However, in a recent study on 200 adults, it has been shown that although circulating resistin may not correlate with insulin resistance, it does remain positively associated with BMI (Owecki et al. 2010).

Leptin

Leptin is an adipocyte-secreted 16-kDa polypeptide with structural homology to cytokines. Leptin expression levels correlate positively with both adipose tissue mass and nutritional status. Receptors for leptin are class I cytokine receptors that are present in peripheral tissues and also in the hypothalamus (Bjorbaek and Kahn 2004). The main function of leptin is to bind to hypothalamic receptors and inhibit appetite by suppressing orexigenic peptides such as neuropeptide Y while elevating the levels of anorexigenic peptides such as pro-opiomelanocortin (Ahima and Flier 2000). A deficiency of leptin in both mice and humans leads to obesity and insulin resistance; leptin treatment reverses these conditions (Farooqi and O'Rahilly 2004). The limitations of using leptin as an antiobesity drug, however, became apparent when it was found that, in obese individuals, leptin levels are already characteristically high and, furthermore, administration of recombinant leptin failed to lessen obesity, indicating the onset of leptin resistance (Zelissen et al. 2005). More recently, it has been found that a target gene of leptin, IGF binding protein 2 (IGFBP2), although not directly causing weight loss, can improve insulin sensitivity and glucose metabolism when infused into obese mice (Hedbacker et al. 2010).

Adiponectin

Adiponectin is a 30-kDa adipocytokine also known as apM1, Acrp30, adipoQ, and GBP28 (Maeda et al. 2007; Scherer et al. 1995; Nakano et al. 1996; Hu et al. 1996), which is secreted from differentiated adipocytes and circulates systemically at high levels (Chandran et al. 2003). Adiponectin receptors are present on both muscle and liver tissues (Yamauchi et al. 2003). An inverse correlation exists between adiponectin levels and insulin resistance (Chandran et al. 2003; Diez and Iglesias 2003). Low levels of adiponectin have been shown to predict the onset of components of the metabolic syndrome that characterize type 2 diabetes, such as insulin resistance, hyperinsulinemia, and hyperglycemia (Yamamoto et al. 2004; Nakashima et al. 2006). Administration of adiponectin can reverse these effects (Kinlaw and Marsh 2004); similarly, weight loss precedes an increase in circulating adiponectin and a subsequent reduction of insulin resistance (Matsuzawa et al. 2004). Adiponectin regulates insulin resistance by its promotion of glucose uptake in muscle cells, suppression of gluconeogeneis in hepatic cells and increased fatty acid oxidation in both muscle and hepatic tissue, largely via increased IR phosphorylation and by activation of p38 MAP kinase, adenosine monophosphate-activated protein kinase (AMPK) and PPARα (Kadowaki and Yamauchi 2005). Additionally, adiponectin is a potent anti-inflammatory factor, reducing toll-like receptor (TLR) activation of NFκB (Yamaguchi et al. 2005). During prolonged high fat feeding in obesity, it has been shown that adiponectin resistance gradually occurs in the adiponectin receptor, followed by reduced fatty acid oxidation in muscle cells, reduced insulin signaling, and a propensity for insulin resistance in muscle tissue (Mullen et al. 2009).

Insulin Resistance and Cancer

Obesity-related insulin resistance is characterized by impaired IR signal transduction pathways. Adipocytokine release from excess adipose tissue contributes significantly to this insulin resistance. The IR signaling defects lead to reduced efficacy of the IR in mediating its normal metabolic functions of glucose uptake, glycogen synthesis and lipolytic inhibition. A reduction in glucose uptake into the muscle and liver results in prolonged elevation of postprandial glucose. This leads to the stimulation of pancreatic β cells to secrete more insulin, which is further unable to stimulate glucose uptake into cells, leading to both hyperglycemia and hyperinsulinemia. Owing to insulin resistance in adipose tissue, lipolysis is no longer inhibited by IR signaling. FFA levels then rise and hyperlipidemia ensues. These consequences of insulin resistance begin gradually and are usually present for a considerable time before diagnosis. It is well established that they are involved in the progression of disorders such as cardiovascular disease and hypertension; however, there is also evidence that hyperinsulinemia, hyperglycemia, and hyperlipidemia also have an impact on cancer development or progression.

Hyperinsulinemia and Cancer

In contrast to IR-B, elevated circulating adipocytokine and FFA levels do not antagonize signaling by IR-A (Serrano et al. 2005). Thus, the IR-A form is functional throughout insulin resistance and its associated insulin, glucose, and lipid imbalances. During hyperinsulinemia, the role of IR-A may be central in initiating the atypical proliferation of various cells, leading to a potential risk of tumors. Over 30 years ago, binding sites for insulin were discovered on human breast cancer cells (Osborne et al. 1978). It was then shown that human breast cancer specimens and breast cancer cell lines expressed elevated levels of functional insulin receptor (Papa et al. 1990; Milazzo et al. 1992). Transfection of the IR into nonmalignant breast epithelial cells, fibroblasts (NIH3T3), or ovary cells resulted in cells that became transformed only when stimulated with insulin (Giorgino et al. 1991; Frittitta et al. 1995). Furthermore, IR expression, as well as now being a strong predictor of poor survival rate for human breast cancer, spans all three subsets of this disease (luminal, Her2 positive, and triple negative) (Mathieu et al. 1997; Law et al. 2008). Human endometrial cancer cell lines that express the IR proliferate in response to insulin (Nagamani and Stuart 1998). Certain ovarian cancer cell lines have demonstrated elevated IR-A expression and greater mitogenesis in response to insulin compared to normal ovarian cells (Kalli et al. 2002). Ovarian cancer tissue, including metastatic lesions, also revealed significantly higher expression of IR in all tissues compared to normal (Beck et al. 1994). In acute myeloid leukemia cells, the expression of IR-A, the activation of Akt, and a mitogenic response to insulin have all been reported (Wahner Hendrickson et al. 2009). In colon, pancreatic, and thyroid cancer cell lines, elevations of the IR and a concomitant increase in cell proliferation have been observed (Koenuma et al. 1989; Cox et al. 2009; Vella et al. 2001).

Several animal models have shed light on the consequences of hyperinsulinemia on cancer development and progression. The transgenic MKR mouse overexpresses a dominant-negative IGF-1 receptor in skeletal muscle. Females are insulin resistant and hyperinsulinemic, yet are nonobese and only mildly hyperglycemic (Fernandez et al. 2001). These properties make these mice very appropriate for studying the effect of hyperinsulinemia on breast cancer development. Orthotopic injection of two different murine mammary tumor cell lines resulted in larger tumors in MKR than control mice. Crossing MKR mice with transgenic mice expressing the polyoma virus middle T antigen (PyVmT) in mammary tissue led to greater mammary tumor burden in these mice compared to those expressing PyVmT with no hyperinsuline-mic background. All of these tumor effects could be abrogated by pharmacological blockade of IR/IGF-IR signaling by the small-molecule tyrosine kinase inhibitor BMS-536924 (Novosyadlyy et al. 2010). Furthermore, decreasing hyperinsulinemia by using the β3 adrenergic receptor agonist CL-316243 prevented the accelerated tumor growth via a reduction in IR and IGF-IR signaling (Fierz et al. 2010).

Hyperinsulinemia as a consequence of insulin resistance has also been induced in rodents by high-fat diet (HFD) feeding. Rats fed a HFD became insulin resistant and demonstrated more aberrant crypt foci, which are putative precursors of colorectal cancer (Tran et al. 2003). Mice on a HFD exhibited higher levels of insulin and IGF-I; this correlated with increased growth of transplanted lung carcinoma and colon adenocarcinoma cells (Yakar et al. 2006). Elevated serum insulin due to high-carbohydrate and high-fat feeding also advances the tumor growth of LNCaP human prostate cancer cells implanted into nude mice (Venkateswaran et al. 2007).

As well as the direct mitogenic effects of insulin on its cognate receptor, there are other indirect and complex effects of hyperinsulinemia which can promote cancer. The insulin receptor is highly homologous to the insulin-like growth factor-1 receptor (IGF-1R) tyrosine kinase that elicits similar signaling pathways to the IR when activated by its ligands IGF-I and IGF-II. The IGF-IR itself may be overexpressed and have a transforming effect in several cancers, and much emphasis has been placed on its therapeutic targeting (Bahr and Groner 2004). Hyperinsulinemia has been shown to upregulate growth hormone receptor (GHR) levels and enhance GHR signaling, thus increasing hepatic IGF-I production (Baxter et al. 1980). Hyperinsulinemia also suppresses the levels of IGF binding protein (IGFBP)-1 and -2, thus increasing IGF1 bioavailability (Wang and Wang 2003). Thus, hyperinsulinemia may accelerate IGF-1R mediated cancers. Hyperinsulinemia also reduces sex hormone binding globulin (SHBG) secretion (Nestler et al. 1991), causing an increase in free circulating estrogen levels, which can contribute to the progression of breast cancer (van Agthoven et al. 1995). Cells that express both IR and IGF-IR can form hybrid receptors (Soos et al. 1990; Pandini et al. 1999). Interestingly, IR-A/IGF-1R hybrids bind IGF-I, IGF-II and insulin whereas IR-B/IGF-IR hybrids mostly bind IGF-1(Pandini et al. 2002). This causes cells expressing IR-A/IGF-1R hybrids to be more responsive to insulin and IGF-I stimulation in terms of migration and proliferation (Pandini et al. 2007; Buck et al. 2010) and indicates a further possible link between hyperinsulinemia and cancer cell proliferation in vivo. Recently, the IR has been included as a target for antitumor therapy due to the nature of its compensatory tyrosine kinase activity during IGF-1R is blockade in a mouse mammary tumor model (Buck et al. 2010).

Hyperglycemia and Cancer

As a consequence of impaired IR signaling in peripheral tissues, GLUT-4 activity is diminished, and the usual rises in postprandial blood glucose cannot be effectively controlled. Indeed, an extreme state of glucose intolerance and hyperglycemia is one of the hallmarks of established type 2 diabetes and can lead to a range of serious metabolic disorders such as stroke, blindness, and renal failure (Yudkin et al. 2010). The role of hyperglycemia in cancer development, however, is not yet clear. A prospective study of around 2,500 Swedish adults with cancer showed that high fasting glucose was associated with increased overall cancer in women, but not in men, although the risk of cancer in individual sites of pancreas and urinary system in men was significantly increased (Stattin et al. 2007). In this study however, it has been noted that these effects were not independent of hyperinsulinemia (Bowker and Johnson 2007; Levine et al. 1990; Smith et al. 1992). Smaller prospective studies that examined both fasting and postchallenge glucose concentration found a positive association between elevated glucose and cancer incidence or mortality (Levine et al. 1990; Smith et al. 1992; Tulinius et al. 1997; Saydah et al. 2003; Rapp et al. 2006). Gastric cancer in a section of the Japanese population has been found to be positively associated with hyperglycemia, possibly by acting as a cofactor in increasing the risk posed by *Helicobacter pylori* (Yamagata et al. 2005). However, another study reported a lack of positive association between pancreatic cancer and glycemic index, glycemic load, or carbohydrate intake (Shikany et al. 2010). It has been recently shown that in a hyperglycemic, hypoinsulinemic rat model of diabetes, forestomach tumors induced chemically by N-methyl-N'-nitro-N-nitrosoguanidine (MNNG) grew more aggressively than those in control mice, suggesting that hyperglycemia in the absence of insulin may enhance tumorigenesis (Kodama et al. 2010). Additionally, two pancreatic cancer cell lines were found to proliferate in vitro more rapidly in the presence of elevated glucose (Liu et al. 2010).

A mechanistic link between high glucose levels and cancer was proposed over half a century ago, when the "Warburg Effect" was named (Warburg 1956), an effect whereby cancer cells use the glycolysis pathway for respiration and cell division rather than oxidative phosphorylation. This results in a shift toward lactate production in cancers, even in the presence of adequate oxygen and is now a well-established hallmark of almost all cancer cells (Gatenby and Gillies 2004; Bui and Thompson 2006). Cancer cells also demonstrate increased glucose transport and both increased glucose uptake and glycolytic rates are found to be correlated with both aggressiveness and overall worse prognosis of tumors (Kunkel et al. 2003; Younes et al. 1996). Several therapeutic strategies have been aimed at reducing glucose uptake, such as the use of glucose analogue 2-deoxyglucose (2DG) (Zhang and Aft 2009). The flavonoid apigenin was reported to decrease glucose uptake and downregulate the GLUT-1 glucose transporter in human pancreatic cancer cells (Melstrom et al. 2008). Also, the use of glucose transporter small molecule inhibitors WZB27 and WZB115 is a recently developed strategy which has shown promise in reducing the in vitro proliferation of both breast and lung tumor cells (Liu et al. 2010). The biochemical switch in cancer cells which allows them to continuously utilize glycolytic pathways may involve pyruvate kinase (PK), an enzyme which catalyzes the dephosphorylation of phosphoenolpyruvate (PEP) to convert it into pyruvate. PK exists as four isoforms; two of these, namely, PKM1 and PKM2, have been implicated in cancer progression. Normally, PKM1 is expressed in most adult tissues whereas PKM2 is found normally only during embryonic development (Jurica et al. 1998). However, it has now been demonstrated that in almost all cancer cell lines the PKM2 isoform completely replaces PKM1 and, furthermore, knockdown of PKM2 in human lung cancer cell line H1299 results in decreased rates of glucose metabolism and reduced cell proliferation (Christofk et al. 2008). A recent study shows that this alternative splicing event is controlled by heterogeneous nuclear ribonucleoprotein (hnRNP) family members hnRNPA1 and hnRNPA2, which may be under the regulation of the oncogene, c-Myc (David et al. 2009), leading to novel insights into how glycolysis and glucose metabolism may be dysregulated in cancer.

Hyperlipidemia and Cancer

Postprandially, insulin usually inhibits the triglyceride lipase component of hormone sensitive lipase (HSL), the enzyme which converts triglycerides stored in adipose cells into free fatty acids. This prevents release of unnecessary FFAs into the plasma. When adipose tissue becomes insulin resistant, insulin no longer suppresses HSL and FFA release into the blood becomes elevated. The high FFA levels cause a host of effects that contribute to further insulin resistance in muscle and liver tissue. Over time, an excess of FFAs are also contributes to the condition of hyperlipidemia. Hyperlipidemia may include elevated triglycerides (hypertryglyceridemia) or raised cholesterol (hypercholesterolemia) or both (combined hyperlipidemia). Characteristically, type 2 diabetes is associated with high circulating triglycerides and reduced high-density lipoprotein (HDL) cholesterol (Reaven 1994). The excessive release of FFAs from adipose tissue contributes to the synthesis and release of very low density lipoprotein (VLDL) particles by the liver and this has been proposed as the main cause of increased circulating triglyceride-rich lipoproteins (Parks 2001). Furthermore, both obesity and type 2 diabetes have been associated with increased cholesterol synthesis and decreased cholesterol absorption (Miettinen and Gylling 2000; Simonen et al. 2002), and it has been demonstrated that these effects which result in a state of hypercholesterolemia are also a result of insulin resistance (Pihlajamaki et al. 2004).

In terms of cancer development, the role of hypertriglyceridemia and hypercholesterolemia are only recently beginning to be understood. Several studies have now established a clear link between high cholesterol levels and prostate cancer. Serum cholesterol levels were reported in one study to be directly associated with cancer grade and thus found that men with high cholesterol (>240 mg/dL) were more likely than men with desirable (<200 mg/dL) or borderline levels (200–240 mg/dL) of cholesterol to develop high-grade or rapidly growing metastatic prostate cancer (Mondul et al. 2010). A significant, positive association between colon carcinoma and total serum cholesterol and triglyceride levels has also been noted (Yamada et al. 1998). A study on superficial esophageal cancer (SEC) in 54 adult patients found a significantly increased rate of lymph node metastasis in patients with hypercholesterolemia and hypertriglyceridemia (Sako et al. 2004). In animal studies, rats fed a high cholesterol diet for 18 weeks showed a higher rate of induction of 1,2-dimethylhydrazine (DMH)-induced colon tumors (Tseng et al. 1996).

Statins are cholesterol-lowering drugs that inhibit 3-hydroxy-3-methylglutaryl-coenzyme A (HMG-CoA) reductase, an enzyme which catalyzes the rate-limiting step in cholesterol synthesis. Some controversy surrounds statins because they have been shown to suppress cancer incidence in some studies but not others (Blais et al. 2000; Coogan et al. 2002; Graaf et al. 2004; Kaye et al. 2002; Olsen et al. 1999; Shannon et al. 2005). However, two recent large prospective cohort studies suggest that prostate cancer progression specifically is clearly inhibited by long-term cholesterol-lowering therapy in the form of statins (Mondul et al. 2010; Platz et al. 2006), suggesting that hypercholesterolemia may directly promote prostate cancer progression. Furthermore, prostate cancer cells are dependent on androgens for proliferation. Thus, the removal of androgen sources is common in the treatment of prostate cancer and is initially very successful (Feldman et al. 2001). However, eventually up to 80% of prostate cancers may emerge later with a more aggressive phenotype (Goldenberg et al. 1999). Cholesterol is a precursor for androgen synthesis and so is a molecule of critical importance in the control of prostate cancer. It has recently been suggested that prostate cancer cells may take up cholesterol and then synthesize de novo androgens resulting in castration-resistant prostrate cancers, which may be more difficult to treat (Leon et al. 2010). One of the major molecules involved in cellular cholesterol influx is the low-density lipoprotein (LDL) receptor. This transporter interacts with other donor lipoproteins to take up cholesterol (Brown and Goldstein 1986). Scavenger receptor class B type I (SR-BI), also known as CLA-1 (CD36 and LIMPII analogous-1) in humans (Calvo et al. 1997) is one such donor lipoprotein which, along with the LDL receptor has been found to be upregulated in castration-resistant prostrate cancers, suggesting that cholesterol requirement is increased in these cells. Furthermore, blocking of SR-BI led to a significant decrease in cholesterol flux into four different cell lines in vitro (Nieland et al. 2002). Estrogen-dependent breast cancer also relies on cholesterol for the synthesis of estrogen from androgens. Using SiRNA to SR-BI in breast cancer cell line MCF-7, cell proliferation was inhibited, suggesting that breast cancer cells, in a similar way to prostate cancer cells, may rely on cholesterol for estrogen-mediated proliferation and tumor development (Cao et al. 2004).

Even in non-androgen-dependent cancers, cholesterol may still prove to be a probable candidate molecule for accelerating malignant cell growth. Cholesterol-rich domains or "lipid rafts" have been shown to be sites where cholesterol sequesters a range of key membrane-bound signaling proteins. Akt, a major signaling protein involved in cell survival, has been identified as localizing to lipid rafts in a cholesterol-dependent manner (Adam et al. 2007). The synthetic alkyl-lysophospholipid analogues (ALPs) are a new class of drugs that have been shown to act at the membrane level by interacting with lipid rafts. In vitro treatment of a range of human tumor cells including Jurkat, THP-1 (human acute monocytic leukemia), Colo-205 (human colon carcinoma), Calu-3 (human lung adenocarcinoma), and A-43 1 (human epidermoid carcinoma) with edelfosine, the ALP prototype, induced apoptosis in all cell lines tested (Mollinedo et al. 1997). Further studies demonstrated that an interaction of the Fas/CD95 death receptor with membrane bound cholesterol rafts was responsible for this effect (Gajate et al. 2007; Gajate et al. 2004). Recently, in vivo studies using a human multiple myeloma cancer model in SCID mice have demonstrated dramatic cholesterol-raft mediated Fas/CD95 – induced apoptosis using edelfosine (Mollinedo and Gajate 2010). These studies suggest promising new therapies for targeting tumors which have become cholesterol-dependent for malignant progression.

Adipocytokines and Cancer

As well as causing insulin resistance, certain adipocytokines have been noted to directly affect cancer progression. In a study on 80 Korean women, elevations in serum resistin were shown to be positively associated with breast cancer, independent of obesity (Kang et al. 2007). A recent case–control study on 1,100 women has also shown that those in the highest quartile for resistin levels had a 2.08 times greater relative risk of developing breast cancer (Sun et al. 2010). Resistin was also found to be expressed at much higher levels in high-grade versus low-grade prostate cancer tissue and caused Akt activation and proliferation of prostate cancer cell lines PC-3 and DU-145 (Kim et al. 2010a). Both colon and gastric cancer progression have also been recently shown to be positively associated with elevated resistin expression (Nakajima et al. 2009, 2010; Wagsater et al. 2008).

Raised leptin levels have also been shown to potentiate cancer risk. Breast cancer cell lines MDA-MB-231, MCF-7, T47-D and ZR-75-1 all respond to leptin with increased proliferation (Somasundar et al. 2003; Ray et al. 2007; Hu et al. 2002; Dieudonne et al. 2002). Animal models have also demonstrated increased human breast tissue growth in mice during leptin exposure (Mauro et al. 2007) and mice which are deficient in either leptin or leptin receptor were unable to develop MMTV-induced mammary tumors (Cleary et al. 2004). In humans, tissue leptin levels have been found to correlate with breast cancer progression in several studies (Caldefie-Chezet et al. 2005; Jarde et al. 2008; Karaduman et al. 2010), and leptin is now being considered a realistic target for therapeutic treatment of breast cancer (Surmacz 2007). Leptin has also been found to be positively associated with colon cancer (Melen-Mucha et al. 1998; Ogunwobi et al. 2006; Slattery et al. 2008) and prostate cancer (Gade-Andavolu et al. 2006; Mistry et al. 2008; Huang et al. 2010; Singh et al. 2010). In accordance with its downregulation during obesity, adiponectin levels have been discovered to correlate inversely with cancer progression, as has been demonstrated in breast cancer (Nkhata et al. 2009; Chen and Wang 2010; Jarde et al. 2010), prostate cancer (Lopez Fontana et al. 2009) and colon cancer (Kim et al. 2010b).

Although in its inflammatory role, it has a typically antitumor effect, TNF itself has been shown to promote cancer, suggesting complex mechanisms in the growth inhibiting and promoting pathways of this cytokine (Mocellin and Nitti 2008; Bertazza and Mocellin 2010). Additionally, IL-6 has also been implicated in the development of several cancers such as prostate cancer (Alcover et al. 2010), breast cancer (Asgeirsson et al. 1998), and colorectal cancer (Ashizawa et al. 2006).

Obesity, Estrogen and Cancer

Estrogen is a steroid hormone whose principal function is to orchestrate the stages of female sexual development and reproduction; however, this hormone has also been identified as a potent stimulator of breast cancer (van Agthoven et al. 1995; Ali and Coombes 2000; Gaforio et al. 2003). Different forms of estrogen predominate depending on menopausal status, with estradiol being the main form premenopausally and estrone postmenopausally (Kirilovas et al. 2007). The final and important rate-limiting step of estrogen synthesis is the aromatization of an androgen molecule. Estradiol and estrone result from the aromatization of testosterone and androstenidione, respectively, and both reactions are dependent on the aromatase, cytochrome P450 (Means et al. 1989). Estradiol is produced mainly in the granulosa cells of the ovary, although lower concentrations are also present in adipose tissue. (Dos Santos et al. 2010). Postmenopausally, ovarian production of estradiol ceases and adipose tissue becomes the primary source of circulating estrogen, as estrone or estrone sulfate, a long-lived derivative of estrone that may also be converted to estradiol (Borkowski et al. 1978).

As noted earlier, epidemiological data has demonstrated a positive association between obesity and breast cancer in postmenopausal women. An explanation for this association may come from other studies that show a correlation between obesity and estrogen levels postmenopausally. A report on 200 American women found that increased BMI specifically led to increases of estrone, estrone sulfate, and estradiol levels (Hankinson et al. 1998). Further similar studies in the USA on postmenopausal women have all shown a correlation between obesity and increased circulating estrone, estrone sulfate, and estradiol (McTiernan et al. 2003, 2006; Castracane et al. 2006), although an EPIC study also suggested that estrogens may only contribute a partial risk to the development of breast cancer in individuals with increased BMI (Rinaldi et al. 2006). Premenopausally, obesity has been shown to play a protective role in the incidence of estrogen related breast cancer, although the mechanism for this is not well understood (Rose and Vona-Davis 2010).

To exacerbate the problem in postmenopausal breast cancer, obesity-related factors actually promote aromatase expression. TNF-α and IL-6 have both been shown to induce aromatase expression (Purohit and Reed 2002). Glucocorticoids such as cortisol can directly increase aromatase levels (Zhao et al. 1995). Positive feedback loops from breast cancer cells themselves, which express the estrogen receptor, also increase levels of aromatase locally in adipose tissue proximal to the tumor site (Mouridsen et al. 2010). Estrone may also be converted in postmenopausal women to the more potent estradiol that can also enhance ovarian tumor growth (Kirilovas et al. 2007). With increased aromatase expression, the rate of estrone synthesis may be enhanced, possibly contributing to the progression of postmenopausal estrogen-mediated breast cancer, specifically.

Current Medications for Type 2 Diabetes: Relationship to Cancer

Insulin and Insulin Analogues

In late-stage type 2 diabetes, pancreatic β-cell exhaustion occurs. Hyperinsulinemia is no longer present but the problem of postprandial hyperglycemia must be adequately addressed. Owing to the increasing evidence that insulin can play a role in cancer cell proliferation as (discussed in earlier sections), several studies have investigated the potential cancer risks of insulin treatment for long-term hyperglycemic control. One retrospective cohort study has compared insulin treatment with metformin, another antidiabetic therapy. In this study, it was found that patients receiving insulin had a 90% increase in relative risk of developing cancer in general compared to metformin (Bowker et al. 2006). It was shown that for specific sites of cancer, insulin therapy was associated with an increased risk of pancreatic and colorectal cancer but no such risk was observed for breast or prostate cancer (Currie 2009). In a study on colorectal cancer specifically, it was found that risk of colorectal tumors was positively correlated with the duration of insulin treatment (Yang et al. 2004).

Genetic engineering has been used to manufacture insulin analogues which can replace human insulin for treatment purposes. Although the mechanism of insulin receptor activation is similar to insulin, the analogues may be designed to differ from insulin structure in amino acid residues so that certain properties such as absorption, distribution, metabolism, and excretion may be altered to suit the particular insulin treatment that is desired. For example, insulin is required in both fast-release and slow-release forms. Some of the common analogues are insulin glargine (long-acting), insulin detemir (long-lasting), insulin lispro (short-acting), and insulin aspart (short-acting). Several of these analogues have been compared to insulin for their ability to cause undesirable cellular mitogenic effects. In rats and mice, mammary tumor growth was compared in a group of glargine-treated and human-insulin-treated animals; no difference was observed (Stammberger et al. 2002). With human cells in vitro, however, the glargine insulin analogue was found to cause more proliferation of osteosarcoma cells than insulin itself, whereas the analogues lispro and aspart caused slightly less proliferation than insulin (Kurtzhals et al. 2000). Breast cancer cell line MCF-7 exhibited higher proliferation rates when stimulated with glargine as compared to insulin (Mayer et al. 2008). Cell lines MCF-7, colorectal cancer cell line HCT-116 and prostate cancer cell line PC-3 all responded more mitogenically to the insulin analogues glargine, detimir, and lispro than to insulin itself (Weinstein et al. 2009). In studies on type 2 diabetic patients the effect of glargine is not so clear, and in fact in vivo may not be more potent than insulin in inducing cells to proliferate. One study has reported a dose-dependent increase in the risk of cancer when patients were treated with glargine rather that insulin (Hemkens et al. 2009). However, this study has created some controversy (de Miguel-Yanes and Meigs 2009), especially since three other recent studies have all found no positive association between glargine use and cancer risk compared to insulin (Currie 2009; Colhoun 2009; Jonasson et al. 2009).

Metformin

Metformin (1,1-dimethylbiguanide hydrochloride) has been used in Europe since 1979 and in the USA since 1994 for the successful treatment of type 2 diabetes. Metformin is an insulin sensitizer and lowers insulin resistance by increasing the number of insulin receptors on skeletal muscle cells and thereby improving glucose uptake in muscle. Metformin also decreases hepatic glucose output by suppressing hepatic gluconeogenesis and plays an important antiproliferative role by activating adenosine monophosphate-dependent protein kinase (AMPK), which then inhibits signaling through the potent driver of cell growth and proliferation, mTOR. Through upregulation of the p53–p21 axis, metformin also reduces cyclin D1 levels and suppresses cyclin dependent kinases leading to cell cycle arrest (Correia et al. 2008; Cazzaniga et al. 2009).

In terms of cancer development, metformin has consistently shown potent anti-tumor properties. In vitro studies have shown that MCF-7 breast cancer cells show reduced proliferation when treated with metformin (Zakikhani et al. 2006). Prostate cancer cell line PC-3, and colon cancer cell line HT-29 underwent a loss of mitogenic potential when exposed to metformin (Zakikhani et al. 2008). A low dose of metformin treatment was also shown in vitro to kill breast cancer stem cells of four genetically different types (Hirsch 1999), and when metformin was combined with the chemotherapy drug doxorubicin, stem cells and differentiated breast tumor cells alike were killed more effectively than in the presence of either drug alone (Jonasson et al. 2009). In a study on prostate cancer cell lines, metformin caused a potent decrease in cyclin D1 levels thereby reducing cell proliferation

(Ben Sahra et al. 2008). In several different breast cancer cell lines (MCF-7, T47D, Hs-578-T, and MDA-MB-231), metformin action was compared with that of rapamycin, a well-known mTOR inhibitor. For all cell lines, increasing rapamycin concentrations up to as high as 500 times normal levels had little effect on cell proliferation, while increasing concentrations of metformin led to growth inhibition of cells in a dose-dependent manner. Metformin increased apoptosis and markedly increased AMPK (Thr172) phosphorylation, effects not observed with rapamycin treatment (de Miguel-Yanes and Meigs 2009).

In a mouse model of prostate cancer, prostate tumor xenografts demonstrated reduced cyclin D1 expression and a reduction in growth following systemic metformin treatment (Correia et al. 2008). In a Her2/Neu transgenic mouse model, less spontaneous mammary tumor formation occurred with metformin treatment, resulting in lengthened survival period of the animals (Anisimov et al. 2005). It has also been shown that metformin acts selectively on p53-deficient colon cancer cells. Since several types of cancer become p53 deficient, this selectivity may suggest a possible mechanism whereby metformin can target malignant cells (Buzzai et al. 2007; Ben Sahra et al. 2010).

In human studies, a dose-dependent relationship of metformin treatment with the reduction of cancer risk in patients with newly diagnosed T2D has been established (Evans et al. 2005). Metformin was also shown to significantly reduce fasting insulin levels in hyperinsulinemic, nondiabetic women with early-stage breast cancer (Goodwin et al. 2006), and additionally, metformin was found to improve insulin resistance in nondiabetic women with breast cancer (Goodwin et al. 2008). Patients receiving metformin were found to have a significantly lower rate of cancer than those patients receiving insulin or sulfonylureas, another type 2 diabetes medication (Currie 2009). A observational cohort study also demonstrated reduced cancer risk with metformin use (Libby et al. 2009) and in another study metformin has been proven, in a dose-dependent manner, to reduce cancer-related mortality of type 2 diabetics to that of the risk of the general population (Landman et al. 2008). A large group of 2,500 patients receiving neoadjuvant chemotherapy for early-stage breast cancer were selected for a trial on metformin efficacy in reducing cancer progression. During the study period, the pathological complete response rate (pCR) was 24% in patients receiving metformin versus 8% in patients receiving insulin or sulfonylureas and a pCR of 16% was observed in nondiabetic breast cancer patients. (Jiralerspong et al. 2009). Recently, a further study has also strengthened the case for the antitumor properties of metformin. It has been shown that long-term metformin use is directly associated with a decreased risk of breast cancer in female patients suffering from type 2 diabetes (Bodmer et al. 2010).

One interesting and extremely relevant finding about metformin and breast cancer is that metformin is active against all variants of human breast cancer (luminal, Her2 positive, and triple negative). Indeed, metformin has been shown to be particularly effective against triple negative breast cancer. This fact has important implications for the treatment of this type of breast cancer, which, due to its lack of known ligand binding sites and highly metastatic phenotype has been traditionally linked to very poor survival rates. In a recent study, it has been demonstrated that metformin inhibits the proliferation and survival and increases the apoptotic rate of triple negative cell line MDA-MB-231 both in vitro and in vivo (Liu et al. 2009).

In breast cancer, metastasis is still a common cause of mortality. A recent study has noted that metformin inhibits important stages of the epithelial to mesenchymal transition (EMT) a critical step in the progression of cell dissemination and intravasation from the primary tumor site (Vazquez-Martin et al. 2010). Furthermore, it has been suggested that rare, tumor-initiating breast cancer stem cells may be responsible for these events (Gupta et al. 2009; Nguyen et al. 2010). Specifically, metformin was found to decrease expression of some of the main drivers of the EMT, including transcription factors such as TWIST1, ZEB1, and Slug (Oliveras-Ferraros et al. 2010).

Owing to its success mostly in treating breast cancer, metformin has now been realized as a potentially powerful therapeutic agent (Gonzalez-Angulo et al. 2010; Wysocki and Wierusz-Wysocka 2010). As such, a large-scale phase III trial breast cancer clinical trial spanning patients from Europe and the USA is being planned. This study, led by the National Cancer Institute of Canada Clinical Trials Group, is being proposed to evaluate the effects of metformin on breast cancer outcomes and plans to obtain information about the efficacy of metformin treatment, both in diabetics/nondiabetics, hyperinsulinemics/nonhyperinsulinemics and in breast tissue with varying levels of insulin receptor expression.

Thiazolidinediones

TZDs (also known as glitazones) are a class of antidiabetic drugs which are insulin sensitizers and which affect adipose, liver, and muscle tissue. TZD action is mediated by binding to peroxisome proliferator-activator receptor (PPAR)-γ, a nuclear hormone receptor belonging to the family of PPAR receptors that also includes PPAR-α and PPAR-δ. The TZD class of compounds includes pioglitazone, rosiglitazone, ciglitazone, and troglitazone (withdrawn from the market due to an increased incidence of hepatic toxicity).

To date, the studies on TZDs and cancer development have provided inconclusive results. In vitro studies mostly show that the TZDs reduce cancer cell growth. Troglitazone was found to inhibit the growth of 19 different colon cancer cell lines in vitro. 15 of these cell lines were found to have very high levels of (PPAR)-γ expression (Sarraf et al. 1998). Studies on breast cancer cells have also demonstrated reduced proliferation in response to TZD treatment (Mueller et al. 2000; Elstner et al. 1998). A reduction or equilibrium of prostate cancer that demonstrate high expression of PPAR-γ has also been observed with troglitazone treatment (Mueller et al. 2000). Lower tumor weights and volume in MCF-7 mediated mammary tumors in mice were observed in the presence of TDZ (Elstner et al. 1998). Prostate tumors growing subcutaneously in a murine prostate cancer model were reduced dramatically in size after TZD treatment (Sarraf et al. 1998). However, other studies have reported that TZDs may in fact increase tumor growth. In particular, both mammary tumors and intestinal neoplasia were increased in mice undergoing TZD treatment (Saez et al. 2004; Lefebvre et al. 1998).

In humans, results of various studies have also led to conflicting results. The prospective Pioglitazone Clinical Trial in Macrovascular Events (PROACTIVE) reported that pioglitazone resulted in a reduction in breast cancer incidence, although this difference did not reach significance (Dormandy et al. 2005). Meanwhile, an analysis of the association between pioglitazone use and bladder cancer has revealed a significant risk for this type of cancer with use of this TDZ (Piccinni et al. 2011). Another study in human patients found that TZDs could significantly reduce lung cancer risk, but this was not the case for either prostrate or colorectal cancer. However, in gastric cancer, evidence is accumulating which demonstrates that the TZDs may have potent antitumor effects and possible mechanisms for these have recently been proposed (Okumura 2010).

Summary

Epidemiology shows that obesity has contributed to the current trend for the rise in type 2 diabetes globally. Furthermore, both obesity and type 2 diabetes are now both linked to several types of cancer development and progression. The common link between obesity, type 2 diabetes, and cancer is the state of insulin resistance, which can be induced by several different factors, the majority of which stem from adipose tissue and include free fatty acids and a range of adipocytokines. Incorporating diet and lifestyle changes that reduce adipose tissue mass and subsequently insulin resistance can correct some of the resulting homeostatic imbalances of hyperinsulinemia, hyperglycemia, and hyperlipidemia. Over time, chronic exposure of healthy cells to these imbalances can lead to changes in cells which may predispose them to become more likely to adopt a transformed phenotype. Therapeutic targeting of cancer cell growth in response to these imbalances is critical. Currently, new therapeutics based on reducing cell proliferation in response to insulin, glucose, and cholesterol are being developed; in combination with changes in dietary habits, these agents may help to significantly reduce cancer incidence and progression in the future.

References

Physical status: the use and interpretation of anthropometry. Report of a WHO Expert Committee. World Health Organ Tech Rep Ser, 1995. 854: p. 1–452.

Kelly, T., et al., *Global burden of obesity in 2005 and projections to 2030.* Int J Obes (Lond), 2008. 32(9): p. 1431–7.

Flegal, K.M., et al., *Prevalence and trends in obesity among US adults, 1999–2008.* Jama. 303(3): p. 235–41.

Wang, Y., et al., *Will all Americans become overweight or obese? estimating the progression and cost of the US obesity epidemic.* Obesity (Silver Spring), 2008. 16(10): p. 2323–30.

Healthy lifestyles: Knowledge, attitudes and behavour, in *Health Survey for England*, NHS, Editor. 2008.

McMichael, A.J., *Food, nutrition, physical activity and cancer prevention. Authoritative report from World Cancer Research Fund provides global update.* Public Health Nutr, 2008. 11(7): p. 762–3.

Finkelstein, E.A., et al., *Annual medical spending attributable to obesity: Payer- and service-specific estimates.* Health Affairs, 2009. 28(5): w822–w831.

Withrow, D. and D.A. Alter, *The economic burden of obesity worldwide: a systematic review of the direct costs of obesity.* Obes Rev, 2010.

Diabetes Research and Statistics. 2007.

Diabetes UK. What is diabetes? 2010.

Alberti, K.G. and P.Z. Zimmet, *Definition, diagnosis and classification of diabetes mellitus and its complications. Part 1: diagnosis and classification of diabetes mellitus provisional report of a WHO consultation.* Diabet Med, 1998. 15(7): p. 539–53.

Van Itallie, T.B., *Health implications of overweight and obesity in the United States.* Ann Intern Med, 1985. 103(6 (Pt 2)): p. 983–8.

Ohlson, L.O., et al., *Risk factors for type 2 (non-insulin-dependent) diabetes mellitus. Thirteen and one-half years of follow-up of the participants in a study of Swedish men born in 1913.* Diabetologia, 1988. 31(11): p. 798–805.

Lundgren, H., et al., *Dietary habits and incidence of noninsulin-dependent diabetes mellitus in a population study of women in Gothenburg, Sweden.* Am J Clin Nutr, 1989. 49(4): p. 708–12.

Perry, I.J., et al., *Prospective study of risk factors for development of non-insulin dependent diabetes in middle aged British men.* Bmj, 1995. 310(6979): p. 560–4.

Colditz, G.A., et al., *Weight gain as a risk factor for clinical diabetes mellitus in women.* Ann Intern Med, 1995. 122(7): p. 481–6.

Arnlov, J., et al., *Impact of body mass index and the metabolic syndrome on the risk of cardiovascular disease and death in middle-aged men.* Circulation, 2009. 121(2): p. 230–6.

Willett, W.C., et al., *Weight, weight change, and coronary heart disease in women. Risk within the 'normal' weight range.* Jama, 1995. 273(6): p. 461–5.

Rimm, E.B., et al., *Body size and fat distribution as predictors of coronary heart disease among middle-aged and older US men.* Am J Epidemiol, 1995. 141(12): p. 1117–27.

Krauss, R.M., et al., *Obesity: impact on cardiovascular disease.* Circulation, 1998. 98(14): p. 1472–6.

Rexrode, K.M., et al., *A prospective study of body mass index, weight change, and risk of stroke in women.* Jama, 1997. 277(19): p. 1539–45.

Kato, I., et al., *Prospective study of clinical gallbladder disease and its association with obesity, physical activity, and other factors.* Dig Dis Sci, 1992. 37(5): p. 784–90.

Anderson, J.J. and D.T. Felson, *Factors associated with osteoarthritis of the knee in the first national Health and Nutrition Examination Survey (HANES I). Evidence for an association with overweight, race, and physical demands of work.* Am J Epidemiol, 1988. 128(1): p. 179–89.

WHO, *International Agency for Research on Cancer. Nutrition and lifestyle: Opportunities for cancer prevention.* 2002.

ACS, *Cancer Facts and Figures.* American Cancer Society, 2010: p. 1–64.

Vainio, H., R. Kaaks, and F. Bianchini, *Weight control and physical activity in cancer prevention: international evaluation of the evidence.* Eur J Cancer Prev, 2002. 11 Suppl 2: p. S94–100.

Calle, E.E., et al., *Overweight, obesity, and mortality from cancer in a prospectively studied cohort of U.S. adults.* N Engl J Med, 2003. 348(17): p. 1625–38.

Lahmann, P.H., et al., *Body size and breast cancer risk: findings from the European Prospective Investigation into Cancer And Nutrition (EPIC).* Int J Cancer, 2004. 111(5): p. 762–71.

Berclaz, G., et al., *Body mass index as a prognostic feature in operable breast cancer: the International Breast Cancer Study Group experience.* Ann Oncol, 2004. 15(6): p. 875–84.

Dossus, L., et al., *Obesity, inflammatory markers and endometrial cancer risk: a prospective case-control study.* Endocr Relat Cancer 2010.

Moore, L.L., et al., *BMI and waist circumference as predictors of lifetime colon cancer risk in Framingham Study adults.* Int J Obes Relat Metab Disord, 2004. 28(4): p. 559–67.

Larsson, S.C. and A. Wolk, *Obesity and colon and rectal cancer risk: a meta-analysis of prospective studies.* Am J Clin Nutr, 2007. 86(3): p. 556–65.

Moghaddam, A.A., M. Woodward, and R. Huxley, *Obesity and risk of colorectal cancer: a meta-analysis of 31 studies with 70,000 events.* Cancer Epidemiol Biomarkers Prev, 2007. 16(12): p. 2533–47.

Larsson, S.C., N. Orsini, and A. Wolk, *Body mass index and pancreatic cancer risk: A meta-analysis of prospective studies.* Int J Cancer, 2007. 120(9): p. 1993–8.

Corley, D.A., A. Kubo, and W. Zhao, *Abdominal obesity and the risk of esophageal and gastric cardia carcinomas.* Cancer Epidemiol Biomarkers Prev, 2008. 17(2): p. 352–8.

Larsson, S.C. and A. Wolk, *Obesity and risk of non-Hodgkin's lymphoma: a meta-analysis.* Int J Cancer, 2007. 121(7): p. 1564–70.

Birmann, B.M., et al., *Body mass index, physical activity, and risk of multiple myeloma.* Cancer Epidemiol Biomarkers Prev, 2007. 16(7): p. 1474–8.

Kubo, A. and D.A. Corley, *Body mass index and adenocarcinomas of the esophagus or gastric cardia: a systematic review and meta-analysis.* Cancer Epidemiol Biomarkers Prev, 2006. 15(5): p. 872–8.

Welzel, T.M., et al., *Risk factors for intrahepatic and extrahepatic cholangiocarcinoma in the United States: a population-based case-control study.* Clin Gastroenterol Hepatol, 2007. 5(10): p. 1221–8.

Batty, G.D., et al., *Obesity and overweight in relation to liver disease mortality in men: 38 year follow-up of the original Whitehall study.* Int J Obes (Lond), 2008. 32(11): p. 1741–4.

Bergstrom, A., et al., *Obesity and renal cell cancer--a quantitative review.* Br J Cancer, 2001. 85(7): p. 984–90.

Pan, B.N., et al., *[Clinical analysis of 174 cases of primary ureteral carcinoma].* Zhonghua Wai Ke Za Zhi, 2004. 42(23): p. 1447–9.

Kuriyama, S., et al., *Obesity and risk of cancer in Japan.* Int J Cancer, 2005. 113(1): p. 148–57.

Renehan, A.G., et al., *Body-mass index and incidence of cancer: a systematic review and meta-analysis of prospective observational studies.* Lancet, 2008. 371(9612): p. 569–78.

Gonzalez, C.A. and E. Riboli, *Diet and cancer prevention: Contributions from the European Prospective Investigation into Cancer and Nutrition (EPIC) study.* Eur J Cancer, 2010. 46(14): p. 2555–62.

Ursin, G., et al., *A meta-analysis of body mass index and risk of premenopausal breast cancer.* Epidemiology, 1995. 6(2): p. 137–41.

van den Brandt, P.A., et al., *Pooled analysis of prospective cohort studies on height, weight, and breast cancer risk.* Am J Epidemiol, 2000. 152(6): p. 514–27.

Olsen, C.M., et al., *Obesity and the risk of epithelial ovarian cancer: a systematic review and meta-analysis.* Eur J Cancer, 2007. 43(4): p. 690–709.

Ma, J., et al., *Prediagnostic body-mass index, plasma C-peptide concentration, and prostate cancer-specific mortality in men with prostate cancer: a long-term survival analysis.* Lancet Oncol, 2008. 9(11): p. 1039–47.

Wallstrom, P., et al., *A prospective Swedish study on body size, body composition, diabetes, and prostate cancer risk.* Br J Cancer, 2009. 100(11): p. 1799–805.

Khan, N., F. Afaq, and H. Mukhtar, *Lifestyle as risk factor for cancer: Evidence from human studies.* Cancer Lett 2010. 293(2): p. 133–43.

Coughlin, S.S., et al., *Diabetes mellitus as a predictor of cancer mortality in a large cohort of US adults.* Am J Epidemiol, 2004. 159(12): p. 1160–7.

Jee, S.H., et al., *Fasting serum glucose level and cancer risk in Korean men and women.* Jama, 2005. 293(2): p. 194–202.

Inoue, M., et al., *Diabetes mellitus and the risk of cancer: results from a large-scale population-based cohort study in Japan.* Arch Intern Med, 2006. 166(17): p. 1871–7.

Noto, H., et al., *Substantially increased risk of cancer in patients with diabetes mellitus: a systematic review and meta-analysis of epidemiologic evidence in Japan.* J Diabetes Complications 2010. 24(5): p. 345–53.

Bruning, P.F., et al., *Insulin resistance and breast-cancer risk.* Int J Cancer, 1992. 52(4): p. 511–6.

Weiderpass, E., et al., *Risk of endometrial and breast cancer in patients with diabetes mellitus.* Int J Cancer, 1997. 71(3): p. 360–3.

Michels, K.B., et al., *Type 2 diabetes and subsequent incidence of breast cancer in the Nurses' Health Study.* Diabetes Care, 2003. 26(6): p. 1752–8.

Pisani, P., *Hyper-insulinaemia and cancer, meta-analyses of epidemiological studies.* Arch Physiol Biochem, 2008. 114(1): p. 63–70.

Verheus, M., et al., *Serum C-peptide levels and breast cancer risk: results from the European Prospective Investigation into Cancer and Nutrition (EPIC).* Int J Cancer, 2006. 119(3): p. 659–67.

Gunter, M.J., et al., *Insulin, insulin-like growth factor-I, and risk of breast cancer in postmenopausal women.* J Natl Cancer Inst, 2009. 101(1): p. 48–60.

Yancik, R., et al., *Effect of age and comorbidity in postmenopausal breast cancer patients aged 55 years and older.* Jama, 2001. 285(7): p. 885–92.

Verlato, G., et al., *Mortality from site-specific malignancies in type 2 diabetic patients from Verona.* Diabetes Care, 2003. 26(4): p. 1047–51.

Rousseau, M.C., et al., *Diabetes mellitus and cancer risk in a population-based case-control study among men from Montreal, Canada.* Int J Cancer, 2006. 118(8): p. 2105–9.

Kuriki, K., K. Hirose, and K. Tajima, *Diabetes and cancer risk for all and specific sites among Japanese men and women.* Eur J Cancer Prev, 2007. 16(1): p. 83–9.

Michaud, D.S., et al., *Prediagnostic plasma C-peptide and pancreatic cancer risk in men and women.* Cancer Epidemiol Biomarkers Prev, 2007. 16(10): p. 2101–9.

Permert, J., et al., *Islet amyloid polypeptide in patients with pancreatic cancer and diabetes.* N Engl J Med, 1994. 330(5): p. 313–8.

Isaksson, B., et al., *Impaired insulin action on phosphatidylinositol 3-kinase activity and glucose transport in skeletal muscle of pancreatic cancer patients.* Pancreas, 2003. 26(2): p. 173–7.

Hu, F.B., et al., *Prospective study of adult onset diabetes mellitus (type 2) and risk of colorectal cancer in women.* J Natl Cancer Inst, 1999. 91(6): p. 542–7.

Yang, Y.X., S. Hennessy, and J.D. Lewis, *Type 2 diabetes mellitus and the risk of colorectal cancer.* Clin Gastroenterol Hepatol, 2005. 3(6): p. 587–94.

Sturmer, T., et al., *Metabolic abnormalities and risk for colorectal cancer in the physicians' health study.* Cancer Epidemiol Biomarkers Prev, 2006. 15(12): p. 2391–7.

Folsom, A.R., et al., *Diabetes as a risk factor for death following endometrial cancer.* Gynecol Oncol, 2004. 94(3): p. 740–5.

Borugian, M.J., et al., *Prediagnostic C-peptide and risk of prostate cancer.* Cancer Epidemiol Biomarkers Prev, 2007. 16(10): p. 2164–5.

Chen, C., et al., *Prostate carcinoma incidence in relation to prediagnostic circulating levels of insulin-like growth factor I, insulin-like growth factor binding protein 3, and insulin.* Cancer, 2005. 103(1): p. 76–84.

Hubbard, J.S., et al., *Association of prostate cancer risk with insulin, glucose, and anthropometry in the Baltimore longitudinal study of aging.* Urology, 2004. 63(2): p. 253–8.

Bonovas, S., K. Filioussi, and A. Tsantes, *Diabetes mellitus and risk of prostate cancer: a meta-analysis.* Diabetologia, 2004. 47(6): p. 1071–8.

Kasper, J.S. and E. Giovannucci, *A meta-analysis of diabetes mellitus and the risk of prostate cancer.* Cancer Epidemiol Biomarkers Prev, 2006. 15(11): p. 2056–62.

Kershaw, E.E. and J.S. Flier, *Adipose tissue as an endocrine organ.* J Clin Endocrinol Metab, 2004. 89(6): p. 2548–56.

Grundy, S.M., *Atherosclerosis imaging and the future of lipid management.* Circulation, 2004. 110(23): p. 3509–11.

Chang, X., et al., *Solution structures of the R6 human insulin hexamer.* Biochemistry, 1997. 36(31): p. 9409–22.

Mosthaf, L., et al., *Functionally distinct insulin receptors generated by tissue-specific alternative splicing.* Embo J, 1990. 9(8): p. 2409–13.

Van Obberghen, E., et al., *Insulin receptor: receptor activation and signal transduction.* Adv Second Messenger Phosphoprotein Res, 1993. 28: p. 195–201.

Lizcano, J.M. and D.R. Alessi, *The insulin signalling pathway.* Curr Biol, 2002. 12(7): p. R236-8.

Puigserver, P., et al., *Insulin-regulated hepatic gluconeogenesis through FOXO1-PGC-1alpha interaction.* Nature, 2003. 423(6939): p. 550–5.

Castan, I., et al., *Mechanisms of inhibition of lipolysis by insulin, vanadate and peroxovanadate in rat adipocytes.* Biochem J, 1999. 339 (Pt 2): p. 281–9.

Sciacca, L., et al., *Insulin receptor activation by IGF-II in breast cancers: evidence for a new autocrine/paracrine mechanism.* Oncogene, 1999. 18(15): p. 2471–9.

Uhles, S., et al., *Isoform-specific insulin receptor signaling involves different plasma membrane domains.* J Cell Biol, 2003. 163(6): p. 1327–37.

Frasca, F., et al., *Insulin receptor isoform A, a newly recognized, high-affinity insulin-like growth factor II receptor in fetal and cancer cells.* Mol Cell Biol, 1999. 19(5): p. 3278–88.

Sacco, A., et al., *Differential signaling activation by insulin and insulin-like growth factors I and II upon binding to insulin receptor isoform A.* Endocrinology, 2009. 150(8): p. 3594–602.

Galbaugh, T., et al., *EGF-induced activation of Akt results in mTOR-dependent p70S6 kinase phosphorylation and inhibition of HC11 cell lactogenic differentiation.* BMC Cell Biol, 2006. 7: p. 34.

Isotani, S., et al., *Immunopurified mammalian target of rapamycin phosphorylates and activates p70 S6 kinase alpha in vitro.* J Biol Chem, 1999. 274(48): p. 34493–8.

Flynn, A. and G. Proud, *Insulin-stimulated phosphorylation of initiation factor 4E is mediated by the MAP kinase pathway.* FEBS Lett, 1996. 389(2): p. 162–6.

Holz, M.K., et al., *mTOR and S6K1 mediate assembly of the translation preinitiation complex through dynamic protein interchange and ordered phosphorylation events.* Cell, 2005. 123(4): p. 569–80.

Le Marchand-Brustel, Y., et al., *Insulin receptor tyrosine kinase is defective in skeletal muscle of insulin-resistant obese mice.* Nature, 1985. 315(6021): p. 676–9.

Pessin, J.E. and A.R. Saltiel, *Signaling pathways in insulin action: molecular targets of insulin resistance.* J Clin Invest, 2000. 106(2): p. 165–9.

Brassard, P., et al., *Impaired plasma nonesterified fatty acid tolerance is an early defect in the natural history of type 2 diabetes.* J Clin Endocrinol Metab, 2008. 93(3): p. 837–44.

Boden, G., et al., *FFA cause hepatic insulin resistance by inhibiting insulin suppression of glycogenolysis.* Am J Physiol Endocrinol Metab, 2002. 283(1): p. E12–9.

Patti, M.E., et al., *Coordinated reduction of genes of oxidative metabolism in humans with insulin resistance and diabetes: Potential role of PGC1 and NRF1.* Proc Natl Acad Sci USA, 2003. 100(14): p. 8466–71.

Peterson, L.R., et al., *Effect of obesity and insulin resistance on myocardial substrate metabolism and efficiency in young women.* Circulation, 2004. 109(18): p. 2191–6.

Taylor, S.I. and E. Arioglu, *Syndromes associated with insulin resistance and acanthosis nigricans.* J Basic Clin Physiol Pharmacol, 1998. 9(2–4): p. 419–39.

Stern, M.P., *Strategies and prospects for finding insulin resistance genes.* J Clin Invest, 2000. 106(3): p. 323–7.

Gulli, G., et al., *The metabolic profile of NIDDM is fully established in glucose-tolerant offspring of two Mexican-American NIDDM parents.* Diabetes, 1992. 41(12): p. 1575–86.

Kashyap, S., et al., *A sustained increase in plasma free fatty acids impairs insulin secretion in nondiabetic subjects genetically predisposed to develop type 2 diabetes.* Diabetes, 2003. 52(10): p. 2461–74.

McGarry, J.D., *What if Minkowski had been ageusic? An alternative angle on diabetes.* Science, 1992. 258(5083): p. 766–70.

Coppack, S.W., *Pro-inflammatory cytokines and adipose tissue.* Proc Nutr Soc, 2001. 60(3): p. 349–56.

Hotamisligil, G.S., *Inflammatory pathways and insulin action.* Int J Obes Relat Metab Disord, 2003. 27 Suppl 3: p. S53–5.

Hotamisligil, G.S., *Role of endoplasmic reticulum stress and c-Jun NH2-terminal kinase pathways in inflammation and origin of obesity and diabetes.* Diabetes, 2005. 54 Suppl 2: p. S73–8.

Levinger, I., et al., *Akt, AS160, metabolic risk factors and aerobic fitness in middle-aged women.* Exerc Immunol Rev 2010. 16: p. 98–104.

Zhang, H.H., et al., *Tumor necrosis factor-alpha stimulates lipolysis in differentiated human adipocytes through activation of extracellular signal-related kinase and elevation of intracellular cAMP.* Diabetes, 2002. 51(10): p. 2929–35.

Ruan, H., et al., *Tumor necrosis factor-alpha suppresses adipocyte-specific genes and activates expression of preadipocyte genes in 3T3-L1 adipocytes: nuclear factor-kappaB activation by TNF-alpha is obligatory.* Diabetes, 2002. 51(5): p. 1319–36.

Ye, J., *Regulation of PPARgamma function by TNF-alpha.* Biochem Biophys Res Commun, 2008. 374(3): p. 405–8.

Fain, J.N., et al., *Comparison of the release of adipokines by adipose tissue, adipose tissue matrix, and adipocytes from visceral and subcutaneous abdominal adipose tissues of obese humans.* Endocrinology, 2004. 145(5): p. 2273–82.

Vozarova, B., et al., *Circulating interleukin-6 in relation to adiposity, insulin action, and insulin secretion.* Obes Res, 2001. 9(7): p. 414–7.

Esposito, K., et al., *Effect of weight loss and lifestyle changes on vascular inflammatory markers in obese women: a randomized trial.* Jama, 2003. 289(14): p. 1799–804.

Stith, R.D. and J. Luo, *Endocrine and carbohydrate responses to interleukin-6 in vivo.* Circ Shock, 1994. 44(4): p. 210–5.

Tsigos, C. and G.P. Chrousos, *Physiology of the hypothalamic-pituitary-adrenal axis in health and dysregulation in psychiatric and autoimmune disorders.* Endocrinol Metab Clin North Am, 1994. 23(3): p. 451–66.

Lagathu, C., et al., *Chronic interleukin-6 (IL-6) treatment increased IL-6 secretion and induced insulin resistance in adipocyte: prevention by rosiglitazone.* Biochem Biophys Res Commun, 2003. 311(2): p. 372–9.

Rieusset, J., et al., *Suppressor of cytokine signaling 3 expression and insulin resistance in skeletal muscle of obese and type 2 diabetic patients.* Diabetes, 2004. 53(9): p. 2232–41.

Emanuelli, B., et al., *SOCS-3 is an insulin-induced negative regulator of insulin signaling.* J Biol Chem, 2000. 275(21): p. 15985–91.

Klover, P.J., et al., *Chronic exposure to interleukin-6 causes hepatic insulin resistance in mice.* Diabetes, 2003. 52(11): p. 2784–9.

Banerjee, R.R. and M.A. Lazar, *Resistin: molecular history and prognosis.* J Mol Med, 2003. 81(4): p. 218–26.

Steppan, C.M., et al., *The hormone resistin links obesity to diabetes.* Nature, 2001. 409(6818): p. 307–12.

Li, J., et al., *Gene expression profile of rat adipose tissue at the onset of high-fat-diet obesity.* Am J Physiol Endocrinol Metab, 2002. 282(6): p. E1334–41.

Juan, C.C., et al., *Suppressed gene expression of adipocyte resistin in an insulin-resistant rat model probably by elevated free fatty acids.* Biochem Biophys Res Commun, 2001. 289(5): p. 1328–33.

Le Lay, S., et al., *Decreased resistin expression in mice with different sensitivities to a high-fat diet.* Biochem Biophys Res Commun, 2001. 289(2): p. 564–7.

Haugen, F., et al., *Inhibition by insulin of resistin gene expression in 3T3-L1 adipocytes.* FEBS Lett, 2001. 507(1): p. 105–8.

Owecki, M., et al., *Serum Resistin Concentrations are Higher in Human Obesity but Independent from Insulin Resistance.* Exp Clin Endocrinol Diabetes, 2010.

Bjorbaek, C. and B.B. Kahn, *Leptin signaling in the central nervous system and the periphery.* Recent Prog Horm Res, 2004. 59: p. 305–31.

Ahima, R.S. and J.S. Flier, *Leptin.* Annu Rev Physiol, 2000. 62: p. 413–37.

Farooqi, I.S. and S. O'Rahilly, *Monogenic human obesity syndromes.* Recent Prog Horm Res, 2004. 59: p. 409–24.

Zelissen, P.M., et al., *Effect of three treatment schedules of recombinant methionyl human leptin on body weight in obese adults: a randomized, placebo-controlled trial.* Diabetes Obes Metab, 2005. 7(6): p. 755–61.

Hedbacker, K., et al., *Antidiabetic effects of IGFBP2, a leptin-regulated gene.* Cell Metab, 2010. 11(1): p. 11–22.

Maeda, R., et al., *[Genetic analysis of left-right asymmetry in Drosophila melanogaster].* Seikagaku, 2007. 79(12): p. 1131–4.

Scherer, P.E., et al., *A novel serum protein similar to C1q, produced exclusively in adipocytes.* J Biol Chem, 1995. 270(45): p. 26746–9.

Nakano, Y., et al., *Isolation and characterization of GBP28, a novel gelatin-binding protein purified from human plasma.* J Biochem, 1996. 120(4): p. 803–12.

Hu, E., P. Liang, and B.M. Spiegelman, *AdipoQ is a novel adipose-specific gene dysregulated in obesity.* J Biol Chem, 1996. 271(18): p. 10697–703.

Chandran, M., et al., *Adiponectin: more than just another fat cell hormone?* Diabetes Care, 2003. 26(8): p. 2442–50.

Yamauchi, T., et al., *Dual roles of adiponectin/Acrp30 in vivo as an anti-diabetic and anti-atherogenic adipokine.* Curr Drug Targets Immune Endocr Metabol Disord, 2003. 3(4): p. 243–54.

Diez, J.J. and P. Iglesias, *The role of the novel adipocyte-derived hormone adiponectin in human disease.* Eur J Endocrinol, 2003. 148(3): p. 293–300.

Yamamoto, Y., et al., *Adiponectin, an adipocyte-derived protein, predicts future insulin resistance: two-year follow-up study in Japanese population.* J Clin Endocrinol Metab, 2004. 89(1): p. 87–90.

Nakashima, R., et al., *Decreased total and high molecular weight adiponectin are independent risk factors for the development of type 2 diabetes in Japanese-Americans.* J Clin Endocrinol Metab, 2006. 91(10): p. 3873–7.

Kinlaw, W.B. and B. Marsh, *Adiponectin and HIV-lipodystrophy: taking HAART.* Endocrinology, 2004. 145(2): p. 484–6.

Matsuzawa, Y., et al., *Adiponectin and metabolic syndrome.* Arterioscler Thromb Vasc Biol, 2004. 24(1): p. 29–33.

Kadowaki, T. and T. Yamauchi, *Adiponectin and adiponectin receptors.* Endocr Rev, 2005. 26(3): p. 439–51.

Yamaguchi, N., et al., *Adiponectin inhibits Toll-like receptor family-induced signaling.* FEBS Lett, 2005. 579(30): p. 6821–6.

Mullen, K.L., et al., *Adiponectin resistance precedes the accumulation of skeletal muscle lipids and insulin resistance in high-fat-fed rats.* Am J Physiol Regul Integr Comp Physiol, 2009. 296(2): p. R243–51.

Serrano, R., et al., *Differential gene expression of insulin receptor isoforms A and B and insulin receptor substrates 1, 2 and 3 in rat tissues: modulation by aging and differentiation in rat adipose tissue.* J Mol Endocrinol, 2005. 34(1): p. 153–61.

Osborne, C.K., et al., *Correlation among insulin binding, degradation, and biological activity in human breast cancer cells in long-term tissue culture.* Cancer Res, 1978. 38(1): p. 94–102.

Papa, V., et al., *Elevated insulin receptor content in human breast cancer.* J Clin Invest, 1990. 86(5): p. 1503–10.

Milazzo, G., et al., *Insulin receptor expression and function in human breast cancer cell lines.* Cancer Res, 1992. 52(14): p. 3924–30.

Giorgino, F., et al., *Overexpression of insulin receptors in fibroblast and ovary cells induces a ligand-mediated transformed phenotype.* Mol Endocrinol, 1991. 5(3): p. 452–9.

Frittitta, L., et al., *Insulin receptor overexpression in 184B5 human mammary epithelial cells induces a ligand-dependent transformed phenotype.* J Cell Biochem, 1995. 57(4): p. 666–9.

Mathieu, M.C., et al., *Insulin receptor expression and clinical outcome in node-negative breast cancer.* Proc Assoc Am Physicians, 1997. 109(6): p. 565–71.

Law, J.H., et al., *Phosphorylated insulin-like growth factor-i/insulin receptor is present in all breast cancer subtypes and is related to poor survival.* Cancer Res, 2008. 68(24): p. 10238–46.

Nagamani, M. and C.A. Stuart, *Specific binding and growth-promoting activity of insulin in endometrial cancer cells in culture.* Am J Obstet Gynecol, 1998. 179(1): p. 6–12.

Kalli, K.R., et al., *Functional insulin receptors on human epithelial ovarian carcinoma cells: implications for IGF-II mitogenic signaling.* Endocrinology, 2002. 143(9): p. 3259–67.

Beck, E.P., et al., *Identification of insulin and insulin-like growth factor I (IGF I) receptors in ovarian cancer tissue.* Gynecol Oncol, 1994. 53(2): p. 196–201.

Wahner Hendrickson, A.E., et al., *Expression of insulin receptor isoform A and insulin-like growth factor-1 receptor in human acute myelogenous leukemia: effect of the dual-receptor inhibitor BMS-536924 in vitro.* Cancer Res, 2009. 69(19): p. 7635–43.

Koenuma, M., T. Yamori, and T. Tsuruo, *Insulin and insulin-like growth factor 1 stimulate proliferation of metastatic variants of colon carcinoma 26.* Jpn J Cancer Res, 1989. 80(1): p. 51–8.

Cox, M.E., et al., *Insulin receptor expression by human prostate cancers.* Prostate, 2009. 69(1): p. 33–40.

Vella, V., et al., *The IGF system in thyroid cancer: new concepts.* Mol Pathol, 2001. 54(3): p. 121–4.

Fernandez, A.M., et al., *Functional inactivation of the IGF-1 and insulin receptors in skeletal muscle causes type 2 diabetes.* Genes Dev, 2001. 15(15): p. 1926–34.

Novosyadlyy, R., et al., *Insulin-mediated acceleration of breast cancer development and progression in a nonobese model of type 2 diabetes.* Cancer Res, 2010. 70(2): p. 741–51.

Fierz, Y., et al., *Insulin-sensitizing therapy attenuates type 2 diabetes-mediated mammary tumor progression.* Diabetes, 2010. 59(3): p. 686–93.

Tran, T.T., et al., *Direct measure of insulin sensitivity with the hyperinsulinemic-euglycemic clamp and surrogate measures of insulin sensitivity with the oral glucose tolerance test: correlations with aberrant crypt foci promotion in rats.* Cancer Epidemiol Biomarkers Prev, 2003. 12(1): p. 47–56.

Yakar, S., et al., *Increased tumor growth in mice with diet-induced obesity: impact of ovarian hormones.* Endocrinology, 2006. 147(12): p. 5826–34.

Venkateswaran, V., et al., *Association of diet-induced hyperinsulinemia with accelerated growth of prostate cancer (LNCaP) xenografts.* J Natl Cancer Inst, 2007. 99(23): p. 1793–800.

Bahr, C. and B. Groner, *The insulin like growth factor-1 receptor (IGF-1R) as a drug target: novel approaches to cancer therapy.* Growth Horm IGF Res, 2004. 14(4): p. 287–95.

Baxter, R.C., J.M. Bryson, and J.R. Turtle, *Somatogenic receptors of rat liver: regulation by insulin.* Endocrinology, 1980. 107(4): p. 1176–81.

Wang, H.S. and T.H. Wang, *Polycystic ovary syndrome (PCOS), insulin resistance and insulin-like growth factors (IGfs)/IGF-binding proteins (IGFBPs).* Chang Gung Med J, 2003. 26(8): p. 540–53.

Nestler, J.E., et al., *A direct effect of hyperinsulinemia on serum sex hormone-binding globulin levels in obese women with the polycystic ovary syndrome.* J Clin Endocrinol Metab, 1991. 72(1): p. 83–9.

van Agthoven, T., et al., *Expression of estrogen, progesterone and epidermal growth factor receptors in primary and metastatic breast cancer.* Int J Cancer, 1995. 63(6): p. 790–3.

Soos, M.A., et al., *Receptors for insulin and insulin-like growth factor-I can form hybrid dimers. Characterisation of hybrid receptors in transfected cells.* Biochem J, 1990. 270(2): p. 383–90.

Pandini, G., et al., *Insulin and insulin-like growth factor-I (IGF-I) receptor overexpression in breast cancers leads to insulin/IGF-I hybrid receptor overexpression: evidence for a second mechanism of IGF-I signaling.* Clin Cancer Res, 1999. 5(7): p. 1935–44.

Pandini, G., et al., *Insulin/insulin-like growth factor I hybrid receptors have different biological characteristics depending on the insulin receptor isoform involved.* J Biol Chem, 2002. 277(42): p. 39684–95.

Pandini, G., et al., *Functional responses and in vivo anti-tumour activity of h7C10: a humanised monoclonal antibody with neutralising activity against the insulin-like growth factor-1 (IGF-1) receptor and insulin/IGF-1 hybrid receptors.* Eur J Cancer, 2007. 43(8): p. 1318–27.

Buck, E., et al., *Compensatory insulin receptor (IR) activation on inhibition of insulin-like growth factor-1 receptor (IGF-1R): rationale for cotargeting IGF-1R and IR in cancer.* Mol Cancer Ther, 2010. 9(10): p. 2652–64.

3 Obesity, Type 2 Diabetes and Cancer

Yudkin, J.S., B. Richter, and E.A. Gale, *Intensive treatment of hyperglycaemia: what are the objectives?* Lancet, 2010. 376(9751): p. 1462–3.

Stattin, P., et al., *Prospective study of hyperglycemia and cancer risk.* Diabetes Care, 2007. 30(3): p. 561–7.

Bowker, S.L. and J.A. Johnson, *Prospective study of hyperglycemia and cancer risk: response to Stattin et al.* Diabetes Care, 2007. 30(7): p. e77; author reply e78.

Levine, W., et al., *Post-load plasma glucose and cancer mortality in middle-aged men and women. 12-year follow-up findings of the Chicago Heart Association Detection Project in Industry.* Am J Epidemiol, 1990. 131(2): p. 254–62.

Smith, G.D., et al., *Post-challenge glucose concentration, impaired glucose tolerance, diabetes, and cancer mortality in men.* Am J Epidemiol, 1992. 136(9): p. 1110–4.

Tulinius, H., et al., *Risk factors for malignant diseases: a cohort study on a population of 22,946 Icelanders.* Cancer Epidemiol Biomarkers Prev, 1997. 6(11): p. 863–73.

Saydah, S.H., et al., *Abnormal glucose tolerance and the risk of cancer death in the United States.* Am J Epidemiol, 2003. 157(12): p. 1092–100.

Rapp, K., et al., *Fasting blood glucose and cancer risk in a cohort of more than 140,000 adults in Austria.* Diabetologia, 2006. 49(5): p. 945–52.

Yamagata, H., et al., *Impact of fasting plasma glucose levels on gastric cancer incidence in a general Japanese population: the Hisayama study.* Diabetes Care, 2005. 28(4): p. 789–94.

Shikany, J.M., et al., *Association of glycemic load with cardiovascular disease risk factors: the Women's Health Initiative Observational Study.* Nutrition, 2010. 26(6): p. 641–7.

Kodama, Y., et al., *Enhanced tumorigenesis of forestomach tumors induced by N-Methyl-N'-nitro-N-nitrosoguanidine in rats with hypoinsulinemic diabetes.* Cancer Sci, 2010. 101(7): p. 1604–9.

Liu, H., Q. Ma, and J. Li, *High glucose promotes cell proliferation and enhances GDNF and RET expression in pancreatic cancer cells.* Mol Cell Biochem 2010.

Warburg, O., *On the origin of cancer cells.* Science, 1956. 123(3191): p. 309–14.

Gatenby, R.A. and R.J. Gillies, *Why do cancers have high aerobic glycolysis?* Nat Rev Cancer, 2004. 4(11): p. 891–9.

Bui, T. and C.B. Thompson, *Cancer's sweet tooth.* Cancer Cell, 2006. 9(6): p. 419–20.

Kunkel, M., et al., *Overexpression of Glut-1 and increased glucose metabolism in tumors are associated with a poor prognosis in patients with oral squamous cell carcinoma.* Cancer, 2003. 97(4): p. 1015–24.

Younes, M., et al., *Wide expression of the human erythrocyte glucose transporter Glut1 in human cancers.* Cancer Res, 1996. 56(5): p. 1164–7.

Zhang, F. and R.L. Aft, *Chemosensitizing and cytotoxic effects of 2-deoxy-D-glucose on breast cancer cells.* J Cancer Res Ther, 2009. 5 Suppl 1: p. S41–3.

Melstrom, L.G., et al., *Adenocarcinoma of the gastroesophageal junction after bariatric surgery.* Am J Surg, 2008. 196(1): p. 135–8.

Jurica, M.S., et al., *The allosteric regulation of pyruvate kinase by fructose-1,6-bisphosphate.* Structure, 1998. 6(2): p. 195–210.

Christofk, H.R., et al., *The M2 splice isoform of pyruvate kinase is important for cancer metabolism and tumour growth.* Nature, 2008. 452(7184): p. 230–3.

David, C.J., et al., *HnRNP proteins controlled by c-Myc deregulate pyruvate kinase mRNA splicing in cancer.* Nature, 2009. 463(7279): p. 364–8.

Reaven, G.M., *Syndrome X: is one enough?* Am Heart J, 1994. 127(5): p. 1439–42.

Parks, E.J., *Effect of dietary carbohydrate on triglyceride metabolism in humans.* J Nutr, 2001. 131(10): p. 2772S–2774S.

Miettinen, T.A. and H. Gylling, *Cholesterol absorption efficiency and sterol metabolism in obesity.* Atherosclerosis, 2000. 153(1): p. 241–8.

Simonen, P.P., H.K. Gylling, and T.A. Miettinen, *Diabetes contributes to cholesterol metabolism regardless of obesity.* Diabetes Care, 2002. 25(9): p. 1511–5.

Pihlajamaki, J., et al., *Insulin resistance is associated with increased cholesterol synthesis and decreased cholesterol absorption in normoglycemic men.* J Lipid Res, 2004. 45(3): p. 507–12.

Mondul, A.M., et al., *Association between plasma total cholesterol concentration and incident prostate cancer in the CLUE II cohort.* Cancer Causes Control, 2010. 21(1): p. 61–8.

Yamada, K., et al., *Relation of serum total cholesterol, serum triglycerides and fasting plasma glucose to colorectal carcinoma in situ.* Int J Epidemiol, 1998. 27(5): p. 794–8.

Sako, A., et al., *Hyperlipidemia is a risk factor for lymphatic metastasis in superficial esophageal carcinoma.* Cancer Lett, 2004. 208(1): p. 43–9.

Tseng, T.H., et al., *Promotion of colon carcinogenesis through increasing lipid peroxidation induced in rats by a high cholesterol diet.* Cancer Lett, 1996. 100(1–2): p. 81–7.

Blais, L., A. Desgagne, and J. LeLorier, *3-Hydroxy-3-methylglutaryl coenzyme A reductase inhibitors and the risk of cancer: a nested case-control study.* Arch Intern Med, 2000. 160(15): p. 2363–8.

Coogan, P.F., et al., *Statin use and the risk of breast and prostate cancer.* Epidemiology, 2002. 13(3): p. 262–7.

Graaf, M.R., et al., *Effects of statins and farnesyltransferase inhibitors on the development and progression of cancer.* Cancer Treat Rev, 2004. 30(7): p. 609–41.

Kaye, J.A., et al., *Statin use, hyperlipidaemia, and the risk of breast cancer.* Br J Cancer, 2002. 86(9): p. 1436–9.

Olsen, J.H., et al., *Lipid-lowering medication and risk of cancer.* J Clin Epidemiol, 1999. 52(2): p. 167–9.

Shannon, J., et al., *Statins and prostate cancer risk: a case-control study.* Am J Epidemiol, 2005. 162(4): p. 318–25.

Platz, E.A., et al., *Statin drugs and risk of advanced prostate cancer.* J Natl Cancer Inst, 2006. 98(24): p. 1819–25.

Feldman, B.J. and D. Feldman, *The development of androgen-independent prostate cancer.* Nat Rev Cancer, 2001. 1(1): p. 34–45.

Goldenberg, S.L., et al., *Clinical Experience with Intermittent Androgen Suppression in Prostate Cancer: Minimum of 3 Years' Follow-Up.* Mol Urol, 1999. 3(3): p. 287–292.

Leon, C.G., et al., *Alterations in cholesterol regulation contribute to the production of intratumoral androgens during progression to castration-resistant prostate cancer in a mouse xenograft model.* Prostate, 2010. 70(4): p. 390–400.

Brown, M.S. and J.L. Goldstein, *A receptor-mediated pathway for cholesterol homeostasis.* Science, 1986. 232(4746): p. 34–47.

Calvo, D., et al., *CLA-1 is an 85-kD plasma membrane glycoprotein that acts as a high-affinity receptor for both native (HDL, LDL, and VLDL) and modified (OxLDL and AcLDL) lipoproteins.* Arterioscler Thromb Vasc Biol, 1997. 17(11): p. 2341–9.

Nieland, T.J., et al., *Discovery of chemical inhibitors of the selective transfer of lipids mediated by the HDL receptor SR-BI.* Proc Natl Acad Sci U S A, 2002. 99(24): p. 15422–7.

Cao, W.M., et al., *A mutant high-density lipoprotein receptor inhibits proliferation of human breast cancer cells.* Cancer Res, 2004. 64(4): p. 1515–21.

Adam, R.M., et al., *Cholesterol sensitivity of endogenous and myristoylated Akt.* Cancer Res, 2007. 67(13): p. 6238–46.

Mollinedo, F., et al., *Selective induction of apoptosis in cancer cells by the ether lipid ET-18-OCH3 (Edelfosine): molecular structure requirements, cellular uptake, and protection by Bcl-2 and Bcl-X(L).* Cancer Res, 1997. 57(7): p. 1320–8.

Gajate, C. and F. Mollinedo, *Edelfosine and perifosine induce selective apoptosis in multiple myeloma by recruitment of death receptors and downstream signaling molecules into lipid rafts.* Blood, 2007. 109(2): p. 711–9.

Gajate, C., et al., *Intracellular triggering of Fas aggregation and recruitment of apoptotic molecules into Fas-enriched rafts in selective tumor cell apoptosis.* J Exp Med, 2004. 200(3): p. 353–65.

Mollinedo, F. and C. Gajate, *Lipid rafts and clusters of apoptotic signaling molecule-enriched rafts in cancer therapy.* Future Oncol, 2010. 6(5): p. 811–21.

Kang, J.H., B.Y. Yu, and D.S. Youn, *Relationship of serum adiponectin and resistin levels with breast cancer risk.* J Korean Med Sci, 2007. 22(1): p. 117–21.

Sun, C.A., et al., *Adipocytokine resistin and breast cancer risk.* Breast Cancer Res Treat, 2010. 123(3): p. 869–76.

3 Obesity, Type 2 Diabetes and Cancer

Kim, H.J., et al., *Expression of resistin in the prostate and its stimulatory effect on prostate cancer cell proliferation.* BJU Int, 2010.

Nakajima, S., et al., *Spectra of functional gastrointestinal disorders diagnosed by Rome III integrative questionnaire in a Japanese outpatient office and the impact of overlapping.* J Gastroenterol Hepatol, 2010. 25 Suppl 1: p. S138–43.

Nakajima, T.E., et al., *Adipocytokine levels in gastric cancer patients: resistin and visfatin as biomarkers of gastric cancer.* J Gastroenterol, 2009. 44(7): p. 685–90.

Wagsater, D., et al., *Resistin in human colorectal cancer: increased expression independently of resistin promoter -420C > G genotype.* Cancer Invest, 2008. 26(10): p. 1008–14.

Somasundar, P., et al., *Differential effects of leptin on cancer in vitro.* J Surg Res, 2003. 113(1): p. 50–5.

Ray, A., K.J. Nkhata, and M.P. Cleary, *Effects of leptin on human breast cancer cell lines in relationship to estrogen receptor and HER2 status.* Int J Oncol, 2007. 30(6): p. 1499–509.

Hu, X., et al., *Leptin--a growth factor in normal and malignant breast cells and for normal mammary gland development.* J Natl Cancer Inst, 2002. 94(22): p. 1704–11.

Dieudonne, M.N., et al., *Leptin mediates a proliferative response in human MCF7 breast cancer cells.* Biochem Biophys Res Commun, 2002. 293(1): p. 622–8.

Mauro, L., et al., *Evidences that leptin up-regulates E-cadherin expression in breast cancer: effects on tumor growth and progression.* Cancer Res, 2007. 67(7): p. 3412–21.

Cleary, M.P., et al., *Diet-induced obesity and mammary tumor development in MMTV-neu female mice.* Nutr Cancer, 2004. 50(2): p. 174–80.

Caldefie-Chezet, F., et al., *Troglitazone reduces leptinemia during experimental dexamethasone-induced stress.* Horm Metab Res, 2005. 37(3): p. 164–71.

Jarde, T., et al., *Leptin and leptin receptor involvement in cancer development: a study on human primary breast carcinoma.* Oncol Rep, 2008. 19(4): p. 905–11.

Karaduman, M., et al., *Tissue leptin levels in patients with breast cancer.* J BUON, 2010. 15(2): p. 369–72.

Surmacz, E., *Obesity hormone leptin: a new target in breast cancer?* Breast Cancer Res, 2007. 9(1): p. 301.

Melen-Mucha, G., K. Winczyk, and M. Pawlikowski, *Somatostatin analogue octreotide and melatonin inhibit bromodeoxyuridine incorporation into cell nuclei and enhance apoptosis in the transplantable murine colon 38 cancer.* Anticancer Res, 1998. 18(5A): p. 3615–9.

Ogunwobi, O.O. and I.L. Beales, *Glycine-extended gastrin stimulates proliferation and inhibits apoptosis in colon cancer cells via cyclo-oxygenase-independent pathways.* Regul Pept, 2006. 134(1): p. 1–8.

Slattery, M.L., et al., *Leptin and leptin receptor genotypes and colon cancer: gene-gene and gene-lifestyle interactions.* Int J Cancer, 2008. 122(7): p. 1611–7.

Gade-Andavolu, R., et al., *Molecular interactions of leptin and prostate cancer.* Cancer J, 2006. 12(3): p. 201–6.

Mistry, T., et al., *Leptin and adiponectin interact in the regulation of prostate cancer cell growth via modulation of p53 and bcl-2 expression.* BJU Int, 2008. 101(10): p. 1317–22.

Huang, C.Y., et al., *Leptin increases motility and integrin up-regulation in human prostate cancer cells.* J Cell Physiol, 2010.

Singh, S.K., et al., *Serum leptin: A marker of prostate cancer irrespective of obesity.* Cancer Biomark, 2010. 7(1): p. 11–5.

Nkhata, K.J., et al., *Effects of adiponectin and leptin co-treatment on human breast cancer cell growth.* Oncol Rep, 2009. 21(6): p. 1611–9.

Chen, X. and Y. Wang, *Adiponectin and breast cancer.* Med Oncol, 2010.

Jarde, T., et al., *Molecular mechanisms of leptin and adiponectin in breast cancer.* Eur J Cancer, 2010.

Lopez Fontana, C.M., et al., *[Influence of leptin and adiponectin on prostate cancer].* Arch Esp Urol, 2009. 62(2): p. 103–8.

Kim, A.Y., et al., *Adiponectin represses colon cancer cell proliferation via AdipoR1- and -R2-mediated AMPK activation.* Mol Endocrinol, 2010. 24(7): p. 1441–52.

Mocellin, S. and D. Nitti, *TNF and cancer: the two sides of the coin.* Front Biosci, 2008. 13: p. 2774–83.

Bertazza, L. and S. Mocellin, *The dual role of tumor necrosis factor (TNF) in cancer biology.* Curr Med Chem, 2010. 17(29): p. 3337–3352.

Alcover, J., et al., *Prognostic value of IL-6 in localized prostatic cancer.* Anticancer Res, 2010. 30(10): p. 4369–72.

Asgeirsson, K.S., et al., *The effects of IL-6 on cell adhesion and e-cadherin expression in breast cancer.* Cytokine, 1998. 10(9): p. 720–8.

Ashizawa, T., et al., *Study of interleukin-6 in the spread of colorectal cancer: the diagnostic significance of IL-6.* Acta Med Okayama, 2006. 60(6): p. 325–30.

Ali, S. and R.C. Coombes, *Estrogen receptor alpha in human breast cancer: occurrence and significance.* J Mammary Gland Biol Neoplasia, 2000. 5(3): p. 271–81.

Gaforio, J.J., et al., *Detection of breast cancer cells in the peripheral blood is positively correlated with estrogen-receptor status and predicts for poor prognosis.* Int J Cancer, 2003. 107(6): p. 984–90.

Kirilovas, D., et al., *Conversion of circulating estrone sulfate to 17beta-estradiol by ovarian tumor tissue: a possible mechanism behind elevated circulating concentrations of 17beta-estradiol in postmenopausal women with ovarian tumors.* Gynecol Endocrinol, 2007. 23(1): p. 25–8.

Means, G.D., et al., *Structural analysis of the gene encoding human aromatase cytochrome P-450, the enzyme responsible for estrogen biosynthesis.* J Biol Chem, 1989. 264(32): p. 19385–91.

Dos Santos, E., et al., *Effects of 17beta-estradiol on preadipocyte proliferation in human adipose tissue: Involvement of IGF1-R signaling.* Horm Metab Res, 2010. 42(7): p. 514–20.

Borkowski, A., et al., *Estrone to estradiol conversion by blood mononuclear cells in normal subjects and in patients with mammary and nonmammary carcinomas.* Cancer Res, 1978. 38(7): p. 2174–9.

Hankinson, S.E., et al., *Plasma sex steroid hormone levels and risk of breast cancer in postmenopausal women.* J Natl Cancer Inst, 1998. 90(17): p. 1292–9.

McTiernan, A., et al., *Recreational physical activity and the risk of breast cancer in postmenopausal women: the Women's Health Initiative Cohort Study.* JAMA, 2003. 290(10): p. 1331–6.

Castracane, V.D., et al., *Interrelationships of serum estradiol, estrone, and estrone sulfate, adiposity, biochemical bone markers, and leptin in post-menopausal women.* Maturitas, 2006. 53(2): p. 217–25.

McTiernan, A., et al., *Relation of BMI and physical activity to sex hormones in postmenopausal women.* Obesity (Silver Spring), 2006. 14(9): p. 1662–77.

Rinaldi, S., et al., *IGF-I, IGFBP-3 and breast cancer risk in women: The European Prospective Investigation into Cancer and Nutrition (EPIC).* Endocr Relat Cancer, 2006. 13(2): p. 593–605.

Rose, D.P. and L. Vona-Davis, *Interaction between menopausal status and obesity in affecting breast cancer risk.* Maturitas, 2010. 66(1): p. 33–8.

Purohit, A. and M.J. Reed, *Regulation of estrogen synthesis in postmenopausal women.* Steroids, 2002. 67(12): p. 979–83.

Zhao, Y., C.R. Mendelson, and E.R. Simpson, *Characterization of the sequences of the human CYP19 (aromatase) gene that mediate regulation by glucocorticoids in adipose stromal cells and fetal hepatocytes.* Mol Endocrinol, 1995. 9(3): p. 340–9.

Mouridsen, H.T., et al., *Use of aromatase inhibitors and bisphosphonates as an anticancer therapy in postmenopausal breast cancer.* Expert Rev Anticancer Ther, 2010.

Bowker, S.L., et al., *Increased cancer-related mortality for patients with type 2 diabetes who use sulfonylureas or insulin: Response to Farooki and Schneider.* Diabetes Care, 2006. 29(8): p. 1990–1.

Currie, C.J., *The longest ever randomised controlled trial of insulin glargine: study design and HbA(1c) findings.* Diabetologia, 2009. 52(10): p. 2234–5; author reply 2236–9.

Yang, Y.X., S. Hennessy, and J.D. Lewis, *Insulin therapy and colorectal cancer risk among type 2 diabetes mellitus patients.* Gastroenterology, 2004. 127(4): p. 1044–50.

Stammberger, I., et al., *Evaluation of the carcinogenic potential of insulin glargine (LANTUS) in rats and mice.* Int J Toxicol, 2002. 21(3): p. 171–9.

3 Obesity, Type 2 Diabetes and Cancer

Kurtzhals, P., et al., *Correlations of receptor binding and metabolic and mitogenic potencies of insulin analogs designed for clinical use.* Diabetes, 2000. 49(6): p. 999–1005.

Mayer, D., A. Shukla, and H. Enzmann, *Proliferative effects of insulin analogues on mammary epithelial cells.* Arch Physiol Biochem, 2008. 114(1): p. 38–44.

Weinstein, D., et al., *Insulin analogues display IGF-I-like mitogenic and anti-apoptotic activities in cultured cancer cells.* Diabetes Metab Res Rev, 2009. 25(1): p. 41–9.

Hemkens, L.G., et al., *Insulin glargine and cancer.* Lancet, 2009. 374(9703): p. 1743–4; author reply 1744.

de Miguel-Yanes, J.M. and J.B. Meigs, *When "flawed" translates into "flood": the unproven association between cancer incidence and glargine insulin therapy.* Oncologist, 2009. 14(12): p. 1175–7.

Colhoun, H.M., *Use of insulin glargine and cancer incidence in Scotland: a study from the Scottish Diabetes Research Network Epidemiology Group.* Diabetologia, 2009. 52(9): p. 1755–65.

Jonasson, J.M., et al., *Insulin glargine use and short-term incidence of malignancies-a population-based follow-up study in Sweden.* Diabetologia, 2009. 52(9): p. 1745–54.

Correia, S., et al., *Metformin protects the brain against the oxidative imbalance promoted by type 2 diabetes.* Med Chem, 2008. 4(4): p. 358–64.

Cazzaniga, M., et al., *Is it time to test metformin in breast cancer clinical trials?* Cancer Epidemiol Biomarkers Prev, 2009. 18(3): p. 701–5.

Zakikhani, M., et al., *Metformin is an AMP kinase-dependent growth inhibitor for breast cancer cells.* Cancer Res, 2006. 66(21): p. 10269–73.

Zakikhani, M., et al., *The effects of adiponectin and metformin on prostate and colon neoplasia involve activation of AMP-activated protein kinase.* Cancer Prev Res (Phila), 2008. 1(5): p. 369–75.

Hirsch, I.B., *Metformin added to insulin therapy in poorly controlled type 2 diabetes.* Diabetes Care, 1999. 22(5): p. 854.

Ben Sahra, I., et al., *The antidiabetic drug metformin exerts an antitumoral effect in vitro and in vivo through a decrease of cyclin D1 level.* Oncogene, 2008. 27(25): p. 3576–86.

Anisimov, V.N., et al., *Effect of metformin on life span and on the development of spontaneous mammary tumors in HER-2/neu transgenic mice.* Exp Gerontol, 2005. 40(8–9): p. 685–93.

Buzzai, M., et al., *Systemic treatment with the antidiabetic drug metformin selectively impairs p53-deficient tumor cell growth.* Cancer Res, 2007. 67(14): p. 6745–52.

Ben Sahra, I., et al., *Metformin in cancer therapy: a new perspective for an old antidiabetic drug?* Mol Cancer Ther, 2010. 9(5): p. 1092–9.

Evans, J.M., et al., *Metformin and reduced risk of cancer in diabetic patients.* BMJ, 2005. 330(7503): p. 1304–5.

Goodwin, S.S., et al., *Breast cancer screening in Rockland County, New York: a survey of attitudes and behaviors.* Ethn Dis, 2006. 16(2): p. 428–34.

Goodwin, P.J., et al., *Insulin-lowering effects of metformin in women with early breast cancer.* Clin Breast Cancer, 2008. 8(6): p. 501–5.

Libby, G., et al., *New users of metformin are at low risk of incident cancer: a cohort study among people with type 2 diabetes.* Diabetes Care, 2009. 32(9): p. 1620–5.

Landman, G.W., et al., *Increased cancer mortality in type 2 diabetes (ZODIAC-3).* Anticancer Res, 2008. 28(2B): p. 1373–5.

Jiralerspong, S., et al., *Metformin and pathologic complete responses to neoadjuvant chemotherapy in diabetic patients with breast cancer.* J Clin Oncol, 2009. 27(20): p. 3297–302.

Bodmer, M., et al., *Long-term metformin use is associated with decreased risk of breast cancer.* Diabetes Care, 2010. 33(6): p. 1304–8.

Liu, B., et al., *Metformin induces unique biological and molecular responses in triple negative breast cancer cells.* Cell Cycle, 2009. 8(13): p. 2031–40.

Vazquez-Martin, A., et al., *The anti-diabetic drug metformin suppresses self-renewal and proliferation of trastuzumab-resistant tumor-initiating breast cancer stem cells.* Breast Cancer Res Treat, 2010.

Gupta, R., P. Vyas, and T. Enver, *Molecular targeting of cancer stem cells.* Cell Stem Cell, 2009. 5(2): p. 125–6.

Nguyen, N.P., et al., *Molecular biology of breast cancer stem cells: potential clinical applications.* Cancer Treat Rev, 2010. 36(6): p. 485–91.

Oliveras-Ferraros, C., et al., *Dynamic emergence of the mesenchymal CD44(pos)CD24(neg/low) phenotype in HER2-gene amplified breast cancer cells with de novo resistance to trastuzumab (Herceptin).* Biochem Biophys Res Commun, 2010. 397(1): p. 27–33.

Gonzalez-Angulo, A.M. and F. Meric-Bernstam, *Metformin: a therapeutic opportunity in breast cancer.* Clin Cancer Res, 2010. 16(6): p. 1695–700.

Wysocki, P.J. and B. Wierusz-Wysocka, *Obesity, hyperinsulinemia and breast cancer: novel targets and a novel role for metformin.* Expert Rev Mol Diagn, 2010. 10(4): p. 509–19.

Sarraf, P., et al., *Differentiation and reversal of malignant changes in colon cancer through PPARgamma.* Nat Med, 1998. 4(9): p. 1046–52.

Mueller, E., et al., *Effects of ligand activation of peroxisome proliferator-activated receptor gamma in human prostate cancer.* Proc Natl Acad Sci USA, 2000. 97(20): p. 10990–5.

Elstner, E., et al., *Ligands for peroxisome proliferator-activated receptorgamma and retinoic acid receptor inhibit growth and induce apoptosis of human breast cancer cells in vitro and in BNX mice.* Proc Natl Acad Sci USA, 1998. 95(15): p. 8806–11.

Saez, E., et al., *PPAR gamma signaling exacerbates mammary gland tumor development.* Genes Dev, 2004. 18(5): p. 528–40.

Lefebvre, A.M., et al., *Activation of the peroxisome proliferator-activated receptor gamma promotes the development of colon tumors in C57BL/6J-APCMin/+ mice.* Nat Med, 1998. 4(9): p. 1053–7.

Dormandy, J.A., et al., *Secondary prevention of macrovascular events in patients with type 2 diabetes in the PROactive Study (PROspective pioglitAzone Clinical Trial In macroVascular Events): a randomised controlled trial.* Lancet, 2005. 366(9493): p. 1279–89.

Piccinni et al., *Assessing the association of pioglitazone use and bladder cancer through drug adverse event reporting.* Diabetes Care, 2011. (34): p. 1369–71.

Okumura, T., *Mechanisms by which thiazolidinediones induce anti-cancer effects in cancers in digestive organs.* J Gastroenterol, 2010.

Chapter 4
IGF System and Breast Cancer

Marc A. Becker and Douglas Yee

Current Diagnostic and Therapeutic Options in Breast Cancer

In 2009, approximately 250,000 women in the USA were diagnosed with in situ or invasive breast cancer, and it represents the second leading cause of cancer death in women (Jemal et al. 2010). Fortunately, advances in screening (mammography, ultrasound, MRI) and therapy (radiation and systemic hormonal and/or chemotherapy) have led to continued decreases in mortality. These developments have improved diagnosis, reduced recurrences, and have increased the number of women surviving the diagnosis of breast cancer; approximately 85% of women will survive the disease compared with approximately 50% just several decades ago.

The contribution of cytotoxic and hormonal therapy is noteworthy, as clear patient benefit has been demonstrated in all stages of disease. However, growing bodies of evidence suggest the advent and progress of targeted therapy has the potential to decrease cancer mortality rates beyond conventional therapeutics. Specifically, since the 1990s, breast cancer deaths have decreased steadily at an annual rate of roughly 2%. Further decreases will likely occur because of the benefit of additional targeted therapies beyond the estrogen receptor-α (ERα). These benefits are due to the widespread investment, development, adoption, and application of molecularly targeted agents designed to block oncogenic factors and aberrant signaling pathways thought to drive breast tumor malignancy.

D. Yee (✉)
Masonic Cancer Center, University of Minnesota,
Minneapolis, MN, USA

Department of Pharmacology, University of Minnesota,
Minneapolis, MN, USA

Department of Medicine, University of Minnesota,
Minneapolis, MN, USA
e-mail: yeexx006@umn.edu

D. LeRoith (ed.), *Insulin-like Growth Factors and Cancer: From Basic Biology to Therapeutics*, Cancer Drug Discovery and Development,
DOI 10.1007/978-1-4614-0598-6_4, © Springer Science+Business Media, LLC 2012

The anti-HER2 therapies, trastuzumab and lapatinib, are examples of new targeted therapies that are functioning to decrease breast cancer mortality.

These successes have led to the development of a plethora of monoclonal antibodies and small molecule tyrosine kinase inhibitors emerging from preclinical studies. The clinical efficacy of these agents is ultimately dependent upon target identification and appropriate patient selection. As a result, clinical assays have been designed as a means of assessing tumor heterogeneity via the expression and/ or activity of tumor-dependent factors previously linked to breast tumorigenesis and metastasis. For example, Oncotype® DX was developed as a diagnostic test to analyze the expression levels of 21 genes in ERα positive tumors. A recurrence score is derived from this set of genes and then used to determine the potential benefit of chemotherapy compared to tamoxifen. In a similar vein, the MammaPrint® assay measures the expression of 70 genes and quantifies the probability of distant recurrence independent of estrogen receptor status.

In addition to adjuvant systemic benefit, expression indices from these tests offer evidence of growth factor pathway influence and further justify the use of molecular-targeted therapeutics. However, which pathway should be targeted and when over the course of the disease should such therapy be implemented remain an active area of investigation. With an established role in tumor cell transformation and propagation, the IGF pathway represents one such target.

IGF System and Breast Cancer

The IGF system functions in normal developmental and physiology. A host of ligands (insulin, IGF-I, IGF-II), binding proteins (IGF binding proteins 1–6), and proteases mediate receptor (IGF-1R, IR, IGF-1R/IR) binding and activation (LeRoith 1997). Upon ligand-induced receptor autophosphorylation, a number of intermediate docking proteins are recruited to the membrane at the level of the receptor, including Shc, p85, Grb2, and insulin receptor substrate (IRS-1, IRS-2) isoforms. These events trigger a myriad of intracellular events, most notably the activation of various downstream oncogenic pathways such as the mitogen-activated protein kinase (MAPK) and phosphatidylinositol-3 kinase (PI3K) signaling cascades and expression of numerous genes linked to cellular proliferation, growth, and motile behavior.

As a result of its potent mitogenic, antiapoptotic, and promigratory properties, the IGF system is also involved in the pathophysiology of numerous childhood and adult malignancies (Favoni et al. 1994; Hassan and Macaulay 2002; Lee et al. 1998; LeRoith and Roberts 1993; Zofkova 2003). In breast tumors, aberrant IGF signaling induces angiogenesis, proliferation, migration, invasion, and resistance to apoptosis. The targeted disruption of IGF signaling has antitumorigenic properties in mammary, prostate, hepatic, pancreatic, ovarian, colorectal, and non-small-cell lung cancer (NSCLC) (Alexia et al. 2004; Bermont et al. 2000; Bonnette and Hadsell 2001; Damon et al. 2001; Hopfner et al. 2006; Stoeltzing et al. 2003; Sueoka et al. 2000).

This blockade of IGF signaling is additive and potentially synergistic when combined with other anticancer therapies, including cytotoxic chemotherapy, radiation, and non-IGF-targeted therapeutics (Sachdev and Yee 2007). However, the question of which signaling components of the IGF cascade represent the most viable targets in patients has garnered the attention of investigators throughout the field of breast cancer.

IGF Ligands and Bindings Proteins in Breast Cancer

Cognate IGF ligand binds IGF receptor to initiate downstream signaling, and as multiple in vitro models have shown, the presence and bioavailability of extracellular ligand and binding proteins serve as markers of IGF signal strength and duration (Perks and Holly 2008). Therefore, efforts to block IGF pathway activation via ligand sequestration and binding protein regulation have been pursued (Clemmons 2007). However, establishing a direct correlation between IGF pathway activity and ligand/binding protein expression has proven more complex in patient tumors compared to in vitro models. Increases in IGF-I, reduced IGFBP-3, or an increased ratio of IGF-I to IGFBP-3 in the circulation have been linked with development of breast cancer, and as a result, efforts to monitor and assess their contribution in breast cancer patients have received great attention (Camirand et al. 2002; Goetsch et al. 2005; Jerome et al. 2003).

Nearly 90% of all IGF-I circulates throughout the body bound as a ternary complex between IGF-I, IGFBP-3, and an acid-labile subunit (ALS). The complex regulates ligand half-life, modulates receptor access, and influences target cell signaling in a ligand-independent fashion; prospective data analyses examining large-scale breast cancer patient cohorts have uncovered a number of intriguing findings (Jones et al. 1993; McKinnon et al. 2001; Mohan and Baylink 2002; Perks et al. 1999). On the one hand, studies have not shown an association between total IGF-I and IGFBP-3 levels and increased risk of postmenopausal breast cancer incidence (Fletcher et al. 2005; Renehan et al. 2004, 2005; Shi et al. 2004; Sugumar et al. 2004). On the other hand, prospective analysis of women that were either premenopausal or younger than 50 years of age revealed a positive association between total IGF-I and IGFBP-3 levels and an increased risk of breast cancer (Baglietto et al. 2007; Rinaldi et al. 2006; Sugumar et al. 2004). Moreover, numerous reports reveal that high circulating levels of IGF-I in younger women increases the risk of developing breast cancer (Bohlke et al. 1998; Bruning et al. 1995; Hankinson et al. 1998; Muti et al. 2002; Peyrat et al. 1993; Toniolo et al. 2000; Yu et al. 2002).

The correlative absence reported in postmenopausal women may stem from a lack of accurate biomarker assessment and/or patient stratification. For example, a significant association between circulating IGF-I levels and increased risk of breast cancer was reported in nonusers of hormonal therapy (Gunter et al. 2009). The aforementioned study measured circulating IGF-I levels in its free form. While only a small fraction of total IGF-I circulates in this state, it is considered to be biologically active and may represent a form more directly reflective of IGF-I ligand tissue activity (Juul et al. 1997). Furthermore, independent studies have reported that levels of free, and not total IGF-I levels are significantly associated with increased breast cancer risk in postmenopausal women (Li et al. 2001; Muti et al. 2002).

With an estimated 97% of the 370,000 women included in a large population database (EPIC – European Prospective Investigation into Cancer and Nutrition) are Caucasian, it is imperative that high risk and underrepresented groups receive proper inquiry (Bingham and Riboli 2004). Interestingly, more recent epidemiological data highlight differences between groups when distinguished by ethnic affiliation. In the case of African-American and Hispanic women, elevations in plasma IGF-I and serum IGFBP-3 levels were correlated with a number of factors (e.g., tumor histopathology, menopausal status) and were significantly associated with breast cancer progression and served as predictors for both risk of recurrence and probability of survival (Vadgama et al. 1999).

Although IGF-I and IGFBP-3 are of special interest, investigation into the roles of IGF-II, IGFBP-1, IGFBP-2, IGFBP-5, and IGFBP-7 in breast cancer has shown promise (Ahn et al. 2010; Amemiya et al. 2010; Probst-Hensch et al. 2010; So et al. 2008; Taverne et al. 2010). IGF-II is highly expressed in tumors and has been recognized as an important angiogenic factor during solid tumor progression (Bae et al. 1998; Osborne et al. 1989; Volpert et al. 1996). In addition to rapid tumor growth induction, apoptotic blockade, and metastatic promotion, IGF-II expression has been linked to an increased risk of relapse (Espelund et al. 2008; Mu et al. 2009). The recent discovery that IGF-II expression was upregulated in breast tissue of African-American women offers a potential explanation for survival disparities when compared to Caucasian patients and presents IGF-II as a population-specific target (Kalla Singh et al. 2010). Moreover, a significant number of breast tumors exhibit altered CpG island methlyation resulting in the subsequent loss of imprinting and biallelic expression of IGF2, thereby further substantiating the utility of IGF-II as a potential biomarker and diagnostic variable (Shetty et al. 2010).

The potential for targeting IGF ligands and binding proteins in breast cancer patients is suggested by these epidemiological studies and in preclinical models. While endogenous IGFBP expression may modulate tumor cell growth in either a positive or negative manner, exogenous application serves as a pharmacological inhibitor in breast cancer cells, as the addition of IGFBP-1 greatly reduces IGF-I-induced mitogenesis, motility, and xenograft tumor growth (McGuire et al. 1992; Van den Berg et al. 1997; Zhang and Yee 2002). In addition, altered IGF signaling dynamics via IGFBPs can improve the efficacy of other agents. For example, the development and characterization of recombinant human IGF binding protein 3 (rhIGFBP-3) reveals that it can act as an antagonist of IGF-1R signaling by neutralizing IGF ligand and potentiating the activity of trastuzumab (targets HER2) in breast cancer cells (Jerome et al. 2006). Furthermore, ligand-neutralizing strategies, such as bevacizumab was initially FDA approved in breast cancer in combination with chemotherapy (Haines and Miklos 2008). The successful clinical translation of a neutralization strategy is currently being tested in phase I trial with a neutralizing monoclonal antibody to IGF-I and IGF-II (MEDI-573, NCT00816361). Additional data from this trial will be needed to prove if direct IGF ligand and/or binding protein modulation will prove successful.

IGF-1 Receptor and Adaptor Proteins in Breast Cancer

A primary means of IGF regulation occurs at the level of receptor and the effects of IGF-1R blockade on malignant transformation, growth, and metastasis have remained a continued area of interest since the discovery of IGF-1R expression in breast cancer cells (Arteaga et al. 1989; Furlanetto and DiCarlo 1984; Pollak et al. 1987). Circumstantial evidence has shown that patient outcome is linked to elevated IGF-1R expression in breast tumors that have become refractory to standard treatment and acquired resistance. For example, immunohistochemical analysis of primary breast tumors revealed that high IGF-1R levels significantly correlated with ipsilateral tumor recurrence (IBTR) and radioresistance following lumpectomy and radiation therapy (Turner et al. 1997). Conversely, elevated IGF-1R levels in low-risk breast cancer cohorts compared to both normal breast tissue and high-risk breast tumors suggest that increased IGF-1R expression is a favorable prognostic factor (Papa et al. 1993). These data provided rationale for IGF-1R-targeting in select patient cohorts and as a result, a host of inhibitory agents have been developed that block the IGF pathway through IGF-1R antagonism.

When a diverse panel of breast cancer lines and patient tumors were assayed for active (phosphorylated) IGF-1R/IR (insulin receptor; the high degree of receptor homology shared between IGF-1R and IR prevent small molecule inhibitor specificity), it was discovered that active IGF-1R/IR was present in all tumors (Law et al. 2008). Even though active IGF-1R/IR was deemed ubiquitously expressed and its presence significantly correlated to poor survival, this occurred regardless of breast cancer subtype. A number of tyrosine kinase inhibitors have been shown to simultaneously block IGF-1R and IR, but more evidence is needed to determine the full effect of dual inhibition on clinical outcome (Carboni et al. 2009; Sabbatini et al. 2009). While both IGF-1R and IR represent viable targets in the targeted disruption of IGF signaling, attempts to concretely link IGF-1R expression with patient outcome have not succeeded as no definitive evidence exists to support that IGF-1R alone is of predictive value (Kostler et al. 2006). As a result, efforts to enhance the prediction of tumors driven by IGF-1R signaling are underway.

If IGF-1R functions as the gatekeeper of signaling activation, then IRS proteins may be regarded as the director of cellular resources and expenditures of IGF-induced malignancy. As previously mentioned, activation of IGF-1R by IGF initiates the association of the intracellular IRS signaling molecules to IGF-1R. With at least six IRS isoforms known to exist, studies involving IRS-1 and IRS-2 knockout mice greatly emphasize the overall impact of these two isoforms on normal physiologic function as well as on tumor biology (Araki et al. 1994; Tamemoto et al. 1994;

Withers et al. 1998). Upon association with activated IGF-1R, IRS-1 and IRS-2 are rapidly phosphorylated at key tyrosine residues and present as docking sites for a multitude of Src homology 2 domain-containing proteins (Grb2, Nck/Crk, SHP2, Syp, PI3K, etc.) (White 1998).

As a result of their role in downstream signal activation, IRS proteins mediate distinct aspects of breast tumor cell biology. Recent evidence has identified IRS-2 as a novel hypoxia-responsive gene (Mardilovich and Shaw 2009). Hypoxia triggered aggressive behavior in terms of increased invasion and improved survival of breast cancer cells in an IRS-2-dependent manner. In addition to IRS-2, IRS-1 has been identified as a key regulator of PI3K signaling and its expression has been shown to activate transcriptional promoters involved in driving cell growth, proliferation, and ultimately a more transformed phenotype (Dalmizrak et al. 2007; Houghton et al. 2010). Moreover, assessment of nuclear IRS-1 expression has been postulated as a predictive marker of tamoxifen response in patients with early breast cancer (Migliaccio et al. 2009). Although further evidence is needed, these data suggest that IRS proteins may represent potential biomarkers for anti-IGF therapy.

IGF Cross Talk and Resistance in Breast Cancer

Primary and acquired resistance to conventional and targeted therapies in breast cancer is a significant clinical problem. Cross talk between the IGF system, steroid receptors, and other growth factor pathways is well documented in breast cancer (Yee and Lee 2000). Specifically, a causal link between the IGF pathway and both ERα and the epidermal growth factor (EGF) pathway represents mechanisms of resistance in refractory tumors, as early studies reveal a coregulation and dependence among pathways. Estrogen is known to upregulate gene expression of IGF-1R, IRS-1, and IGF-II, and selective estrogen receptor modulators can in turn reduce both circulatory and microenvironmental IGF levels to result in suppressed IGF-I-induced growth (Fagan and Yee 2008; Winston et al. 1994). In ERα-positive breast tumor cells, PTEN knockdown increased both basal and ligand-mediated IGR-1R and ErbB3 signaling (Miller et al. 2009). These studies further suggest that cotargeting ERα, IGF-1R, and ErbB3 may be advantageous in select patient cohorts.

IGF Gene Signatures in Breast Cancer

Effective implementation of anti-IGF therapies hinges upon accurate target patient identification and population stratification. As previously mentioned, Oncotype DX® and MammaPrint® correlate gene expression to outcome. Moreover, IGF-I has been identified as a potent inducer of gene expression in numerous tissues (Palsgaard et al. 2009). In patients with advanced epithelial ovarian cancer (EOC), the expression patterns of many genes related to the IGF axis correlated with patient survival and may be of potential prognostic value (Spentzos et al. 2007). Perhaps the most intriguing evidence stems from the gene patterns derived from IGF-I-treated breast cancer cells (Creighton et al. 2008). This study revealed that manifestation of an IGF-I-derived gene expression pattern in both ERα-positive and negative tumors was a strong indicator of poor survival, as measured by a number of prognostic factors. In colorectal cancer (CRC), a novel IGF inhibitor (OSI-906) was used to develop an integrated genomic classifier, incorporating multiple variables that could accurately predict response of patient-derived CRC xenografts (Pitts et al. 2010). This comprehensive study simultaneously advocates for individualized therapy and argues for the use of IGF system components as a means of predicting benefit and improving patient prognosis.

Future IGF Targeting

For years, scientists and clinicians alike have sought to identify the complex regulatory signaling networks that drive tumor cell growth and metastasis in hopes of halting pathological progression and prolong survival in breast cancer patients. However, the heterogeneous nature of breast cancer tumors makes them a constantly evolving and formidable disease. As a pioneer of oncology, Sir George Thomas Beatson recognized early on that many factors are involved in tumorigenesis when he asked, "Could the disease be attacked in any other way and by any other channels?" (Beatson 1896). Today, that answer is clear and there may be multiple "channels." Therefore, novel scientific avenues and therapeutic practices are needed if the mechanistic elucidation and resolution of this disease is to be achieved one day. The IGF system functions as a critical pathway in multiple breast tumor cohorts and may represent one as yet untapped channel.

References

Ahn, B. Y., A. N. Elwi, B. Lee, D. L. Trinh, A. C. Klimowicz, A. Yau, J. A. Chan, A. Magliocco, and S. W. Kim. 2010. Genetic screen identifies insulin-like growth factor binding protein 5 as a modulator of tamoxifen resistance in breast cancer. Cancer Res 70:3013–9.

Alexia, C., G. Fallot, M. Lasfer, G. Schweizer-Groyer, and A. Groyer. 2004. An evaluation of the role of insulin-like growth factors (IGF) and of type-I IGF receptor signalling in hepatocarcinogenesis and in the resistance of hepatocarcinoma cells against drug-induced apoptosis. Biochem Pharmacol 68:1003–15.

Amemiya, Y., W. Yang, T. Benatar, S. Nofech-Mozes, A. Yee, H. Kahn, C. Holloway, and A. Seth. 2010. Insulin like growth factor binding protein-7 reduces growth of human breast cancer cells and xenografted tumors. Breast Cancer Res Treat.

Araki, E., M. A. Lipes, M. E. Patti, J. C. Bruning, B. Haag, 3rd, R. S. Johnson, and C. R. Kahn. 1994. Alternative pathway of insulin signalling in mice with targeted disruption of the IRS-1 gene. Nature 372:186–90.

Arteaga, C. L., L. J. Kitten, E. B. Coronado, S. Jacobs, F. C. Kull, Jr., D. C. Allred, and C. K. Osborne. 1989. Blockade of the type I somatomedin receptor inhibits growth of human breast cancer cells in athymic mice. J Clin Invest 84:1418–23.

Bae, M. H., M. J. Lee, S. K. Bae, O. H. Lee, Y. M. Lee, B. C. Park, and K. W. Kim. 1998. Insulin-like growth factor II (IGF-II) secreted from HepG2 human hepatocellular carcinoma cells shows angiogenic activity. Cancer Lett 128:41–6.

Baglietto, L., D. R. English, J. L. Hopper, H. A. Morris, W. D. Tilley, and G. G. Giles. 2007. Circulating insulin-like growth factor-I and binding protein-3 and the risk of breast cancer. Cancer Epidemiol Biomarkers Prev 16:763–8.

Beatson, G. T. 1896. On the treatment of inoperable cases of carcinoma of the mamma. Suggestions for a new method of treatment with illustrative cases. Lancet 2:104–107.

Bermont, L., S. Fauconnet, F. Lamielle, and G. L. Adessi. 2000. Cell-associated insulin-like growth factor-binding proteins inhibit insulin-like growth factor-I-induced endometrial cancer cell proliferation. Cell Mol Biol (Noisy-le-grand) 46:1173–82.

Bingham, S., and E. Riboli. 2004. Diet and cancer--the European Prospective Investigation into Cancer and Nutrition. Nat Rev Cancer 4:206–15.

Bohlke, K., D. W. Cramer, D. Trichopoulos, and C. S. Mantzoros. 1998. Insulin-like growth factor-I in relation to premenopausal ductal carcinoma in situ of the breast. Epidemiology 9:570–3.

Bonnette, S. G., and D. L. Hadsell. 2001. Targeted disruption of the IGF-I receptor gene decreases cellular proliferation in mammary terminal end buds. Endocrinology 142:4937–45.

Bruning, P. F., J. Van Doorn, J. M. Bonfrer, P. A. Van Noord, C. M. Korse, T. C. Linders, and A. A. Hart. 1995. Insulin-like growth-factor-binding protein 3 is decreased in early-stage operable pre-menopausal breast cancer. Int J Cancer 62:266–70.

Camirand, A., Y. Lu, and M. Pollak. 2002. Co-targeting HER2/ErbB2 and insulin-like growth factor-1 receptors causes synergistic inhibition of growth in HER2-overexpressing breast cancer cells. Med Sci Monit 8:BR521–6.

Carboni, J. M., M. Wittman, Z. Yang, F. Lee, A. Greer, W. Hurlburt, S. Hillerman, C. Cao, G. H. Cantor, J. Dell-John, C. Chen, L. Discenza, K. Menard, A. Li, G. Trainor, D. Vyas, R. Kramer, R. M. Attar, and M. M. Gottardis. 2009. BMS-754807, a small molecule inhibitor of insulin-like growth factor-1R/IR. Mol Cancer Ther 8:3341–9.

Clemmons, D. R. 2007. Modifying IGF1 activity: an approach to treat endocrine disorders, atherosclerosis and cancer. Nat Rev Drug Discov 6:821–33.

Creighton, C. J., A. Casa, Z. Lazard, S. Huang, A. Tsimelzon, S. G. Hilsenbeck, C. K. Osborne, and A. V. Lee. 2008. Insulin-like growth factor-I activates gene transcription programs strongly associated with poor breast cancer prognosis. J Clin Oncol 26:4078–85.

Dalmizrak, O., A. Wu, J. Chen, H. Sun, F. E. Utama, D. Zambelli, T. H. Tran, H. Rui, and R. Baserga. 2007. Insulin receptor substrate-1 regulates the transformed phenotype of BT-20 human mammary cancer cells. Cancer Res 67:2124–30.

Damon, S. E., S. R. Plymate, J. M. Carroll, C. C. Sprenger, C. Dechsukhum, J. L. Ware, and C. T. Roberts, Jr. 2001. Transcriptional regulation of insulin-like growth factor-I receptor gene expression in prostate cancer cells. Endocrinology 142:21–7.

Espelund, U., S. Cold, J. Frystyk, H. Orskov, and A. Flyvbjerg. 2008. Elevated free IGF2 levels in localized, early-stage breast cancer in women. Eur J Endocrinol 159:595–601.

Fagan, D. H., and D. Yee. 2008. Crosstalk between IGF1R and estrogen receptor signaling in breast cancer. J Mammary Gland Biol Neoplasia 13:423–9.

Favoni, R. E., A. de Cupis, F. Ravera, C. Cantoni, P. Pirani, A. Ardizzoni, D. Noonan, and R. Biassoni. 1994. Expression and function of the insulin-like growth factor I system in human non-small-cell lung cancer and normal lung cell lines. Int J Cancer 56:858–66.

Fletcher, O., L. Gibson, N. Johnson, D. R. Altmann, J. M. Holly, A. Ashworth, J. Peto, and S. Silva Idos. 2005. Polymorphisms and circulating levels in the insulin-like growth factor system and risk of breast cancer: a systematic review. Cancer Epidemiol Biomarkers Prev 14:2–19.

Furlanetto, R. W., and J. N. DiCarlo. 1984. Somatomedin-C receptors and growth effects in human breast cells maintained in long-term tissue culture. Cancer Res 44:2122–8.

4 IGF System and Breast Cancer

Goetsch, L., A. Gonzalez, O. Leger, A. Beck, P. J. Pauwels, J. F. Haeuw, and N. Corvaia. 2005. A recombinant humanized anti-insulin-like growth factor receptor type I antibody (h7C10) enhances the antitumor activity of vinorelbine and anti-epidermal growth factor receptor therapy against human cancer xenografts. Int J Cancer 113:316–28.

Gunter, M. J., D. R. Hoover, H. Yu, S. Wassertheil-Smoller, T. E. Rohan, J. E. Manson, J. Li, G. Y. Ho, X. Xue, G. L. Anderson, R. C. Kaplan, T. G. Harris, B. V. Howard, J. Wylie-Rosett, R. D. Burk, and H. D. Strickler. 2009. Insulin, insulin-like growth factor-I, and risk of breast cancer in postmenopausal women. J Natl Cancer Inst 101:48–60.

Haines, I. E., and G. L. Miklos. 2008. Paclitaxel plus bevacizumab for metastatic breast cancer. N Engl J Med 358:1637; author reply 1637–8.

Hankinson, S. E., W. C. Willett, G. A. Colditz, D. J. Hunter, D. S. Michaud, B. Deroo, B. Rosner, F. E. Speizer, and M. Pollak. 1998. Circulating concentrations of insulin-like growth factor-I and risk of breast cancer. Lancet 351:1393–6.

Hassan, A. B., and V. M. Macaulay. 2002. The insulin-like growth factor system as a therapeutic target in colorectal cancer. Ann Oncol 13:349–56.

Hopfner, M., A. P. Sutter, A. Huether, V. Baradari, and H. Scherubl. 2006. Tyrosine kinase of insulin-like growth factor receptor as target for novel treatment and prevention strategies of colorectal cancer. World J Gastroenterol 12:5635–43.

Houghton, A. M., D. M. Rzymkiewicz, H. Ji, A. D. Gregory, E. E. Egea, H. E. Metz, D. B. Stolz, S. R. Land, L. A. Marconcini, C. R. Kliment, K. M. Jenkins, K. A. Beaulieu, M. Mouded, S. J. Frank, K. K. Wong, and S. D. Shapiro. 2010. Neutrophil elastase-mediated degradation of IRS-1 accelerates lung tumor growth. Nat Med 16:219–23.

Jemal, A., R. Siegel, J. Xu, and E. Ward. Cancer Statistics, 2010. CA Cancer J Clin.

Jerome, L., N. Alami, S. Belanger, V. Page, Q. Yu, J. Paterson, L. Shiry, M. Pegram, and B. Leyland-Jones. 2006. Recombinant human insulin-like growth factor binding protein 3 inhibits growth of human epidermal growth factor receptor-2-overexpressing breast tumors and potentiates herceptin activity in vivo. Cancer Res 66:7245–52.

Jerome, L., L. Shiry, and B. Leyland-Jones. 2003. Deregulation of the IGF axis in cancer: epidemiological evidence and potential therapeutic interventions. Endocr Relat Cancer 10:561–78.

Jones, J. I., A. Gockerman, W. H. Busby, Jr., G. Wright, and D. R. Clemmons. 1993. Insulin-like growth factor binding protein 1 stimulates cell migration and binds to the alpha 5 beta 1 integrin by means of its Arg-Gly-Asp sequence. Proc Natl Acad Sci USA 90:10553–7.

Juul, A., K. Holm, K. W. Kastrup, S. A. Pedersen, K. F. Michaelsen, T. Scheike, S. Rasmussen, J. Muller, and N. E. Skakkebaek. 1997. Free insulin-like growth factor I serum levels in 1430 healthy children and adults, and its diagnostic value in patients suspected of growth hormone deficiency. J Clin Endocrinol Metab 82:2497–502.

Kalla Singh, S., Q. W. Tan, C. Brito, M. De Leon, C. Garberoglio, and D. De Leon. 2010. Differential insulin-like growth factor II (IGF-II) expression: A potential role for breast cancer survival disparity. Growth Horm IGF Res 20:162–70.

Kostler, W. J., G. Hudelist, W. Rabitsch, K. Czerwenka, R. Muller, C. F. Singer, and C. C. Zielinski. 2006. Insulin-like growth factor-1 receptor (IGF-1R) expression does not predict for resistance to trastuzumab-based treatment in patients with Her-2/neu overexpressing metastatic breast cancer. J Cancer Res Clin Oncol 132:9–18.

Law, J. H., G. Habibi, K. Hu, H. Masoudi, M. Y. Wang, A. L. Stratford, E. Park, J. M. Gee, P. Finlay, H. E. Jones, R. I. Nicholson, J. Carboni, M. Gottardis, M. Pollak, and S. E. Dunn. 2008. Phosphorylated insulin-like growth factor-i/insulin receptor is present in all breast cancer subtypes and is related to poor survival. Cancer Res 68:10238–46.

LeRoith, D. 1997. Seminars in medicine of the Beth Israel Deaconess Medical Center. Insulin-like growth factors. N Engl J Med 336:633–40.

Lee, A. V., S. G. Hilsenbeck, and D. Yee. 1998. IGF system components as prognostic markers in breast cancer. Breast Cancer Res Treat 47:295–302.

LeRoith, D., and C. T. Roberts, Jr. 1993. Insulin-like growth factors and their receptors in normal physiology and pathological states. J Pediatr Endocrinol 6:251–5.

Li, B. D., M. J. Khosravi, H. J. Berkel, A. Diamandi, M. A. Dayton, M. Smith, and H. Yu. 2001. Free insulin-like growth factor-I and breast cancer risk. Int J Cancer 91:736–9.

Mardilovich, K., and L. M. Shaw. 2009. Hypoxia regulates insulin receptor substrate-2 expression to promote breast carcinoma cell survival and invasion. Cancer Res 69:8894–901.

McGuire, W. L., Jr., J. G. Jackson, J. A. Figueroa, S. Shimasaki, D. R. Powell, and D. Yee. 1992. Regulation of insulin-like growth factor-binding protein (IGFBP) expression by breast cancer cells: use of IGFBP-1 as an inhibitor of insulin-like growth factor action. J Natl Cancer Inst 84:1336–41.

McKinnon, T., C. Chakraborty, L. M. Gleeson, P. Chidiac, and P. K. Lala. 2001. Stimulation of human extravillous trophoblast migration by IGF-II is mediated by IGF type 2 receptor involving inhibitory G protein(s) and phosphorylation of MAPK. J Clin Endocrinol Metab 86:3665–74.

Migliaccio, I., M. F. Wu, C. Gutierrez, L. Malorni, S. K. Mohsin, D. C. Allred, S. G. Hilsenbeck, C. K. Osborne, H. Weiss, and A. V. Lee. 2009. Nuclear IRS-1 predicts tamoxifen response in patients with early breast cancer. Breast Cancer Res Treat.

Miller, T. W., M. Perez-Torres, A. Narasanna, M. Guix, O. Stal, G. Perez-Tenorio, A. M. Gonzalez-Angulo, B. T. Hennessy, G. B. Mills, J. P. Kennedy, C. W. Lindsley, and C. L. Arteaga. 2009. Loss of Phosphatase and Tensin homologue deleted on chromosome 10 engages ErbB3 and insulin-like growth factor-I receptor signaling to promote antiestrogen resistance in breast cancer. Cancer Res 69:4192–201.

Mohan, S., and D. J. Baylink. 2002. IGF-binding proteins are multifunctional and act via IGF-dependent and -independent mechanisms. J Endocrinol 175:19–31.

Mu, L., D. Katsaros, A. Wiley, L. Lu, I. A. de la Longrais, S. Smith, S. Khubchandani, O. Sochirca, R. Arisio, and H. Yu. 2009. Peptide concentrations and mRNA expression of IGF-I, IGF-II and IGFBP-3 in breast cancer and their associations with disease characteristics. Breast Cancer Res Treat 115:151–62.

Muti, P., T. Quattrin, B. J. Grant, V. Krogh, A. Micheli, H. J. Schunemann, M. Ram, J. L. Freudenheim, S. Sieri, M. Trevisan, and F. Berrino. 2002. Fasting glucose is a risk factor for breast cancer: a prospective study. Cancer Epidemiol Biomarkers Prev 11:1361–8.

Osborne, C. K., E. B. Coronado, L. J. Kitten, C. I. Arteaga, S. A. Fuqua, K. Ramasharma, M. Marshall, and C. H. Li. 1989. Insulin-like growth factor-II (IGF-II): a potential autocrine/paracrine growth factor for human breast cancer acting via the IGF-I receptor. Mol Endocrinol 3:1701–9.

Palsgaard, J., A. E. Brown, M. Jensen, R. Borup, M. Walker, and P. De Meyts. 2009. Insulin-like growth factor I (IGF-I) is a more potent regulator of gene expression than insulin in primary human myoblasts and myotubes. Growth Horm IGF Res 19:168–78.

Papa, V., B. Gliozzo, G. M. Clark, W. L. McGuire, D. Moore, Y. Fujita-Yamaguchi, R. Vigneri, I. D. Goldfine, and V. Pezzino. 1993. Insulin-like growth factor-I receptors are overexpressed and predict a low risk in human breast cancer. Cancer Res 53:3736–40.

Perks, C. M., and J. M. Holly. 2008. IGF binding proteins (IGFBPs) and regulation of breast cancer biology. J Mammary Gland Biol Neoplasia 13:455–69.

Perks, C. M., P. V. Newcomb, M. R. Norman, and J. M. Holly. 1999. Effect of insulin-like growth factor binding protein-1 on integrin signalling and the induction of apoptosis in human breast cancer cells. J Mol Endocrinol 22:141–50.

Peyrat, J. P., J. Bonneterre, B. Hecquet, P. Vennin, M. M. Louchez, C. Fournier, J. Lefebvre, and A. Demaille. 1993. Plasma insulin-like growth factor-1 (IGF-1) concentrations in human breast cancer. Eur J Cancer 29A:492–7.

Pitts, T. M., A. C. Tan, G. N. Kulikowski, J. J. Tentler, A. M. Brown, S. A. Flanigan, S. Leong, C. D. Coldren, F. R. Hirsch, M. Varella-Garcia, C. Korch, and S. G. Eckhardt. 2010. Development of an integrated genomic classifier for a novel agent in colorectal cancer: approach to individualized therapy in early development. Clin Cancer Res 16:3193–204.

Pollak, M. N., J. F. Perdue, R. G. Margolese, K. Baer, and M. Richard. 1987. Presence of somatomedin receptors on primary human breast and colon carcinomas. Cancer Lett 38:223–30.

Probst-Hensch, N. M., J. H. Steiner, P. Schraml, Z. Varga, U. Zurrer-Hardi, M. Storz, D. Korol, M. K. Fehr, D. Fink, B. C. Pestalozzi, U. M. Lutolf, J. P. Theurillat, and H. Moch. 2010. IGFBP2 and IGFBP3 protein expressions in human breast cancer: association with hormonal factors and obesity. Clin Cancer Res 16:1025–32.

Renehan, A. G., M. Egger, C. Minder, S. T. O'Dwyer, S. M. Shalet, and M. Zwahlen. 2005. IGF-I, IGF binding protein-3 and breast cancer risk: comparison of 3 meta-analyses. Int J Cancer 115:1006–7; author reply 1008.

Renehan, A. G., M. Zwahlen, C. Minder, S. T. O'Dwyer, S. M. Shalet, and M. Egger. 2004. Insulin-like growth factor (IGF)-I, IGF binding protein-3, and cancer risk: systematic review and meta-regression analysis. Lancet 363:1346–53.

Rinaldi, S., P. H. Peeters, F. Berrino, L. Dossus, C. Biessy, A. Olsen, A. Tjonneland, K. Overvad, F. Clavel-Chapelon, M. C. Boutron-Ruault, B. Tehard, G. Nagel, J. Linseisen, H. Boeing, P. H. Lahmann, A. Trichopoulou, D. Trichopoulos, M. Koliva, D. Palli, S. Panico, R. Tumino, C. Sacerdote, C. H. van Gils, P. van Noord, D. E. Grobbee, H. B. Bueno-de-Mesquita, C. A. Gonzalez, A. Agudo, M. D. Chirlaque, A. Barricarte, N. Larranaga, J. R. Quiros, S. Bingham, K. T. Khaw, T. Key, N. E. Allen, A. Lukanova, N. Slimani, R. Saracci, E. Riboli, and R. Kaaks. 2006. IGF-I, IGFBP-3 and breast cancer risk in women: The European Prospective Investigation into Cancer and Nutrition (EPIC). Endocr Relat Cancer 13:593–605.

Sabbatini, P., J. L. Rowand, A. Groy, S. Korenchuk, Q. Liu, C. Atkins, M. Dumble, J. Yang, K. Anderson, B. J. Wilson, K. A. Emmitte, S. K. Rabindran, and R. Kumar. 2009. Antitumor activity of GSK1904529A, a small-molecule inhibitor of the insulin-like growth factor-I receptor tyrosine kinase. Clin Cancer Res 15:3058–67.

Sachdev, D., and D. Yee. 2007. Disrupting insulin-like growth factor signaling as a potential cancer therapy. Mol Cancer Ther 6:1–12.

Shetty, P. J., S. Movva, N. Pasupuleti, B. Vedicherlla, K. K. Vattam, S. Venkatasubramanian, Y. R. Ahuja, and Q. Hasan. 2010. Regulation of IGF2 transcript and protein expression by altered methylation in breast cancer. J Cancer Res Clin Oncol.

Shi, R., H. Yu, J. McLarty, and J. Glass. 2004. IGF-I and breast cancer: a meta-analysis. Int J Cancer 111:418–23.

So, A. I., R. J. Levitt, B. Eigl, L. Fazli, M. Muramaki, S. Leung, M. C. Cheang, T. O. Nielsen, M. Gleave, and M. Pollak. 2008. Insulin-like growth factor binding protein-2 is a novel therapeutic target associated with breast cancer. Clin Cancer Res 14:6944–54.

Spentzos, D., S. A. Cannistra, F. Grall, D. A. Levine, K. Pillay, T. A. Libermann, and C. S. Mantzoros. 2007. IGF axis gene expression patterns are prognostic of survival in epithelial ovarian cancer. Endocr Relat Cancer 14:781–90.

Stoeltzing, O., W. Liu, N. Reinmuth, F. Fan, A. A. Parikh, C. D. Bucana, D. B. Evans, G. L. Semenza, and L. M. Ellis. 2003. Regulation of hypoxia-inducible factor-1alpha, vascular endothelial growth factor, and angiogenesis by an insulin-like growth factor-I receptor autocrine loop in human pancreatic cancer. Am J Pathol 163:1001–11.

Sueoka, N., H. Y. Lee, S. Wiehle, R. J. Cristiano, B. Fang, L. Ji, J. A. Roth, W. K. Hong, P. Cohen, and J. M. Kurie. 2000. Insulin-like growth factor binding protein-6 activates programmed cell death in non-small cell lung cancer cells. Oncogene 19:4432–6.

Sugumar, A., Y. C. Liu, Q. Xia, Y. S. Koh, and K. Matsuo. 2004. Insulin-like growth factor (IGF)-I and IGF-binding protein 3 and the risk of premenopausal breast cancer: a meta-analysis of literature. Int J Cancer 111:293–7.

Tamemoto, H., T. Kadowaki, K. Tobe, T. Yagi, H. Sakura, T. Hayakawa, Y. Terauchi, Y. Ueki, Y. Kaburagi, S. Satoh, and et al. 1994. Insulin resistance and growth retardation in mice lacking insulin receptor substrate-1. Nature 372:182–6.

Taverne, C. W., M. Verheus, J. D. McKay, R. Kaaks, F. Canzian, D. E. Grobbee, P. H. Peeters, and C. H. van Gils. 2010. Common genetic variation of insulin-like growth factor-binding protein 1 (IGFBP-1), IGFBP-3, and acid labile subunit in relation to serum IGF-I levels and mammographic density. Breast Cancer Res Treat.

Toniolo, P., P. F. Bruning, A. Akhmedkhanov, J. M. Bonfrer, K. L. Koenig, A. Lukanova, R. E. Shore, and A. Zeleniuch-Jacquotte. 2000. Serum insulin-like growth factor-I and breast cancer. Int J Cancer 88:828–32.

Turner, B. C., B. G. Haffty, L. Narayanan, J. Yuan, P. A. Havre, A. A. Gumbs, L. Kaplan, J. L. Burgaud, D. Carter, R. Baserga, and P. M. Glazer. 1997. Insulin-like growth factor-I receptor overexpression mediates cellular radioresistance and local breast cancer recurrence after lumpectomy and radiation. Cancer Res 57:3079–83.

Vadgama, J. V., Y. Wu, G. Datta, H. Khan, and R. Chillar. 1999. Plasma insulin-like growth factor-I and serum IGF-binding protein 3 can be associated with the progression of breast cancer, and predict the risk of recurrence and the probability of survival in African-American and Hispanic women. Oncology 57:330–40.

Van den Berg, C. L., G. N. Cox, C. A. Stroh, S. G. Hilsenbeck, C. N. Weng, M. J. McDermott, D. Pratt, C. K. Osborne, E. B. Coronado-Heinsohn, and D. Yee. 1997. Polyethylene glycol conjugated insulin-like growth factor binding protein-1 (IGFBP-1) inhibits growth of breast cancer in athymic mice. Eur J Cancer 33:1108–13.

Volpert, O., D. Jackson, N. Bouck, and D. I. Linzer. 1996. The insulin-like growth factor II/mannose 6-phosphate receptor is required for proliferin-induced angiogenesis. Endocrinology 137:3871–6.

White, M. F. 1998. The IRS-signaling system: a network of docking proteins that mediate insulin and cytokine action. Recent Prog Horm Res 53:119–38.

Winston, R., P. C. Kao, and D. T. Kiang. 1994. Regulation of insulin-like growth factors by antiestrogen. Breast Cancer Res Treat 31:107–15.

Withers, D. J., J. S. Gutierrez, H. Towery, D. J. Burks, J. M. Ren, S. Previs, Y. Zhang, D. Bernal, S. Pons, G. I. Shulman, S. Bonner-Weir, and M. F. White. 1998. Disruption of IRS-2 causes type 2 diabetes in mice. Nature 391:900–4.

Yee, D., and A. V. Lee. 2000. Crosstalk between the insulin-like growth factors and estrogens in breast cancer. J Mammary Gland Biol Neoplasia 5:107–15.

Yu, H., F. Jin, X. O. Shu, B. D. Li, Q. Dai, J. R. Cheng, H. J. Berkel, and W. Zheng. 2002. Insulin-like growth factors and breast cancer risk in Chinese women. Cancer Epidemiol Biomarkers Prev 11:705–12.

Zhang, X., and D. Yee. 2002. Insulin-like growth factor binding protein-1 (IGFBP-1) inhibits breast cancer cell motility. Cancer Res 62:4369–75.

Zofkova, I. 2003. Pathophysiological and clinical importance of insulin-like growth factor-I with respect to bone metabolism. Physiol Res 52:657–79.

Chapter 5
The Role of Insulin-Like Growth Factor Signaling in Prostate Cancer Development and Progression

Bruce Montgomery, James Dean, and Stephen Plymate

IGF Signaling Networks in Prostate Cancer

An excellent and detailed review of IGF signaling can be found in Chap. 1 of this text, and a brief overview of relevant signaling networks is provided here to inform discussion of novel aspects of IGF signaling in prostate cancer.

An excellent and detailed review of IGF signaling can be found in Chap. 1 of this text (Samani et al. 2007), and a brief overview of relevant signaling networks is provided here, Fig. 5.1.

The insulin-like growth factor type I receptor (IGF-IR) has been suggested to play an important role in prostate cancer progression and possibly in the progression to androgen-independent (AI) disease. The term AI is not be entirely correct, in that recent data suggest that expression of androgen receptor (AR) and androgen-regulated genes is the primary association with prostate cancer progression after hormone ablation. Therefore, signaling through other growth factors has been thought to play a role in AR-mediated prostate cancer progression to AI disease in the absence of androgen ligand. However, existing data on how IGF-IR signaling interacts with AR activation in prostate cancer are conflicting. In this chapter, we review some of the published data on the mechanisms of IGF-IR/AR interaction and present new evidence that IGF-IR signaling may modulate AR compartmentation and thus alter AR activity in prostate cancer cells. Inhibition of IGF-IR signaling can result in cytoplasmic AR retention and a significant change in androgen-regulated

---

S. Plymate (✉)
VA Puget Sound Health Care System,
1660 S. Columbian Way, Seattle, WA, USA

Division of Geriatrics and Gerontology, Department of Medicine,
University of Washington School of Medicine, Seattle, WA, USA
e-mail: splymate@u.washington.edu

D. LeRoith (ed.), *Insulin-like Growth Factors and Cancer: From Basic Biology to Therapeutics*, Cancer Drug Discovery and Development,
DOI 10.1007/978-1-4614-0598-6_5, © Springer Science+Business Media, LLC 2012

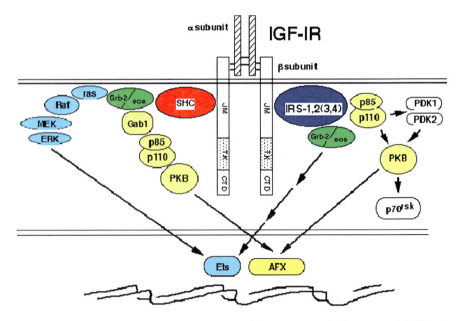

Fig. 5.1 IGF-IR signaling pathways and the role of Shc as a potential integrator of PI3K and MAPK pathway activation

gene expression. Translocation of AR from the cytoplasm to the nucleus may be associated with IGF-induced dephosphorylation. Since fully humanized antibodies targeting the IGF-IR are now in clinical trials, this review is intended to reveal the mechanisms of potential therapeutic effects of these antibodies on AI prostate cancers.

It has been shown that the androgen receptor (AR) is the common factor associated with progression of prostate cancer either before castration or in the setting of castrate-resistant disease (Scher and Sawyers 2005). The caveat here is that the tumors are not neuroendocrine in which case they are AR negative, these cases make up only <10% of all prostate cancers. Classically, in the absence of androgen ligand, AR remains in the cytosol and is not active. Thus, it is of particular interest that malignant prostate cancer progression occurs frequently in men who have been surgically or chemically castrated. The progression of prostate cancer after castration has been termed castrate-resistant prostate cancer (CRPC). However, this is again somewhat of a misnomer since it has been shown by our group and others that following castration, either surgical or medical, that in most tumors there is still a significant concentration of testosterone (T) and dihydrotestosterone (DHT) that remains in the prostate, and are in sufficient concentration to transactivate the AR. However, compounds now in phase III clinical trials that inhibit androgen synthesis, abiraterone, or are very effective blockers of ligand binding to the LBD of the AR, e.g., MDV3100, although effective at inhibiting androgen activity in the tumor still ultimately fail with tumor recurrence approximately 12–18 months after the treatment is started. With recurrence following these drugs there continues to be an increase in PSA, an AR regulated gene, indicating that the AR continues to be the driving force for tumor progression. More interestingly, animal studies showed that when the expression of AR was disrupted, prostate cancer ceased to progress (Taplin and Balk 2004). Together, these data indicate that the genomic activity of the AR is the driving force for prostate cancer progression. If so, it would suggest that the AR is functioning in a nonclassical manner in the absence of steroid ligand. Although nongenomic mechanisms for AR function have been proposed through an interaction with SRC–Raf–Ras–Map kinase in the cytosol rather than the nucleus, this "traditional" nongenomic mechanism also requires the presence of androgen ligand and would not explain progression of disease in a ligand-independent manner (Pandini et al. 2005).

The concept of AR functioning in CRPC was first proposed by Mohler et al. (2004). In relevant studies, tumor biopsies were taken from prostate cancer patients who had been androgen ablated and presented with progression of the cancer (Mohler et al. 2004; Gregory et al. 2001). In these samples, the AR primarily resided in a nuclear location, contrary to what had been expected in a castrated environment. This may in part due to residual levels of androgen in the prostate tissue. When tissue levels of androgen, testosterone, and DHT were measured, although lower than in noncastrated men, they were still detected in the nanomolar range in many of the castrated men (Titus et al. 2005). This subtle level of tissue androgen may account for the nuclear localization of the AR and signal to activate an AR transcriptional program. The failure of castration to completely abolish intraprostatic androgens has also been seen in a study where normal men were placed on a GnRH antagonist for 4 weeks and in whom serum levels of testosterone (T) and DHT were clearly in the castrate range (Page et al. 2006). The source of the androgens in these castrate men has yet to be determined; however, likely sources include conversion from adrenal androgens via 3β hydroxysteroid dehydrogenase from androstanediol or dehydroepiandrosterone or de novo steroid synthesis by tumor. The prostate has active 5α-reductase systems for both isoforms I and II, ensuring that circulating T can be readily converted to DHT in the prostate (Titus et al. 2005). In addition, recent microarray data has shown that the prostate contains mRNAs for the enzymes necessary for the conversion of cholesterol precursor into DHT; however, this conversion has not been demonstrated in the prostate (Mostaghel et al. 2007).

Castration studies on prostate cancer xenograft and transgenic mouse models support the speculation that residual androgen production following castration is only the partial driving force for tumor progression. Since mice do not produce adrenal androgens to any significant degree, castration in a mouse results in "complete androgen ablation" (van Weerden et al. 1992). In these models, tumors progress from androgen-dependent (AD) to CRPC in spite of the fact that prostate-specific androgen levels decrease to nearly undetectable levels, suggesting that residual androgens are unlikely to play a part in postcastration tumor progression (Corey et al. 2003; Thalmann et al. 2000). We and others have shown that, in these models, the majority of tumor nuclei still contain AR after castration although some of the AR moves from the nucleus to the cytoplasm (Fig. 5.2). Furthermore, androgen-regulated genes continue to be expressed in CRPC disease (Corey et al. 2003).

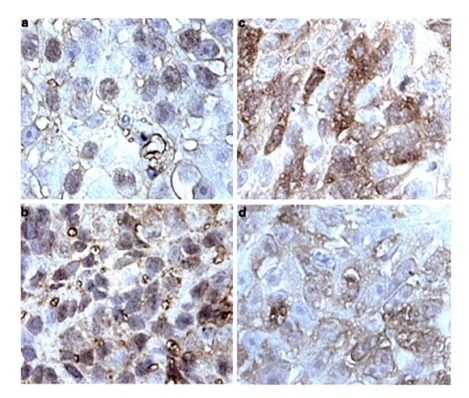

Fig. 5.2 IGF-IR signaling-induced translocation of AR into the nucleus in xenograft human prostate tumors. (**a**) AR compartmentalization in the nucleus in intact animals. (**b**) Blocking IGF-IR signaling with antibody A12 caused cytoplasmic retention of AR in intact animals. (**c**) AR in the nucleus in castrated animals. (**d**) A12 induced marked AR retention in the cytosol in castrated animals (Wu et al. 2006)

Together, these data suggest that other mechanisms beyond the traditional ligand–receptor interaction of AR signaling are responsible for AD to AI prostate cancer progression.

Alterations in co-regulators of the AR, which may enhance ligand-independent AR translocation to the nucleus and binding to DNA, have been suggested as one of the mechanisms for ligand-independent AR (Fujimoto et al. 1999; Kang et al. 1999; Sadar 1999; Sadar and Gleave 2000). It has been suggested that some peptide growth factors can act directly at the androgen-binding domain of the AR or indirectly through modifying the phosphorylation status of the AR or its co-regulators to initiate AR signaling (Sadar 1999; Culig et al. 1994, 1995; Lin et al. 2001). Among peptide growth factor-induced cell signaling, IGF-activated IGF-IR signaling is a potential driving force for the growth of CRPC prostate cancer for several reasons as listed in Table 5.1. In the following sections, we examine the evidence for each of these components of potential interaction between the IGF-IR and AR.

Table 5.1 Evidence for interaction of the IGF-IR and AR in prostate cancer (from Wu et al. 2006)

1. The IGF-IR is necessary for cell transformation
2. Clinical data, although somewhat controversial suggest that higher levels of IGF-I in the serum of men predict men at risk for developing clinical prostate cancer
3. Androgens increase IGF-IR levels in prostate epithelial cells
4. IGF-IR signaling alters AR phosphorylation
5. IGF-IR signaling alters the AR transcriptional profile
6. IGF-IR signaling effects translocation of the AR to the nucleus
7. IGF-IR ligands increase in the progression of prostate cancer and are particularly abundant in bone where prostate cancer metastases are most abundant
8. Xenograft models of prostate cancer respond differently to IGF-IR inhibition depending on the presence or absence of androgens
9. IGF binding proteins (IGFBP) that enhance signaling of IGF ligands through the IGF-IR are increased in the period immediately after castration
10. Inhibition of the IGF-IR in conjunction with castration
11. Transcription factors that stimulate the IGF-IR promoter are also regulated by androgens

IGF-IR Is Necessary for Cell Transformation

Fibroblasts from IGF-IR knockout mice R^- do not transform spontaneously when compared to R^{wt} control cells. When the IGF-IR is re-expressed in these fibroblasts, transformation takes place. In SV40T immortalized prostate epithelial cells, inhibition of IGF-IR expression with an antisense construct significantly decreases colony formation in soft agar, a marker of transformation. In studies when growth hormone and IGF-1 deficient LID mice were crossed with the transgenic prostate cancer (TRAMP) mouse, tumor development was significantly delayed (Majeed et al. 2005). All these studies suggest an essential role of IGF-IR in cellular transformation. Hongo et al. have identified specific tyrosine residues on the β-subunit of the IGF-IR that are crucial for the transforming actions of the IGF-IR (1998; O'Connor et al. 1997).

Since prostate cancer rarely develops in the absence of androgens, it is suspected that androgens are at least permissive in the transformation process of prostate epithelial cells. However, it should be noted that expression of the AR is necessary for normal luminal prostate epithelium to develop. It is suggested that maintaining certain levels of IGF-IR expression in the prostate may be necessary in normal prostate differentiation, increased levels of IGF-IR expression may be required for the prostate epithelia transformation process, and decreased IGF-IR expression may be required for prostate cancer malignant progression. This is consistent with the clinical findings that the levels of IGF-IR decrease following the initial transformation of the epithelium (Tennant et al. 1996). This concept has been corroborated by the decrease in tumor metastases and increase in apoptosis associated with the re-expression IGF-IR in prostate cancer xenograft cell lines (Plymate et al. 1997a, b).

Androgen Modulation of IGF-IR Expression

We had initially detected an increase in IGF-IR expression at protein and mRNA levels in androgen-responsive prostate epithelial cell lines (Plymate et al. 2004). This observation was subsequently confirmed by other investigators (Pandini et al. 2005). The mechanism by which androgens increase the IGF-IR expression has been a topic of controversy. Pandini et al. have shown in their models that the increase in IGF-IR protein induced by androgens does not require nuclear translocation of the AR and is only partially blocked by biclutamide (2005). On the other hand, this effect of AR on IGF-IR expression was completely inhibited by the ERK1/2 inhibitor PD980259 (Pandini et al. 2005). These data suggested a "nongenomic" effect of androgen. This group further confirmed their findings using a mutated AR that will not translocate to the nucleus and demonstrated that the mutated AR can activate the cytoplasmic Src–Raf–Ras–Map kinase pathway and enhance the transcriptional activity of IGF-IR promoter. Other mechanisms including an increase in KFL6 (Kruppel factor like 6) in response to androgens have been suggested from the study in LnCaP lines (Rubinstein et al. 2004). We have shown that KFL6 increases IGF-IR expression by binding to the IGF-IR promoter (Rubinstein et al. 2004). We have also shown in prostate cell lines that androgens can increase IGF-IR protein expression without an increase in its mRNA expression level, suggesting a post-transcriptional modification of IGF-IR expression, such as mRNA stability (Plymate et al. 2004). Despite the existing controversial on the mechanisms, all the studies have consistently showed that androgens signaling through the AR result in increased IGF-IR protein expression in prostate epithelium, which is associated with increased phosphorylation of IGF-IR and increased cell proliferation in response to IGF ligands. However, it is not understood whether the induction of increased IGF-IR is part of the differentiation process of prostate epithelium or part of the mechanism for tumor progression. Since both IGF and androgens are necessary for epithelial differentiation, induction of increase in IGF-IR expression as part of the differentiating function of androgens may appear reasonable. On the other hand, increasing IGF-IR expression would be a mechanism by which androgens could enhance transformation and progression of prostate cancer.

IGF-IR Activation Alters AR Phosphorylation

One mechanism by which IGF-IR signaling could directly affect the function of the AR would be to alter AR phosphorylation. Studies by Lin et al. (2001) first suggested a role of IGF signaling in AR function. They observed that androgen induced apoptosis in AR transiently transfected DU-145 cells and treatment with IGF-1 decreased the transcriptional activity of the AR and inhibited apoptosis. We subsequently found that the effects on IGF-IR signaling on AR activity depended on whether the cells were from an orthotopic or a metastatic lesion (Plymate et al. 2004). If the tumor was in the orthotopic site, IGF-IR activation inhibited AR transcription under a probasin promoter (AAR3). In contrast, when the tumor was in the metastatic site, IGF-IR activation enhanced AR transcriptional activity on the AAR3 promoter. Interestingly, the effect of IGF-IR activation on the AR transcriptional activity in both primary and metastatic tumors appears to be mediated through the PI3K/AKT pathway. Lin et al. subsequently demonstrated that the effects of IGF on AR activity occurred in a biphasic manner in LnCaP cells: suppressing AR transcriptional activity at low passage numbers but enhancing AR transcriptional activity at high passage numbers (2001). Whether the effect is due to IGF-initiated phosphorylation of AR is rather controversial. Lin et al. described that IGF-I phosphorylates AR at serines 210 and 790, whereas Gioeli et al. failed to find any sites on the AR that were phosphorylated by IGF through a peptide terminal degeneration technique (2002; Lin et al. 2001). We examined the effect of IGF-IR activation on AR phosphorylation in AR-transfected M12 (M12AR) cells. We showed that AR phosphorylation was decreased in the presence of IGF-I and that this effect was blocked by an inhibitory IGF-IR antibody A12. We have also shown that serine 16 on the AR is a potential site of dephosphorylation whereas serine 81 on the AR is a potential site of phosphorylation by IGF (Wu et al. 2006). The reasons for discrepancies between studies are not entirely clear. One possible reason for differences in phosphorylation would be differential expression of PP2A in different cell types.

IGF-IR Signaling Modulates Nuclear Translocation of the AR

Phosphorylation of the AR may result in several changes that could alter the AR transcriptional functions. One of these effects could be translocation of the AR to the nucleus. Whereas AR phosphorylation was thought to be necessary for nuclear translocation, recent data have shown that phosphorylation of AR at serine 650, which takes place after the AR is in the nucleus and bound to DNA, results in the export of AR from the nucleus (Gioeli et al. 2006). Thus, the process of dephosphorylation of specific serines on the AR may account for retention of AR in the nucleus and accentuated signaling. As we have shown in Fig. 5.2, IGF decreases phosphorylation of the AR in our M12AR cells. We also have evidence that IGF can enhance AR nuclear translocation in the absence of androgens and that this effect can be inhibited by an IGF-IR inhibitory antibody (Fig. 5.3a). We have also demonstrated the changes in AR compartmentalization in nuclear and cytoplasmic fractions in response to IGF using Western blot analyses (Fig. 5.3b). Using the AAR3 probasin reporter assay, we show a significant transactivation of the AR in the absence of androgen and enhanced AR activation in the presence of androgen by IGF-I in M12AR cells. The AR transactivation response to IGFs can be blocked by the IGF-IR antibody A12. These data indicate that even in the absence of androgen, IGFs can induce transactivation of the AR. Whether this is attributed to changes in

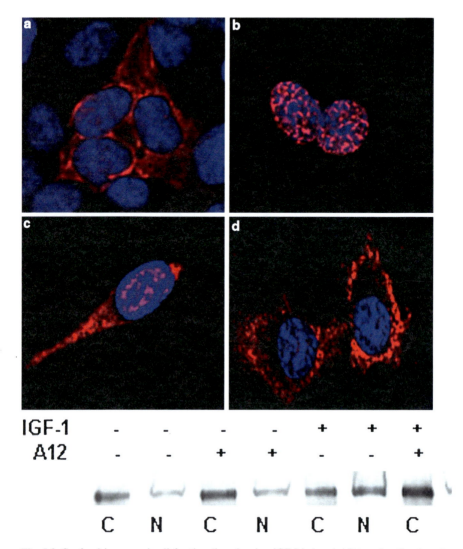

Fig. 5.3 Confocal image and cell fractionation showing IGF-I-induced AR translocation into the nucleus in M12AR cell lines. (a) M12AR cells in IGF-I, DHT-free medium. (b) M12AR cells in medium containing 10^{-8} M of DHT. (c) M12AR cells in medium containing 10 ng/ml of IGF-I. (d) Medium containing 10 ng/ml of IGF-I and 10 μg/ml of anti-IGF-IR antibody A12. (e) AR in cytosol and nuclear fractions of M12AR cells under various culture conditions. Red fluorescence. *AR* androgen receptor, *IGF-I* insulin-like growth factor I, *DHT* dihydrotestosterone (Plymate et al. 2007)

phosphorylation of the AR as we have discussed or to the recruitment of AR cofactors, or to both has yet to be determined. Regardless, these studies suggest that, in castrated patients, the increase in AR expression coupled with intact IGF-IR signaling can lead to AR-mediated AI prostate cancer progression. This marks the IGF-IR a potential therapeutic target in postcastrated prostate cancer.

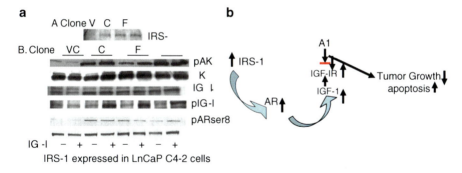

Fig. 5.4 *Panel* (**a**) shows Western blot of effects on AR and IGF-IR following the introduction of IRS-1 into LnCaP C4-2 cells. *Panel* (**b**) is a schematic representation of the autocrine loop generated by introduction of IRS-1 into the LnCaP cell line

IRS-1 Is Necessary for IGF Activation of AR

We have shown that in the LnCaP cell line where the IRS-1 is suppressed due to promoter methylation, it has been demonstrated that re-expression of IRS-1 results in AR phosphorylation at ser81. Following serine phosphorylation of the AR, an increase in both IGF-I and IGF-I receptor is seen along with activation of the IGF-IR as indicated by phosphorylation of IGF-IR. This autocrine proliferation loop is shown in Fig. 5.4.

Differential modulation of prostate cancer xenografts in the presence and absence of androgen. We have reported in prostate cancer human xenograft models that inhibition of the IGF-IR with A12 results in a decreased rate of tumor growth in AD and AI tumors (Wu et al. 2005). However, when we examined the mechanisms by which A12 caused decrease in growth rate, we noted marked differences depending on whether the tumors were AD or AI. In the AD tumors, we found that A12 treatment resulted in a combination of apoptosis and G1 cell cycle arrest, whereas in the AI tumors we found that tumor cells arrested in G2 with no occurrence of apoptosis (Wu et al. 2005). The question arose as to whether these differences in responses were due to a change in the character of the tumor or the absence of androgen. In order to address this issue, we implanted the AI tumor into intact animals. As predicted, tumor growth was inhibited in the A12-treated animals compared to vehicle-treated controls. Interestingly, a majority of these tumors displayed an apoptotic response and G1 cell cycle arrest as opposed to the lack of apoptosis when implanted in the castrated animals. To determine the potential mechanisms for this effect of androgen on the tumors, we performed cDNA microarray analyses of A12-treated AI tumors from castrated and intact animals and found marked differences in the gene expression profiles (Plymate et al. 2007; Sprenger et al. 2009). Some genes such as PP2A and TSC-22 were regulated in opposite direction with A12 treatment, depending on the presence or absence of androgens. It is of interest that TSC-22 has been shown to be androgen-regulated and its expression decreases from benign prostate luminal epithelium to cancer. Another interesting gene differentiation expressed is IGFBP-5, which has been demonstrated to increase postcastration and is associated with recovery from castration-induced apoptosis (Miyake et al. 2000a, b; Sprenger et al. 2009).

Castration induces IGF-binding proteins (IGFBPs) and signaling through IGF-IR. Following castration, IGFBP-2 and IGFBP-5 have been shown to increase significantly in both human prostate and mouse models of prostate cancer. Both of these IGFBPs can increase IGF-ligand signaling through the IGF-IR and enhance recovery from castration-induced apoptosis and cell cycle arrest. These two IGFBPs accomplish this task by binding to extracelluar matrix and maintaining a higher concentration of IGF ligand in the proximity of the IGF-IR (Mohler et al. 2004; Jones and Clemmons 1995; Kiyama et al. 2003; Russo et al. 2005). The functional importance of these changes has been demonstrated by the studies of Miyake et al. (2000a, b) in which overexpression of these IGFBPs in LnCaP cells markedly enhances cell growth following androgen withdrawal. Using antisense oligonucleotides to IGFBP-2 or IGFBP-5, this group was able to demonstrate the stimulatory effects of the IGFBPs on tumor growth (Kiyama et al. 2003).

Combined Inhibition of the IGF-IR and Androgen Signaling in Prostate Cancer

These studies suggest that blocking IGF-IR signaling at the time of castration would enhance the effects of androgen withdraw. Potential mechanisms of the augmented effect of A12 on androgen withdraw may include suppression of Survivin, a member of the inhibitor of apoptosis (IAP) family of proteins that has been shown to play a role in the recovery process of anti-androgen therapy (Zhang et al. 2005). We have shown in multiple human xenograft models of human prostate cancer that a short period of IGF-IR inhibition with the human IGF-IR mab A12 results in a marked prolongation of time to cancer regrowth when compared to castration by itself, Fig. 5.5 (Plymate et al. 2007). The delay in tumor regrowth besides being associated with a decrease in survivin also correlated with a decrease in nuclear androgen receptor, Fig. 5.3.

IGF-IR Activation Induces AR Cofactors that Enhance AR Signaling

IGF may also influence AR signaling by increasing the expression of AR co-stimulatory factors. Given the known 100 or more AR co-regulatory factors, it is not surprising that IGF-IR activation would enhance the expression or activation of one or more co-regulators of the AR. Among them, TIF-2 (GRIP-1) and insulin degrading enzyme

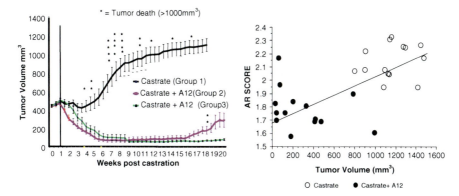

Fig. 5.5 *Top panel* demonstrated the effects of the addition of an IGF-IR mab to castration for 2 weeks beginning 1 or 2 weeks after castration (groups 2 and 3, respectively, compared to castration alone, group 1). *Bottom panel* shows the relationship between nuclear AR score and treatment with A12 from (Plymate et al. 2007)

(IDE) are of particular interest. Studies in a series of human prostate specimens from men with prostate cancer, Mohler and Wilson have demonstrated an increased expression of TIF-2 in most of the recurrent AI prostate cancers that also have high levels of AR in the nucleus (Gregory et al. 2001). The same group has also shown the coincidence of increased TIF-2 expression with the recurrence of AI human prostate cancer in xenograft models. Mohler has also demonstrated that overexpression of TIF-2 in vitro can increase AR transcriptional activity in the presence of the physiological concentrations of adrenal androgen. Studies have shown that IDE is a potent co-stimulator of AR transcriptional activity and the ability of IDE to bind to the AR can be regulated by insulin and IGF ligands (Kupfer et al. 1994). In addition, as the name implies, IDE can degrade insulin, IGF-I, and IGF-II (Udrisar et al. 2005).

The Role of IGF Signaling in Prostate Carcinogenesis

IGFs mediate proliferation and differentiation in multiple tissues, including prostate epithelium. Xenograft models provide clear evidence that dysregulated IGF and IGF-IR mediate progression to carcinoma particularly in the context of aberrant estrogen and testosterone levels (DiGiovanni et al. 2000; Wang et al. 1998). In an attempt to determine the relevance of this preclinical data in humans, prospective cohort studies have attempted to correlate circulating IGF and IGFBP levels with subsequent risk of developing prostate carcinoma. Perhaps the most compelling data were provided by the Physician's Health Study, a prospective case–control study of otherwise healthy men who provided plasma and were followed for a minimum of 10 years after registration. In this cohort, men with serum IGF-1 levels in the highest quartile had a 4.3-fold increased risk of developing prostate cancer compared with men with levels in the lowest quartile. In multivariate analysis, IGFBP-3 and IGF-II did not independently modulate risk of cancer (Chan et al. 1998). Additional analyses combining results from multiple studies confirmed the increased risk of prostate cancer with increasing IGF-1 levels, although pooled analysis suggested a lower relative risk of 1.38 in men with the highest quintile of IGF-I levels compared to those men with levels in the lowest quintile (Roddam et al. 2008). Additional meta-analysis has confirmed the modest increase in risk with increasing IGF-I (Rowlands et al. 2009). Circulating IGF-I levels primarily increase the risk of developing lower grade prostate cancer, and there has been very limited evidence that levels of any of the other IGF or IGFBP peptides add additional information regarding risk.

The role of IGFs in carcinogenesis led to interrogation of single nucleotide polymorphisms (SNPs) in the IGF-I gene, given their potential to regulate the levels and function of IGF-I. Among the various IGF-I SNPs interrogated, one SNP encodes different numbers of cytosine–adenine repeats in the promoter of IGF-I, potentially modulating levels. The presence of the allele encoding 19 repeats increased the hazard ratio of developing prostate cancer between 1.78 and 3.36 (heterozygous or homozygous) in a case–control study in Japanese men (Tsuchiya et al. 2005). Assessment of the same SNP in men with metastatic prostate cancer demonstrated shorter survival if one of the alleles contained at least 18 repeats, referred to as a long allele, with a median survival of 41 months in the presence of a long allele, and 61 months if neither allele contained at least 18 repeats (Tsuchiya et al. 2006).

The role of IGFs in the recurrence and progression of prostate cancer remains an area of ongoing investigation, with implications for how modulation of ligand and receptor might improve therapy. As reviewed above, IGF ligands and receptors can mediate proliferation, modulate differentiation, and interact with other growth hormone pathways to support prostate cancer growth and progression. Paradoxically, although elevated IGF-1 appears to promote carcinogenesis, there has been limited data that serum IGFs or tissue IGF-I receptor expression in clinical specimens predict relapse after definitive therapy. In one series, serum levels of IGF-1, IGFBP-2, or IGFBP-3 were not predictive of relapse in patients followed after radical prostatectomy (Yu et al. 2001). Low preoperative levels of IGFBP-2 and IGFBP-3 were predictors for subsequent PSA progression after prostatectomy and within the group of men who developed progression, lower IGFBP-3 levels predicted for a more aggressive clinical course (Shariat et al. 2002). In this limited series, IGF-1 levels did not add predictive or prognostic information.

In addition to a clear role for IGF signaling in carcinogenesis, multiple lines of evidence suggest that IGFS and IGF receptors play a critical part in the establishment and maintenance of the transformed and metastatic phenotype (Molife et al. 2010; Sachdev 2010; Sachdev et al. 2009). In both hormone naïve and resistant prostate cancer, IGF1-R signaling drives survival and progression through the canonical ERK and PI-3-kinase pathways, as well as through interactions with the AR (Nickerson et al. 2001). Silencing of IGF1-R through antisense and siRNA suppresses

5 The Role of Insulin-Like Growth Factor Signaling in Prostate Cancer Development... 97

Table 5.2 IGF-IR expression in prostate carcinoma

References	No. of samples	Stage	Methods	Treatment	IGFR expression (epithelium) (%)
Chott et al. (1999)	7	Bone CRPC	IHC	ADT	0
Hellawell et al. (2002)	12	Metastatic CRPC	IHC	ADT	100
	22	Localized	IHC	None	95
Krueckl et al. (2004)	21	Localized	IHC	None	75
	13	Metastatic CRPC	IHC	ADT	100
Ryan et al. (2007)	31	Localized	IHC	None	97
	9	Localized CRPC	IHC	ADT	44
	5	Nodal CRPC	IHC	ADT	80
Schmitz et al. (2007)	9	Localized	PCR	None	89 (low level)

tumor growth in castration-sensitive and castration-resistant cell lines (Burfeind et al. 1996; Rochester et al. 2005). Sensitization of prostate cancer lines is achieved in both PTEN wild type and PTEN null cell lines, and IGF1-R knockdown induced sensitivity to DNA damaging agents in castration resistant cells. Work from our group and reviewed previously has also demonstrated that inhibition of IGF1-R function with the monoclonal antibody IMC-A12 sensitizes castration-resistant and castration-sensitive xenografts to chemotherapy and androgen suppression (Wu et al. 2005; Montgomery et al. 2008). As tumors metastasize and become castration resistant, the change in IGF-IR levels has been somewhat controversial. Some studies have suggested a significant decline in IGF-IR with progression whereas others seem to show a general increase compared to untreated localized disease (Chott et al. 1999; Hellawell et al. 2002; Krueckl et al. 2004; Ryan et al. 2007; Schmitz et al. 2007) (Table 5.2).

As discussed above, a proportion of castration-resistant prostate cancer is fueled by tumoral production and metabolism of androgens (Mostaghel et al. 2007) or by upregulation or mutation of the androgen receptor (Scher and Sawyers 2005). The concurrent upregulation of AR and IGF-IR signaling and the defined cross talk between these pathways strongly support the hypothesis that IGF1-R cooperates with AR to support castration-resistant tumor growth. These studies support targeting the IGF pathway in advanced prostate cancer as one of the most promising modalities for improving both hormonal manipulation and chemotherapy sensitivity.

Strategies to target IGF-IR signaling include inhibiting upstream regulators of ligand (growth hormone), the ligands (IGF-I, IGF-II) for IGF-IR, IGF binding proteins, and receptor activation, expression and localization. Each of these approaches exploits potentially important biology, and unique opportunities exist for therapeutic interventions which leverage the prostate cancer-specific interdependence of androgen and IGF signaling, as well as the potential to improve drug sensitivity. Although a large number of agents have been tested in vitro and in preclinical models, a limited number have come to clinical study in men with prostate cancer.

All of the agents in clinical studies for men with prostate cancer have been reported are monoclonal antibodies to the IGF-IR. The humanized monoclonal antibodies to IGF-IR block binding of IGFs to the receptor and downregulate cell surface receptor to varying degrees. These agents include cixutumumab (previously IMC-A12 – ImClone), Figitumumab (previously CP-751871 – Pfizer), dalotuzumab (previously MK0646 – Merck), AMG 479 (Amgen), and BIIB022 (Biogen Idec). The majority of these antibodies have moved into phase II or phase III studies for different indications, many in combination with chemotherapy or agents targeting other pathways. In the phase I setting, the primary toxicity has been hyperglycemia which occurs in 10–30% of patients in most studies. The majority of first-in-man studies with this class of agent did not reach a maximum tolerated dose, and dosing in phase II and III studies has been determined by pharmacokinetics and evidence of IGF-IR inhibition in surrogate tissues.

For patients with untreated, hormone naïve prostate cancer, both cixutumumab and figitumumab have been used in neoadjuvant studies prior to prostatectomy to assess efficacy of the drugs both with and without androgen deprivation. In the study reported by Chi et al. (2010), 16 patients with clinically localized prostate cancer were treated with three doses of figitumumab at 20 mg/kg administered every 3 weeks, and prostatectomy performed within 1 week of the last dose of drug. Five patients demonstrated a 50% or greater decline in PSA during therapy, and 15 patients demonstrated some decline in PSA. Figitumumab therapy significantly decreased phosphorylated IGF-IR and phosphorylated AKT. An ongoing study at the University of Washington aims to leverage the remarkable data for the combination of androgen deprivation with cixutumumab and in this study men with high risk localized disease are administered neoadjuvant cixutumumab every 2 weeks, with LHRH agonist and bicalutamide for 3 months prior to prostatectomy (Dean et al. 2010). Results will await completion of the study. The same rationale exists for IGF-IR inhibition with castration in the setting of newly diagnosed metastatic disease, and a phase II study of cixutumumab with androgen deprivation is planned through the Southwest Oncology Group.

In the setting of CRPC, figitumumab was combined with docetaxel 75 mg/m^2 every 3 weeks in a phase Ib study which included 22 patients with CRPC. Within that group of patients, PSA declines $\geq$30% were seen in 54% of patients and a PSA decline of $\geq$50% in 41% of patients (Molife et al. 2010). This has led to a planned phase III study comparing docetaxel to docetaxel with figitumumab for patients with metastatic CRPC who have not received prior docetaxel. A phase II multicenter study coordinated through the University of Washington treated a similar group of patients with cixutumumab administered either every other week (31 patients) or every three weekly (10 patients) (Higano et al. 2010). The median time to progression in this study ranged from 3.2 to 3.8 months with grade 3 toxicities of fatigue and hyperglycemia. A phase II study combining cixutumumab with mitoxantrone in the second-line treatment of docetaxel-refractory metastatic CRPC is currently underway.

The studies of monoclonal antibodies targeting IGF-IR demonstrate significant activity against hormone naïve and castration-resistant prostate cancer without causing undue or unmanageable toxicity. Defining the settings and combinations of agents most appropriate for these drugs will be the challenge for the next series of studies.

5 The Role of Insulin-Like Growth Factor Signaling in Prostate Cancer Development...   99

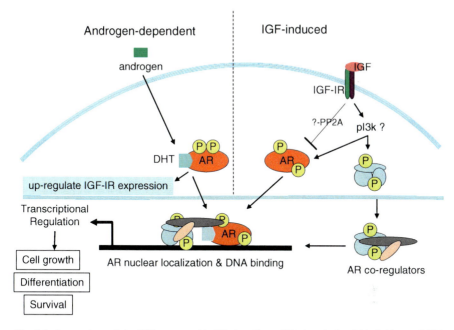

Fig. 5.6 Interactions of the IGF system with AR signaling. *pl3k* phosphoinositide 3-kinase, *PP2A* protein phosphotase 2A

Conclusion

In this chapter, we have summarized our current understandings of the interactions between the IGF system and the AR (Fig. 5.6). The ability of IGF signaling to potentiate the transcriptional activity of the AR in the face of low to no androgen makes the IGF system, especially the IGF-IR, a strong candidate that leads progression of AI prostate cancer through AR signaling.

Acknowledgements Supported by P01-CA85859, Pacific Northwest Prostate Cancer SPORE P50 CA 097186 and Veterans Affairs Research Program (SRP).

References

Samani AA, Yakar S, LeRoith D, Brodt P. The role of the IGF system in cancer growth and metastasis: overview and recent insights. Endocr Rev 2007;28(1):20–47.
Scher H, Sawyers C. Biology of progressive, castration-resistant prostate cancer: directed therapies targeting the androgen-receptor signaling axis. J Clin Oncol 2005;23(32):8235–61.
Taplin M, Balk S. Androgen receptor: a key molecule in the progression of prostate cancer to hormone independence. J Cell Biochem 2004;15:483–90.

Pandini G, Mineo R, Frasca F, Roberts CT, Jr., Marcelli M, Vigneri R, Belfiore A. Androgens up-regulate the insulin-like growth factor-I receptor in prostate cancer cells. Cancer Res 2005;65(5):1849–57.

Mohler J, Gregory C, Ford III O, Kim D, Weaver C, Petrusz P, Wilson E, French F. The Androgen Axis in Recurrent Prostate Cancer. Clinical Cancer Res 2004;10(2):440–8.

Gregory C, He B, Johnson R, Ford O, Mohler J, French F, Wilson E. A mechanism for androgen receptor-mediated prostate cancer recurrence after androgen deprivation therapy. Cancer Res 2001;61:4315–9.

Titus M, Schell M, Lih F, Tomer K, Mohler J. Testosterone and dihydrotestosterone tissue levels in recurrent prostate cancer. Clin Cancer Res 2005;11(13):4653–7.

Page ST, Lin DW, Mostaghel EA, Hess DL, True LD, Amory JK, Nelson PS, Matsumoto AM, Bremner WJ. Persistent intraprostatic androgen concentrations after medical castration in healthy men. J Clin Endocrinol Metab 2006;91(10):3850–6.

Mostaghel EA, Page ST, Lin DW, Fazli L, Coleman IM, True LD, Knudsen B, Hess DL, Nelson CC, Matsumoto AM, Bremner WJ, Gleave ME, Nelson PS. Intraprostatic androgens and androgen-regulated gene expression persist after testosterone suppression: therapeutic implications for castration-resistant prostate cancer. Cancer Res 2007;67(10):5033–41.

van Weerden WM, Bierings HG, van Steenbrugge GJ, de Jong FH, Schroder FH. Adrenal glands of mouse and rat do not synthesize androgens. Life Sci 1992;50(12):857–61.

Corey E, Quinn J, Buhler K, Nelson P, Macoska J, True L, Lange P, Vessella R. LuCaP 35: A New Model of Prostate Cancer Progression to Androgen Independence. Prostate 2003;55(4):239–46.

Thalmann G, Sikes R, Wu T, Degeorges A, Chang S, Ozen M, Pathak S, Chung L. LNCaP progression model of human prostate cancer: androgen-independence and osseous metastasis. The Prostate 2000;44:91–103.

Wu J, Haugk K, Woodke L, Nelson P, Coleman I, Plymate S. Interaction of IGF signaling and the androgen receptor in prostate cancer progression. J Cell Biochem 2006;99:392–401.

Fujimoto N, Yeh S, Kang H, Inui S, Chang H, Mizokami A, Chang C. Cloning and characterization of androgen receptor coactivator, ARA55, in human prostate. Journal of Biological Chemistry 1999;274:8316–21.

Kang J, Bell J, Beard R, Chandraratna R. Mannose 6-phosphate/insulin-like growth factor II receptor mediates the growth-inhibitory effects of retinoids. Cell Growth and Differentiation 1999;10:591–600.

Sadar M. Androgen-independent induction of prostate-specific antigen gene expression via crosstalk between the androgen receptor and protein kinase A signal transduction pathways. J Biol Chem 1999;274(12):7777–83.

Sadar M, Gleave M. Ligand-independent activation of the androgen receptor by the differentiation agent butyrate in human prostate cancer cells. Cancer Res 2000;60(20):5825–31.

Culig Z, Hobisch A, Cronauer M, Radmayr C, Trapman J, Hittmair A, Bartsch G, Klocker H. Androgen receptor activation in prostatic tumor cell lines by insulin-like growth factor-I, keratinocyte growth factor and epidermal growth factor. Eur Urol 1995;27(suppl 2):45–7.

Culig Z, Hobisch A, Cronauer M, Radmayr J, Hittmair A, Bartsch G, Klocker H. Androgen receptor activation in prostatic tumor cell lines by insulin-like growth factor-I, Keratinocyte growth factor, and epidermal growth factor. Cancer Research 1994;54(20):5474–8.

Lin H, Yeh S, Kang H, Chang C. Akt suppresses androgen-induced apoptosis by phosphorylating and inhibiting androgen receptor. PNAS 2001;98:7200–5.

Majeed N, Blouin M, Kaplan-Lefko P, Barry-Shaw J, Greenberg N, Gaudreau P, Bismar T, Pollak M. A germ line mutation that delays prostate cancer progression and prolongs survival in a murine prostate cancer model. Oncogene 2005;24:4736–40.

Hongo A, Yumet G, Resnicoff M, Romano G, O'Connor R, Baserga R. Inhibition of tumorigenesis and induction of apoptosis in human tumor cells by the stable transfection of a myristylated COOH terminus of the insulin-like growth factor 1 receptor. Cancer Research 1998;58:2477–84.

O'Connor R, Kauffmann-Zeh A, Liu Y, Lehar S, Evan G, Baserga R, Blatter W. Identification of domains of the insulin-like growth factor I receptor that are required for protection from apoptosis. mol and cell biol 1997;17:427–35.

Tennant MK, Thrasher JB, Twomey PA, Drivdahl RH, Birnbaum RS, Plymate SR. Protein and messenger ribonucleic acid (mRNA) for the type 1 insulin-like growth factor (IGF) receptor is decreased and IGF-II mRNA is increased in human prostate carcinoma compared to benign prostate epithelium. J Clin Endocrinol Metab 1996;81(10):3774–82.

Plymate SR, Bae VL, Maddison L, Quinn LS, Ware JL. Reexpression of the type 1 insulin-like growth factor receptor inhibits the malignant phenotype of simian virus 40 T antigen immortalized human prostate epithelial cells. Endocrinology 1997;138(4):1728–35.

Plymate SS, Bae VL, Maddison L, Quinn LS, Ware JL. Type-1 insulin-like growth factor receptor reexpression in the malignant phenotype of SV40-T-immortalized human prostate epithelial cells enhances apoptosis. Endocrine 1997;7(1):119–24.

Plymate S, Tennant M, Culp S, Woodke L, Marcelli M, Colman I, Nelson P, Carroll J, Roberts C, Ware J. Androgen receptor (AR) expression in AR-negative prostate cancer cells results in differential effects of DHT and IGF-I on proliferation and AR activity between localized and metastatic tumors. Prostate 2004;61(3):276–90.

Rubinstein M, Idelman G, Plymate SR, Narla G, Friedman SL, Werner H. Transcriptional activation of the insulin-like growth factor I receptor gene by the Kruppel-like factor 6 (KLF6) tumor suppressor protein: potential interactions between KLF6 and p53. Endocrinology 2004;145(8):3769–77.

Gioeli D, Ficarro S, Kwiek J, Aaronson D, Hancock M, Catling A, White F, Christian R, Settlage R, Shabanowitz J, Hunt D, Weber M. Androgen Receptor Phosphorlyation:Regulation and Identification of the phosphorylation sites. J Biol Chem 2002;277:29304–14.

Gioeli D, Black B, Gordon V, Spencer A, Kesler C, Eblen S, Paschal B, Weber M. Stress Kinase Signaling Regulates Androgen Receptor Phosphorylation, Transcription, and Localization. Mol Endocrinol 2006;20:505–15.

Plymate SR, Haugk K, Coleman I, Woodke L, Vessella R, Nelson P, Montgomery RB, Ludwig DL, Wu JD. An antibody targeting the type I insulin-like growth factor receptor enhances the castration-induced response in androgen-dependent prostate cancer. Clin Cancer Res 2007;13(21):6429–39.

Wu JD, Odman A, Higgins LM, Haugk K, Vessella R, Ludwig DL, Plymate SR. In vivo effects of the human type I insulin-like growth factor receptor antibody A12 on androgen-dependent and androgen-independent xenograft human prostate tumors. Clin Cancer Res 2005;11(8):3065–74.

Miyake H, Nelson C, Rennie P, Gleave M. Overexpression of Insulin-Like Growth Factor Binding Protein-5 Helps Accelerate Progression to Androgen-Independence in the Human Prostate LNCaP Tumor Modelthrough Activation of Phosphatidylinositol 3-Kinase Pathway. Endocrinology 2000;141:2257–65.

Miyake H, Pollak M, Gleave M. Castration-induced up-regulation of insulin-like growth fator binding protein-5 potentiates insulin-like growth factor I activity and accelerates progression to androgen independence in prostate cancer models. Cancer Research 2000;60:3058–64.

Sprenger CC, Haugk K, Sun S, Coleman I, Nelson PS, Vessella RL, Ludwig DL, Wu JD, Plymate SR. Transforming Growth Factor-{beta}-Stimulated Clone-22 Is an Androgen-Regulated Gene That Enhances Apoptosis in Prostate Cancer following Insulin-Like Growth Factor-I Receptor Inhibition. Clin Cancer Res 2009;15(24):7634–41.

Jones J, Clemmons D. Insulin-like growth factors and their binding proteins: biological actions. Endoc Rev 1995;16:3–34.

Kiyama S, Morrison K, Zellweger T, Akbari M, Cox M, Yu D, Miyake H, Gleave M. Castration-induced increases in insulin-like growth factor-binding protein 2 promotes proliferation of androgen-independent human prostate LNCaP tumors. Cancer Research 2003;63:3575–84.

Russo V, Schutt B, Andaloro E, Ymer S, Hoeflich A, Ranke M, LA B, Werther G. Insulin-like growth factor binding protein-2 binding to extracellular matrix plays a critical role in neuroblastoma cell proliferation, migration, and invasion. Endocrinology 2005;146:4445–55.

Zhang M, Latham DE, Delaney MA, Chakravarti A. Survivin mediates resistance to antiandrogen therapy in prostate cancer. Oncogene 2005;24(15):2474–82.

Kupfer S, Wilson E, French F. Androgen and glucocorticoid receptors interact with insulin degrading enzyme. J Biol Chem 1994;269:20622–8.

Udrisar D, Wanderley M, Porto R, Cardoso C, Barbosa M, Camberos M, Cresto J. Androgen- and estrogen-dependent regulation of insulin-degrading enzyme in subcellular fractions of rat prostate and uterus. Exp Biol Med 2005;230:479–86.

DiGiovanni J, Kiguchi K, Frijhoff A, Wilker E, Bol D, Beltran L, Moats S, Ramirez A, Jorcano J, Conti C. Deregulated expression of insulin-like growth factor 1 in prostate epithelium leads to neoplasia in transgenic mice. Proc Natl Acad Sci 2000;97:3455–60.

Wang L, Ma W, Markovich R, Lee W, Wang P. IGF-I modulates induction of apoptotic signaling in H9C2 Cardiac muscle cells. endo 1998;139:1354–60.

Chan J, Stampfer M, Giovannucci E, Gann P, Ma J, Wilkinson P, Hennekens C, Pollak M. Plasma Insulin-like Growth Factor-I and Prostate Cancer Risk: A Prospective Study. Science 1998;279:563–71.

Roddam AW, Allen NE, Appleby P, Key TJ, Ferrucci L, Carter HB, Metter EJ, Chen C, Weiss NS, Fitzpatrick A, Hsing AW, Lacey JV, Jr., Helzlsouer K, Rinaldi S, Riboli E, Kaaks R, Janssen JA, Wildhagen MF, Schroder FH, Platz EA, Pollak M, Giovannucci E, Schaefer C, Quesenberry CP, Jr., Vogelman JH, Severi G, English DR, Giles GG, Stattin P, Hallmans G, Johansson M, Chan JM, Gann P, Oliver SE, Holly JM, Donovan J, Meyer F, Bairati I, Galan P. Insulin-like growth factors, their binding proteins, and prostate cancer risk: analysis of individual patient data from 12 prospective studies. Ann Intern Med 2008;149(7):461–71, W83-8.

Rowlands MA, Gunnell D, Harris R, Vatten LJ, Holly JM, Martin RM. Circulating insulin-like growth factor peptides and prostate cancer risk: a systematic review and meta-analysis. Int J Cancer 2009;124(10):2416–29.

Tsuchiya N, Wang L, Horikawa Y, Inoue T, Kakinuma H, Matsuura S, Sato K, Ogawa O, Kato T, Habuchi T. CA repeat polymorphism in the insulin-like growth factor-I gene is associated with increased risk of prostate cancer and benign prostatic hyperplasia. Int J Oncol 2005;26(1):225–31.

Tsuchiya N, Wang L, Suzuki H, Segawa T, Fukuda H, Narita S, Shimbo M, Kamoto T, Mitsumori K, Ichikawa T, Ogawa O, Nakamura A, Habuchi T. Impact of IGF-I and CYP19 gene polymorphisms on the survival of patients with metastatic prostate cancer. J Clin Oncol 2006;24(13):1982–9.

Yu H, Nicar MR, Shi R, Berkel HJ, Nam R, Trachtenberg J, Diamandis EP. Levels of insulin-like growth factor I (IGF-I) and IGF binding proteins 2 and 3 in serial postoperative serum samples and risk of prostate cancer recurrence. Urology 2001,57(3):471–5.

Shariat SF, Lamb DJ, Kattan MW, Nguyen C, Kim J, Beck J, Wheeler TM, Slawin KM. Association of preoperative plasma levels of insulin-like growth factor I and insulin-like growth factor binding proteins-2 and -3 with prostate cancer invasion, progression, and metastasis. J Clin Oncol 2002;20(3):833–41.

Molife LR, Fong PC, Paccagnella L, Reid AH, Shaw HM, Vidal L, Arkenau HT, Karavasilis V, Yap TA, Olmos D, Spicer J, Postel-Vinay S, Yin D, Lipton A, Demers L, Leitzel K, Gualberto A, de Bono JS. The insulin-like growth factor-I receptor inhibitor figitumumab (CP-751,871) in combination with docetaxel in patients with advanced solid tumours: results of a phase Ib dose-escalation, open-label study. Br J Cancer 2010;103(3):332–9.

Sachdev D. Targeting the Type I Insulin-Like Growth Factor System for Breast Cancer Therapy. Curr Drug Targets 2010.

Sachdev D, Zhang X, Matise I, Gaillard-Kelly M, Yee D. The type I insulin-like growth factor receptor regulates cancer metastasis independently of primary tumor growth by promoting invasion and survival. Oncogene 2009;29(2):251–62.

Nickerson T, Chang F, Lorimer D, Smeekens SP, Sawyers CL, Pollak M. In vivo progression of LAPC-9 and LNCaP prostate cancer models to androgen independence is associated with increased expression of insulin-like growth factor I (IGF-I) and IGF-I receptor (IGF-IR). Cancer Res 2001;61(16):6276–80.

Burfeind P, Chernicky CL, Rininsland F, Ilan J. Antisense RNA to the type I insulin-like growth factor receptor suppresses tumor growth and prevents invasion by rat prostate cancer cells in vivo. Proc Natl Acad Sci USA 1996;93(14):7263–8.

Rochester MA, Riedemann J, Hellawell GO, Brewster SF, Macaulay VM. Silencing of the IGF1R gene enhances sensitivity to DNA-damaging agents in both PTEN wild-type and mutant human prostate cancer. Cancer Gene Ther 2005;12(1):90–100.

Montgomery RB, Mostaghel EA, Vessella R, Hess DL, Kalhorn TF, Higano CS, True LD, Nelson PS. Maintenance of intratumoral androgens in metastatic prostate cancer: a mechanism for castration-resistant tumor growth. Cancer Res 2008;68(11):4447–54.

Chott A, Sun Z, Morganstern D, Pan J, Li T, Susani M, Mosberger I, Upton MP, Bubley GJ, Balk SP. Tyrosine kinases expressed in vivo by human prostate cancer bone marrow metastases and loss of the type 1 insulin-like growth factor receptor. Am J Pathol 1999;155(4):1271–9.

Hellawell GO, Turner GD, Davies DR, Poulsom R, Brewster SF, Macaulay VM. Expression of the type 1 insulin-like growth factor receptor is up-regulated in primary prostate cancer and commonly persists in metastatic disease. Cancer Res 2002;62(10):2942–50.

Krueckl SL, Sikes RA, Edlund NM, Bell RH, Hurtado-Coll A, Fazli L, Gleave ME, Cox ME. Increased insulin-like growth factor I receptor expression and signaling are components of androgen-independent progression in a lineage-derived prostate cancer progression model. Cancer Res 2004;64(23):8620–9.

Ryan CJ, Haqq CM, Simko J, Nonaka DF, Chan JM, Weinberg V, Small EJ, Goldfine ID. Expression of insulin-like growth factor-1 receptor in local and metastatic prostate cancer. Urol Oncol 2007;25(2):134–40.

Schmitz M, Grignard G, Margue C, Dippel W, Capesius C, Mossong J, Nathan M, Giacchi S, Scheiden R, Kieffer N. Complete loss of PTEN expression as a possible early prognostic marker for prostate cancer metastasis. Int J Cancer 2007;120(6):1284–92.

Chi N, al e. A phase II study of preoperative figitumumab (F) in patients (pts) with localized prostate cancer (PCa). J Clin Oncol 2010;28(abstr 4662).

Dean JP, al e. Neoadjuvant IMC-A12 and combined androgen deprivation with prostatectomy for high-risk prostate cancer: J Clin Oncol 2010;28(15s, abstr TPS251).

Higano CS, al e. A phase II study of cixutumumab (IMC-A12), a monoclonal antibody (MAb) against the insulin-like growth factor 1 receptor (IGF-IR), monotherapy in metastatic castration-resistant prostate cancer (mCRPC): Feasibility of every 3-week dosing and updated results. . Proc ASCO GU Cancers Symposium, 2010 2010;abstr 189.

Chapter 6
IGF-1 Cellular Action and its Relationship to Cancer: Evidence from in Vitro and in Vivo Studies

Rosalyn D. Ferguson, Nyosha Alikhani, Archana Vijayakumar, Yvonne Fierz, Dara Cannata, and Shoshana Yakar

Introduction to the IGF System

Insulin-like growth factors (IGFs), which include insulin-like growth factor I (IGF-I) and insulin-like growth factor II (IGF-II) are mitogenic and anti-apoptotic growth factors that regulate cellular proliferation, differentiation and cell death. The mitogenic and anti-apoptotic properties of IGF-I and IGF-II affect both normal and cancerous cells. The effects of the IGFs on cell growth and apoptosis are mediated through binding to a tyrosine kinase receptor, the insulin-like growth factor-I receptor (IGF-IR). The IGF-IIR (the cation-independent mannose-6-phosphate receptor – M6P-R) is a single transmembrane glycoprotein that mediates the uptake and processing of M6P-containing cytokines, enzymes and peptide hormones and is involved in diverse functions related to lysosome biogenesis. IGF-II also binds the insulin receptor isoform-A (IR-A), with high affinity and can trigger mitogenic activity. IR and IGF-IR form hybrid heterodimeric receptors that bind insulin and IGFs. However, the role of the hybrid receptors in physiology and carcinogenesis is not fully understood and remains an area of active investigation.

In the circulation, the IGFs bind to IGF-binding proteins (IGFBPs), which regulate the interaction between the IGFs and IGF-IR. Greater than 95% of circulating IGF-I is complexed with IGFBP-3 and an acid labile subunit (Baxter 1988). IGFBP-3 regulates IGF-I bioavailability and independently affects cell proliferation and survival (Yu and Rohan 2000).

S. Yakar (✉)
Division of Endocrinology, Diabetes and Bone Diseases,
The Samuel Bronfman Department of Medicine, Mount Sinai School of Medicine,
New York, NY, USA
e-mail: shoshana.yakar@mssm.edu

D. LeRoith (ed.), *Insulin-like Growth Factors and Cancer: From Basic Biology to Therapeutics*, Cancer Drug Discovery and Development,
DOI 10.1007/978-1-4614-0598-6_6, © Springer Science+Business Media, LLC 2012

IGF levels are tightly regulated and an imbalance in their production or function is associated with various pathological conditions including type II diabetes/obesity, cachexia, chronic inflammatory conditions, and the reduced mental and physical capacity associated with aging. Because of the central role that the IGF axis plays in the regulation of cell survival, cell cycle progression, growth and differentiation, an imbalance in the expression of the IGF ligand and/or receptor can result in uncontrolled cell division and ultimately in malignant transformation. This review focuses on the role of IGF in cancer.

IGF-Mediated Cell Signaling

The biological activities of IGF-I are mediated via the IGF-I receptor, which belongs to the receptor tyrosine kinase (RTK) family of membrane receptors. The IGF-IR is a heterotetrameric protein that consists of two extracellular alpha (α) subunits linked via disulfide bonds to two transmembrane beta (β) subunits. Upon IGF-I binding to the extracellular pit on the α-subunits, the two intracellular β-subunits undergo auto trans-phosphorylation of tyrosine residues. The IGF-IR shares about 80% structural similarity with the insulin receptor resulting in over-lapping signal transduction pathways and in some instances, intracellular effects for the two factors. Following receptor activation, two canonical signaling cascades are activated: the phospho-inositide-3-kinase (PI3K) and the mitogen-activated protein kinase (MAPK) pathways. Ultimately, the spatio-temporal dynamics of activation of the PI3K and/or MAPK pathways govern their specific effects on cellular behavior.

Activation of the PI3K pathway occurs by the recruitment and tyrosine phosphorylation of adaptor molecules such as the insulin receptor substrates (IRSs), of which there are four isoforms. Depending on the cellular context, the IRS proteins associate with the p85 regulatory subunit of PI3K leading to the activation of its p110 catalytic subunit. Subsequently, there is an increase in the levels of the membrane-bound phospholipid phosphatidyl inositol-3,4,5-triphosphate (PIP_3) and the recruitment of phosphoinositide-dependent kinase 1 (PDK1) and Akt (or protein kinase B) to the membrane. PDK1 phosphorylates Akt at Thr[308], which primes the kinase for the activating phosphorylation by mammalian target of rapamycin (mTOR) complex 2 (mTORC2) at Ser[473]. Akt is a central mediator of the intracellular effects of the IGF-IR and is involved in metabolism, cell survival, cell migration, and proliferation via various mechanisms.

Three effectors are central to the downstream signaling events triggered by Akt: the mTOR complex 1 (mTORC1), forkhead transcription factors (FOXO), and glycogen synthase kinase 3 (GSK3) as shown in Fig. 6.1. mTORC1 is activated by Akt and plays an important role in cell growth and survival by promoting nutrient uptake, storage of energy, and protein translation. mTORC1 stimulates p70 S6 kinase (p70S6K) thereby mediating the release of the eukaryotic translation initiation factor 4E (eIF4E) from its transcriptional repressor eIF4E-BP1. There also exists a negative feedback loop between p70S6K and IRS implicating the mTOR

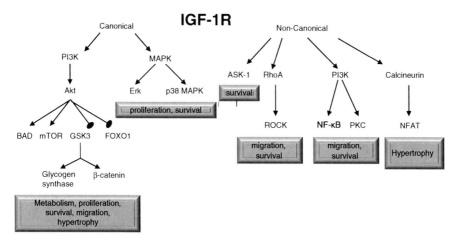

Fig. 6.1 Summary of the canonical and noncanonical signaling pathways activated downstream of the insulin-like growth factor 1 receptor (IGF-1R), demonstrating how the IGF signaling system is involved in mediating a complex range of cellular effects (the figure included in this review is original and created by Dr. Yakar)

pathway in insulin resistance. The mTOR pathway has also been associated with IGF-I-induced cell survival, proliferation, hypertrophy, and cell migration (Park et al. 2005; Leger et al. 2006; Finlay and Cantrell 2010). The FOXO family of transcription factors is a major target of Akt. They promote cell cycle arrest, apoptosis, oxidative stress, and the activation of gluconeogenic enzymes. Thus, their phosphorylation and cytoplasmic retention mediated by Akt has been implicated in IGF-I-induced cell proliferation, survival, and hypertrophy (Burgering and Medema 2003; Stitt et al. 2004; Leger et al. 2006; Elia et al. 2009). GSK3 is inhibited by Akt, resulting in the activation of glycogen synthase and an increase in the rate of glycogenesis. GSK3 also mediates other effects in the cell. It is involved in the Wnt signaling pathway where it phosphorylates β-catenin and primes it for degradation in the cytoplasm. Studies also suggest that GKS3 is involved in IGF-I-induced anti-apoptotic and hypertrophic effects (Vyas et al. 2002; Leger et al. 2006; Schakman et al. 2008). Apart from these pathways, Akt can also promote cell survival via the inactivating phosphorylation of the apoptotic protein Bad, and procaspase 9 (Tseng et al. 2002; Pang et al. 2007).

Activation of the MAPK pathway by IGF-I also occurs downstream of adaptor proteins such as the IRSs and Src homology collagen (SHC) which associate with GrbB2. This is followed by recruitment of the guanine nucleotide exchange factor son of sevenless (SOS) and the sequential activation of the small GTPase Ras, the MAPK kinase kinase (MAPKKK) Raf, the MAPK kinase (MAPKK) MEK and finally the MAPKs, such as extracellular-signal-regulated kinase (Erk1/2), Jun kinase (JNK), and p38 MAPK (Fig. 6.1) which exert mitogenic and inflammatory effects of IGF-1. This mechanism of the sequential activation of several kinases allows for signal amplification and feedback regulation. The MAPK pathway has been associated with the mitogenic effects of IGF-1, although it has also been implicated in cell migration and cell survival (Peruzzi et al. 1999; Zhang et al. 2005; Stoeltzing et al. 2007). The apoptosis signal regulating kinase-1 (ASK-1) is a MAPKKK that activates JNK and p38 MAPK in response to proinflammatory stimuli. Interestingly, it has been demonstrated that activated IGF-IR interacts with, tyrosine phosphorylates and represses ASK-1 thereby promoting cell survival (Galvan et al. 2003). In the 32D hematopoietic cell line, IGF-I treatment resulted in serine phosphorylation and mitochondrial translocation of Raf-1 and the E3 ubiquitin ligase Nedd4 which has previously shown to be a target for caspases (Harvey et al. 1998; Peruzzi et al. 1999, 2001).

While the canonical PI3K/Akt and MAPK pathways mediate a wide range of the intracellular effects initiated by the IGF-IR, several other pathways are also involved in IGF-I signaling (Fig. 6.1). IGF-I-induced migration of human monocytes/macrophages (THP-1 cells) via induction of the PI3K/protein kinase C (PKC)/p38 MAPK pathway has been implicated in the initiation of atherosclerosis (Furundzija et al. 2010). IGF-I inhibited rapamycin-induced apoptosis in human sarcoma cells in a PI3K/PKC-dependent manner (Thimmaiah et al. 2010). Apart from the PI3K/Akt pathway, the calcineurin/NFAT pathway has also been widely implicated in IGF-I-induced muscle hypertrophy. Calcineurin is a calcium-dependent serine/threonine phosphatase which is activated by IGF-I and subsequently dephosphorylates the transcription factor nuclear factor of activated T cells (NFAT) causing its nuclear translocation and the initiation of transcription of hypertrophic genes such as GATA binding protein-2 (GATA-2) (Musaro et al. 1999; Semsarian et al. 1999; Delling et al. 2000; Miyashita et al. 2001; Vyas et al. 2002). However, the role of this pathway in skeletal muscle hypertrophy has been questioned in light of recent studies that suggest that calcineurin may not be involved in IGF-I mediated muscle hypertrophy (Parsons et al. 2004; Quinn et al. 2007).

RhoA belongs to the family of Rho GTPases and has increasingly been implicated in IGF-I-induced cell migration. In human multiple myeloma cells, IGF-I activated RhoA and its downstream effector, Rho-associated kinase (ROCK) in a PI3K-dependent manner. Inhibition of PI3K or ROCK resulted in a decrease in IGF-I-induced migration of the cells through vascular endothelial and bone marrow stromal cell lines (Qiang et al. 2004). Moreover, the involvement of the RhoA/ROCK pathway has been identified in a study on IGF-I-induced cell migration in breast cancer cells where it was specifically shown that ROCK-induced activation of p38 MAPK was involved in IGF-I induced cell motility (Zhang et al. 2005).

Another noncanonical signaling pathway activated by IGF-I is the Wnt/β-catenin pathway, which is downstream of the PI3K/Akt/GSK3 signaling network. IGF-1-mediated stabilization of β-catenin resulted in enhanced cell proliferation of oligodendronal cells (Ye et al. 2010). Moreover, in colonic adenocarcinoma cells, IGF-I promoted the dissociation of cell adhesion complexes by tyrosine phosphorylation of E-cadherin and β-catenin, thereby promoting cell motility (Andre et al. 1999). IGF-I also induced chondrocyte differentiation in a β-catenin-dependent manner (Wang et al. 2010).

IGF-I increased adhesion of monocytes to human umbilical vein endothelial cells (HUVECs) by activation of NFκB-induced gene transcription of intracellular adhesion molecule-1 (ICAM-1) (Balaram et al. 1999). Long-term IGF-I treatment of HUVECs augmented TNF-α-mediated increases in the expression of adhesion molecules via the NFκB and c-Jun pathways. This is believed to be a result of the IGF-1-mediated down-regulation of the adaptor protein Gab 1 which represses the TNF-α proinflammatory pathway (Che et al. 2002). IGF-I also promotes neuronal cell survival by activation of the NFκB pathway downstream of PI3K (Heck et al. 1999).

IGF-I signals also modulate adhesion complexes and integrins in a manner that promotes cell migration. IGF-1 induced the recruitment of α5β3-integrin, the activation of the nonreceptor tyrosine kinase focal adhesion kinase (FAK), and the redistribution of the integrin adaptor protein paxillin to the focal adhesion sites in macrophages, thereby promoting their migration along endothelial cells (Furundzija et al. 2010). IGF-I stimulated the translocation of integrins to the leading edge of migrating human colonic adenocarcinoma cells (Andre et al. 1999); while in breast cancer cells it promoted the redistribution of FAK away from the focal adhesion contacts (Zhang et al. 2005). Moreover, in Schwann cells IGF-I facilitated motility by phosphorylation of FAK and re-organization of the actin cytoskeleton in a PI3K- and Rac1-dependent manner (Cheng et al. 2000).

The spatial localization of the IGF-IR may also influence its intracellular effects. Caveolin-1, a component of invaginations in the plasma membrane known as caveoli, was shown to be important for IGF-IR tyrosine phosphorylation and for the subsequent anti-apoptotic effects of IGF-IR via the PI3K pathway (Salani et al. 2008). Moreover, the localization of IGF-IR to lipid rafts was shown to play a role in the proapoptotic effects that it exerted on colon carcinoma cells (Remacle-Bonnet et al. 2005).

Downregulation of the IGF-1R signaling cascade occurs via inhibitory serine phosphorylation of the receptors as well as of their adaptor proteins, IRS and SHC. The inhibitory serine phosphorylation of IRS-1 is catalyzed by GSK3, PI3K, MAPK, and JNK. Another mechanism of receptor regulation is dephosphorylation by protein tyrosine phosphatase-1B (PTP-1B). Moreover, other tyrosine phosphatases such as phosphatase and tensin homolog (PTEN), SH2 domain-containing protein-tyrosine phosphatase PTPN11 (Shp2) have been implicated in inactivating PI3K and downstream effectors (Dominici et al. 2005; LeRoith 2007).

The Role of IGF-1R in Cell Cycle Progression and Its Regulation by Tumor Suppressor Genes

Tumor suppressor genes are involved in cell cycle control and often regulate checkpoints involving cyclins and cyclin-dependent kinases (CDKs). CDKs are constitutively expressed in the cell while cyclins are synthesized at specific stages of the cell cycle in response to various stimuli. A few tumor suppressor genes have been shown to regulate the IGF-1R gene expression via *cis*-acting and *trans*-acting elements in the promoter region. Activation of the IGF-1R can facilitate G0–G1 transition through activation of p70 S6K and subsequent phosphorylation of the S6 ribosomal protein resulting in increased ribosomal pool, which is necessary for entry into the cycle (Dupont et al. 2003). However, the major effect of IGF-1R is exerted at the G1-S transition, via activation of the PI-3K/Akt and/or the ERK pathways, leading to increased expression of cyclin D1 and CDK4 (Lavoie et al. 1996; Hamelers et al. 2002). The latter results in phosphorylation of retinoblastoma (Rb) protein, release of the transcription factor E2F, and the synthesis of cyclin E (Rosenthal and Cheng 1995; Dupont et al. 2000). The IGF-IR may also exert a regulatory role at the G2-M transition, possibly by increasing cyclins A and B and cdc2 synthesis (Furlanetto et al. 1994). Together, IGF-1R can mediate cell cycle progression via many mechanisms and therefore its expression must be tightly regulated.

p53 is a tumor suppressor gene product encoded by the *tp53* (tumor protein 53) gene (Vousden 2000). It is found in the nucleus and functions as a transcription factor of genes that are involved in cell cycle regulation. Mutations of the p53 gene are the most frequent events in human neoplasia and cancer. One of the target genes of p53 is the IGF-1R. Co-expression of wild type p53 and IGF-1R in osteosarcoma (Saos-2) as well as rhabdomyosarcoma-derived cells led to a suppression of IGF-1R gene expression in a dose-dependent manner. In contrast, mutant forms of p53 (at codons 143, 248, and 273) led to an increased IGF-1R promoter activity as well as an elevation of IGF-1R mRNA levels (Werner et al. 1996). The inhibitory effect of p53 on IGF-1R expression is mediated by its interaction with Sp1, a zinc finger transcription factor (Ohlsson et al. 1998). Using the same cellular system, the tumor suppressor gene *BRCA1* repressed IGF-1R promoter activity in a dose-dependent manner (Maor et al. 2000), while a mutated form of BRCA1 (185delAG) did not reduce IGF-1R promoter activity (Abramovitch et al. 2003). Similar to p53, the mechanism involved in the repression of the IGF-1R by BRCA1 has been shown to involve specific binding to Sp1. Physical association of BRCA1 with Sp1 prevents Sp1 binding to the IGF-1R promoter (Abramovitch et al. 2003). The clinical relevance of these findings was confirmed by a recent study investigating BRCA1-mutated primary breast tumors. In these tumors, IGF-1R levels were significantly elevated as detected by immunohistochemical staining (Maor et al. 2007). IGF-1R promoter activity is also regulated by the tumor suppressor Wilms tumor protein 1 (WT1). Mutations in WT1 have been implicated in the formation of Wilms tumor, a pediatric kidney tumor (Call et al. 1990; Gessler et al. 1990), where IGF-1R mRNA levels are increased around sixfold when compared to normal kidney tissue (Werner et al. 1993). As previously shown for p53 and BRCA1, WT1 is also a negative regulator of IGF-1R (Werner et al. 1993). The binding of WT1 to the IGF-1R promoter includes binding of the zinc finger domain of WT1 to consensus sites on both sides of the initiator element of the IGF-1R promoter (Werner et al. 1994). Chromosomal translocation t(11;22)(p13;q12) (occurring in desmoplastic small round cell tumors) leading to the pathological fusion of the Ewing gene (*EWS*) to *WT1* (Gerald et al. 1995) led to a threefold increase in IGF-1R promoter activity (Karnieli et al. 1996). Interestingly, WT1 has also been shown to be a target for

IGF-1. In Saos-2 cells, IGF-1 reduced WT1 promoter activity as well as protein expression, and the effect seemed to be mediated through the MAPK pathway (Bentov et al. 2003). Lastly, characterization of the highly chemoresistant clear cell renal cell cancer (CC-RCC), in which the von Hippel-Lindau (VHL) tumor suppressor gene is inactivated, revealed that the IGF-1R gene was upregulated and likely implicated in activation of cell survival mechanisms. Similar to the previously described tumor suppressor genes, the VHL protein binds Sp1 sites on the IGF-1R promoter and downregulates its expression as well as reducing the stability of IGF-1R mRNA via sequestration of HuR protein (Yuen et al. 2007).

The phosphatase and tensin homolog (PTEN) is a tumor suppressor gene product that is frequently mutated in human malignancies (Di Cristofano and Pandolfi 2000). PTEN acts as a phosphatase and dephosphorylates PIP3 resulting in inactivation of PI3K, which further leads to inactivation of Akt (Cantley and Neel 1999). In human pancreatic cancer cells (PANC1 and AsPC1 cells) transfected with constitutively active Akt, expression of the IGF-1R gene was increased. PTEN on the other hand reduced IGF-1R expression through its inhibitory effect on Akt (Tanno et al. 2001). Stable overexpression of PTEN in PC3 prostate cancer cells resulted in a decrease of IGF-1R protein levels and cell surface IGF-1R expression by 44–60% and 49–64%, respectively. Furthermore, IGF-1R synthesis was inhibited at the level of precursor translation, whereas IGF-1R mRNA levels were unchanged by PTEN overexpression. Thus, these findings suggest that PTEN regulates IGF-1R expression at the posttranscriptional level. However, unlike in the aforementioned study in pancreatic cancer cells, Akt activity was not associated with IGF-1R expression, suggesting a direct effect of PTEN on IGF-1R translation (Zhao et al. 2004). Furthermore, a recent study showed that PTEN loss is linked with increased phosphorylation of the IGF-1R in primary human breast cancer; however, the mechanism(s) by which PTEN regulates IGF-1R phosphorylation in human breast tumors remains unclear (Miller et al. 2009).

Taken together, various tumor suppressor gene products can repress the IGF-IR either at the transcriptional or the posttranscriptional level, thus inhibiting the effects of IGF-1 on tumor growth and progression. Loss of function of these suppressor genes therefore results in increased IGF-1R levels leading to mitogenic activation by locally produced or circulating IGFs.

The Role of IGF in ER Stress Induced Apoptosis

The endoplasmic reticulum (ER) possesses an important role in normal cellular function as well as in cell survival. In the ER, nascent proteins are folded and modified with the help of molecular chaperones and folding enzymes to achieve their right conformation. The correctly folded proteins are thereafter transported via the Golgi apparatus to reach their final destination. Misfolded and incompletely folded proteins, however, are retained in ER to complete the folding process or to be transported from the organelle to the cytosol for degradation by the proteasome. The ER also has a crucial role in the maintenance of cellular calcium homeostasis as well as lipid membrane and cholesterol biosynthesis. To overcome the ER stress the organelles have a specific set of signaling pathways leading to translational repression, increased folding capacity, and enhanced degradation of the misfolded proteins (van der Kallen et al. 2009). The following responses are mediated by elements of ER stress signaling network: activation of activating transcription factor-6 (ATF6), inositol-requiring ER-to-nucleus signal kinase-1 α (IRE1 α), and PRK (RNA-dependent protein kinase)-like ER kinase (PERK). ATF6 is an ER localized transmembrane protein, which during ER stress undergoes a complex cleavage in the ER and Golgi and is translocated to the nucleus. The processed ATF6 interacts thereafter with the promoter of genes implicated in restoration of ER homeostasis. Activation of IRE1 α, also an ER-resident transmembrane protein, leads to processing of mRNA that encodes X-box-binding protein-1 (XBP-1), a transcription factor resulting in upregulation of XBP-1 protein. XBP-1 protein has an important role in the recovery from ER stress. The ER stress also promotes the activation of PERK, a protein kinase located in ER. The activated PERK is responsible for phosphorylation and thereby inactivation of eukaryotic translation initiation factor-2 α (elF2 α), causing the inhibition of ER protein synthesis followed by translation of transcription factor-4 (ATF4) (Schroder and Kaufman 2005). These signaling pathways can induce the transcription of growth arrest and DNA damage-inducible gene 153/C/EBP homologue protein (GADD153/CHOP), which is known to be a powerful transcription factor with a crucial role in the ER stress response (Oyadomari and Mori 2004).

If the ER dysfunction is prolonged, these recovery mechanisms may fail, leading to apoptosis, which is the major form of programmed cell death. Apoptosis induced by ER stress is implicated in the pathogenesis of a range of disorders, including obesity and diabetes (Harding and Ron 2002; Hotamisligil 2006). Thus, induction of apoptosis by ER stress can be used as an approach against tumor growth and metastasis (Ma and Hendershot 2004).

IGF-I plays an important role in protecting cells from deadly consequences mediated through ER stress. In human MCF-7 breast cancer cells, IGF-I has the capacity to protect cells from severe consequences of ER stress by enhancing the ATF6, IRE1α, and PERK-mediated signaling system. The addition of IGF-I to ER stress induced cells leads to accumulation of cleaved ATF6 in the nucleus, which thereby regulates the genes involved in restoring the function of ER. During induced ER stress, IGF-I has been shown to potentiate IRE1α activation, which in turn stimulates splicing of XBP-1 mRNA and therefore nuclear accumulation of active XBP-1. Lastly, addition of IGF-I to ER stress-induced cells leads to increased phosphorylated PERK resulting in reduced protein synthesis (Novosyadlyy et al. 2008).

The overexpression of molecular chaperones in the ER is associated with an ER stress recovery program since these chaperones are facilitating protein folding and protecting the unfolded segments of the protein from the surrounding environment (Schroder and Kaufman 2005). Grp78/Bip is one of the major chaperones, which under normal conditions, blocks the luminal domains of IRE1α, ATF6, and PERK and thereby inhibits their activation. Induction of ER stress releases the Grp78/BiP into the ER lumen leading to the activation of the IRE1α,

ATF6, and PERK signaling pathways. Also, ER stress has been shown to increase the level of Grp78/BiP. IGF-I has a significant role in enhancing mRNA and protein level of Grp78/BiP (Novosyadlyy et al. 2008).

The intracellular signal transduction mediating the protective effect of IGF-I in ER stress induced cell death needs to be further elucidated. In mouse insulinoma cells, it has been shown that the PI3/Akt/glycagon synthase-3β pathway is partially involved in mediating the protective effect of IGF-I (Srinivasan et al. 2005). A recent investigation has revealed that IGF-I effectively guards neuronal cells against ER stress induced apoptosis through (PI3K)/Akt and p38 MAPK pathway (Zou et al. 2009). However, in MCF-7 breast cancer cells the antiapoptotic role of IGF-I against ER stress induced cell death may be mediated by a novel and unidentified signaling pathway, since the well-known signal transduction pathways used by IGF-IR, MAPK, and PI3K, were shown not to be involved in the IGF-1-mediated protection against ER stress induced apoptosis in these cells (Novosyadlyy et al. 2008).

The Role of IGF in Cell Detachment and Motility

Increased cell motility can lead to increased cell migration and enhanced cancer progression through the formation of metastases. Reduced cell–cell and cell–ECM adhesion facilitates the detachment of tumor cells from their primary site. Increased motility and decreased adhesion are thus important mechanisms which are involved in cancer progression. To find strategies to limit these processes in IGF-1R/IGF-mediated cancer development it is important to decipher the mechanisms involved in motility and adhesion so that they can be targeted with appropriate therapies.

The molecular mechanisms driving cell motility are common to both non-neoplastic and cancer cells. Briefly, cell motility consists of a four-step process consisting of (1) cell polarization characterized by the emergence of a distinct "leading" and "trailing" edge of the cell and the initiation of pseudopodia at the former, (2) adhesions of pseudopodia to the substrate, (3) translocation of the cell body, and (4) retraction of the trailing edge (reviewed in Mitchison and Cramer 1996; Yamazaki et al. 2005). It is important to note that the majority of studies investigating the implication of IGF-1 or IGF-1R in cellular motility were performed in vitro. In many cases, those assays were performed on plastic and not ECM therefore, conclusions must be drawn carefully.

The Rho family binding proteins are members of the Ras superfamily and exist as GDP-bound inactive and GTP-bound active forms, which are interconvertible by GDP/GTP exchange and GTPase reactions (reviewed in Nobes and Hall 1994). Their involvement in signal transduction from the extracellular environment, cell polarization, and cytoskeletal reorganization makes Rho GTPases important molecular switches for the initiation and maintenance of motility (Raftopoulou and Hall 2004). In particular, Rac and cdc42 are important regulators of actin assembly and during cell migration direct the formation of lamellipodia and filopodia, respectively (Etienne-Manneville and Hall 2002), mediated by downstream interactions with the Wiskott–Aldrich syndrome protein (WASP) family and the Arp2/3 complex (Takenawa and Miki 2001; Miki and Takenawa 2003). Activated RhoA, RhoB, and RhoC interact with a number of downstream effectors, the most important being Rho-associated coiled-coil protein kinase, or Rho kinase (ROCK). Activation of ROCK by the IGF-1R leads to phosphorylation of myosin light chain (MLC) and MLC phosphatase. These phosphorylated molecules in turn lead to myosin filament assembly and F-actin bundling, resulting in stress fiber formation (reviewed in Kjoller and Hall 1999; Sah et al. 2000). Rho GTPases are themselves regulated by upstream signaling molecules, one important being PI-3 kinase which plays a critical role in establishing cell polarity by responding to chemoattractants with the release of PIP3 which stimulates Rac and cdc42 one functions (Wang et al. 2002; Weiner et al. 2002).

IGF-1 has been demonstrated to be a potent inducer of motility in several different types of human cancer cells. Melanoma cell line A2058, which endogenously expresses IGF-1R moved chemotactically toward IGF-1, IGF-II, and insulin in motility assays, and this migratory effect could be blocked by incubating A2058 cells with a monoclonal IGF-1-receptor-blocking antibody (αIR-3) (Stracke et al. 1989). Similarly, pancreatic cell line FG demonstrated increased movement toward IGF-1 in migration assays (Klemke et al. 1994). Two breast cancer cell lines MCF7 and MDA-MB-231 which express IGF-1R, showed enhanced motility toward IGF-1 in migration assays, an effect which could be directly inhibited by αIR-3 (Doerr and Jones 1996). Neuroblastoma cell line SH-SY5Y demonstrated increased motility following IGF-1 stimulation in a phagokinetic track assay (Meyer et al. 2001), while a similar neuroblastoma cell line IMR32 migrated toward IGF-1 expressing human bone stromal cells in a transendothelial migration assay (van Golen et al. 2006). In wound assays, seven different IGF-R1-expressing pancreatic cancer cell lines demonstrated efficient migration toward IGF-1, which could be abrogated by picropodophyllin (PPP), a specific inhibitor of the IGF-1R (Tomizawa et al. 2010). IGF-1-induced motility in two head and neck cancer cell lines 183A and TU159, which also could be blocked by the anti-IGF-1R therapeutic antibody A12 (Barnes et al. 2007). Urothelial carcinoma-derived cell lines 5637 and T24 in a wound healing assay undergo migration toward IGF-1 (Metalli et al. 2010). In accordance with this evidence, cells in which IGF-1R activity is diminished showed concomitant decreases in IGF-1-induced cell motility. A dominant negative mutant of the IGF-1R stably expressed in a metastatic variant (LCC6) of the human breast cancer cell line MDA-MB-435 inhibited its typically enhanced migratory response to IGF-1 (Sachdev et al. 2004).

Cell polarization and cytoskeletal rearrangement with formation of adherent pseudopods at the leading edge are the distinguishing properties of a cell undergoing motility. Evidence for involvement of IGF-1 in these events has been described in a study on non-neoplastic cultured rat glomerular mesangial cells. Treatment of quiescent cell cultures with IGF-1 resulted in rearrangement of the cytoskeletal proteins actin, vimentin, and vinculin, formation of a "leading edge" undergoing actin polymerization, and expression of a wound healing phenotype characterized by increased motility, suggesting that IGF-1 can initiate motility-associated cytoskeletal alterations in these cells (Berfield et al. 1997). IGF-1 stimulation of 3T3 cells overexpressing IGF-1R resulted in an elongated cell body with long filopodial extensions and fine microspikes along the cell edges, effects not observed in control 3T3 cells (Sachdev et al. 2001). Immunofluorescence microscopy of head and neck cancer cell lines expressing high levels of IGF-1R demonstrated minimal amounts of thick actin stress fibers typical of nonmotile, growth-inhibited cells, suggesting that cells were motile. Following cell treatment with A12, IGF-1R expression was reduced and stress fibers typical of nonmotile cells began to assemble (Barnes et al. 2007).

Because adhesion complexes continually form and then disassemble as a motile cell undergoes translocation, integrins, which are involved in mediating these complexes, are critical in regulating cell motility. Changes in integrin expression during cancer may facilitate greater motility across a given ECM substrate, thus enhancing tumorogenesis. In breast cancer cell line MDA231-BO, IGF-1-mediated motility was shown to be dependent on expression of $\alpha5\beta1$ integrin (Zhang and Yee 2002), and in MCF-7 breast cancer cell line it was shown that altered integrin expression affected motility response to IGF-1 (Zhang et al. 2004b). Also in MCF-7 cells, an association of IGF-1, $\beta1$ integrin, and the scaffolding protein RACK1 was shown to mediate efficient cell migration (Kiely et al. 2006). In a prostate carcinoma cell line, expression of $\alpha5\beta1$ integrin was critical for the IGF-1-induced motility of cells in culture (Marelli et al. 2006) and in epithelial colonic adenocarcinoma cell line HT29-D4, five out of six of the cell surface-expressed integrins were required for efficient migration mediated by IGF-1 (Andre et al. 1999).

As noted above, several signaling cascades co-operate to induce the complex cytoskeletal reorganizations required for cell motility. There is accumulating evidence that in cancer, these signaling pathways may be altered to enhance cell motility. As an important multifunctional receptor tyrosine kinase, IGF-1R is linked to many different signaling networks, some of which, as described below, may also include pathways mediating cell motility.

In smooth muscle cells, IGF-1R has been shown to tyrosine phosphorylate the adaptor protein p130[cas] which is necessary for Rac1 activation and formation of lamellopodia at the leading edge of the cell (Ceacareanu et al. 2006) while in human trophoblast cells, IGF-1R-mediated migration depends on both RhoA and RhoC activation (Shields et al. 2007). The prostate cancer cell line PC3 expresses high levels of IGF-1R, as well as RhoC, a Rho family member implicated in the progression of several aggressive and invasive types of cancers such as breast, ovary, and pancreatic carcinomas (Suwa et al. 1998; Kleer et al. 2002; van Golen et al. 2002; Horiuchi et al. 2003). Unlike RhoA, RhoC inhibited cytoskeletal changes associated with motility but rather appeared to enhance progression to the invasive phenotype, suggesting that RhoC may be one of the factors responsible for driving highly invasive and metastatic cancer development (Yao et al. 2006). Furthermore, in IGF-1R-transformed 3T3 fibroblast cells, Rho A activation has been suggested to contribute to increased cell colony formation by means of down-regulating contact inhibition during cell motility (Sachdev et al. 2001). Following IGF-1 treatment of MDCKII epithelial cells, IGF-1R formed a complex with LARG (leukemia-associated RhoGEF) which induced the activation of Rho and its effector, ROCK, thereby enhancing formation of actin stress fibers and regulating cytoskeletal arrangements (Taya et al. 2001).

Pancreatic cancer cell lines KP-4 and PANC-1 treated with the PI-3 kinase inhibitor LY294002 showed reduced motility in wound assays, suggesting involvement of this signaling protein in cell motility (Tomizawa et al. 2010). The highly motile, IGF-1R-expressing head and neck cancer cell line 183A was analyzed for upregulated signaling pathways downstream of IGF-IR activation. IGF-1 treatment of 183A cells resulted in ERK1/2 phosphorylation, demonstrating a possible role for this signaling pathway in motility. Differently, Akt phosphorylation was found to be constitutively active in these cells, suggesting a loss of PTEN function and an upregulation/amplification of PI-3 kinase in this cell line which contributes to the observed increase in motility (Barnes et al. 2007). An investigation into IGF-1R involvement in lamellopodia formation in neuroblastoma cell line SH-SY5Y demonstrated that the membrane bound Ca^{2+}-dependent protein myristoylated alanine-rich C kinase substrate (MARCKS) and β-actin were recruited in lipid rafts to the site of lamellopodia formation following IGF-1 stimulation. Furthermore, translocation of lipid rafts and subsequent lamellopodia formation was abolished by the PI-3 kinase inhibitor LY294002 (Yamaguchi et al. 2009). Motility of urothelial carcinoma cells also involves an IGF-1 induced activation of the adaptor protein paxillin. Paxillin associates directly with FAK at the leading edge of the cell, thus suggesting a role for IGF-1 in orchestrating an active "leading edge" during the initiation of motility. Signaling between IGF-1R and paxillin was shown to depend upon ERK1/2 activation although Akt activation was also shown to be involved (Metalli et al. 2010). Interestingly, it has also been demonstrated that paxillin activation leads to upregulation of Rac1, an essential small GTPase for filipodia formation (Nishiya et al. 2005).

Signaling via IGF-1R is implicated in many different cancers and is also relevant to the formation of tumor metastases. An array of different cancer cell types respond with increased motility to IGF-1, signifying that IGF-1R signals to proteins involved in cytoskeletal rearrangement. Here, it has been highlighted that IGF-1R signaling in cancer cells can affect motility by orchestrating changes in actin and myosin assembly through activation of IRS1/2, Akt/MAPK, and Rho GTPase family signaling proteins, as well as through modulation of integrin expression. Several studies have implicated IGF-I induced motility in liver metastasis of different tumor types including human sarcoma (Nanni et al. 2010) and uveal melanoma cells (Girnita et al. 2006) and in the intra and extra-hepatic spread of hepatocarcinoma cells (Nussbaum et al. 2008; Chen et al. 2009).

The Role of IGF in Cell Adhesion

Adhesion between cells and between cells and their extracellular matrix (ECM) is critical for the integrity of all body tissues. Even during wound repair and angiogenesis, migrating cells maintain a certain level of adhesion between each other and

6 IGF-1 Cellular Action and its Relationship to Cancer... 117

move collectively in sheet-like structures (Friedl et al. 2004). During certain stages of cancer, however, reductions in either cell–cell or cell–ECM adhesions may result in separation of individual cells from each other and from the matrix, allowing them to migrate as single cells. This transition from individual to collective migration is termed epithelial to mesenchymal transition (EMT) and is a characteristic indicator of tumor progression (Friedl 2004).

Points where cells contact each other are known as adherence junctions. The core of these junctions consists of E-cadherin, a transmembrane cell–cell adhesion molecule belonging to a large superfamily of Ca^{2+}-dependent homophilic adhesion receptors that play vital roles in cell recognition and sorting during development (reviewed in Takeichi 1991; Gumbiner 2000) and cytoplasmic α-, β-, and γ-catenins which, by means of actin-binding proteins such as α-actinin and vinculin, are coupled directly to microfilaments of the cytoskeleton (Knudsen et al. 1995; Vasioukhin et al. 2000). These cadherin–catenin links with cytoskeletal proteins are critical for the stabilization of intercellular adhesion and the maintenance of epithelial tissue structure and function (Tsukatani et al. 1997). Other important molecules involved in cell–cell adhesion are the Ca^{2+}-dependent selectins, and the Ca^{2+}-independent Ig-superfamily cell adhesion molecules while cell–ECM adhesions are regulated by the integrins (reviewed in Humphries 2000).

Evidence for how the IGF-1R/IGF complex influences cell–cell adhesion has come from studies on NBT-II rat bladder cells which typically possess an epithelial-like polarized cell morphology with extensive cell–cell contacts and demonstrate tight attachment to one another. Upon IGF-1 treatment, cell–cell contacts became weakened and cells became flattened and spread-out, taking on a loosely attached, nonpolarized mesenchymal phenotype (Toyoshima et al. 1971). Various molecular events are now known to be associated with the loss of adhesion mediated by IGF signaling, including the intracellular sequestration and degradation of E-cadherin and desmoplakin, a protein associated with intracellular junctions. IGF-1 also causes β-catenin to dissociate from E-cadherin and become redistributed to the nucleus (Morali et al. 2001). ARCaP prostate cancer cells can be induced to undergo EMT by IGF-1 stimulation and by doing so demonstrate a higher potential than control cells to initiate bone metastasis in vivo (Zhau et al. 2008). ZEB (Zinc finger E-box-binding homeobox) 1 is a zinc finger homeodomain transcriptional repressor that regulates developmental processes such as skeletal patterning and muscle and lymphoid differentiation (reviewed in Peinado et al. 2007) and also represses E-cadherin through interaction with an E-box in its promoter region leading to chromatin condensation and gene silencing (Grooteclaes and Frisch 2000; Chinnadurai 2002; Ohira et al. 2003). Through its silencing of E-cadherin, ZEB1 has been shown to be an important candidate for promoting EMT of prostate cancer cells. IGF-I stimulation of these cells resulted in increased expression of ZEB1 in the epithelial state, suggesting a role of IGF-1R signaling in EMT during cancer progression (Graham et al. 2008). Further evidence for a loss of cell–cell adhesion mediated by IGF-1 is shown in mammary epithelial cells overexpressing a constitutively active IGF-1R. Prolonged signaling via this receptor caused cells to undergo EMT with an induction of the E-cadherin transcriptional repressor Snail and an associated reduction in E-cadherin protein expression (Cano et al. 2000; Kim et al. 2007). Weakening of cell–ECM adhesion in breast cancer cells treated with IGF-1 has also been reported, principally due to a reduction in cell–ECM interactions mediated by α5β1 integrin (Lynch et al. 2005).

Loss of adhesion of tumor cells promotes their mobility and possible release into lymphatic or hematopoetic circulations. IGF-1R signaling has been shown to mediate the transition of epithelial cells to dedifferentiated mesenchymal cells, which promotes this increased motility. Since metastases at distant sites are the major cause of death from most cancers, finding ways of reducing the potential of tumor cells to migrate from one tissue to another is one of the greatest challenges we face in cancer research at present.

The Role of IGF in Tissue Remodeling

Both the ability of tumor cells to disseminate from their primary site and their ability to invade the surrounding tissue or vessel, depends on ECM remodeling. The remodeling process is mediated by proteolytic enzymes, which are secreted by the tumor cells or by activated resident cells within the tissue.

The most studied proteinases associated with liver metastasis are the metalloproteinases (MMPs). Cleavage of ECM components by MMPs can also generate fragments with new functions, for example, cleavage of laminin-5 and collagen type IV results in exposure of sites that promote cell migration (Giannelli et al. 1997; Xu et al. 2001). Similarly, cleavage of insulin-like growth-factor-binding protein (IGF-BP) and perlecan releases IGFs and fibroblast growth factors (FGFs), respectively (Whitelock et al. 1996; Manes et al. 1997; 1999). Recent studies have implicated the matrilysin MMP-7, an enzyme frequently upregulated during malignant progression (Hemers et al. 2005), in proteolytic processing of all six IGFBPs, identifying it as an indirect activator of the IGF-IR via increased IGF bioavailability (Nakamura et al. 2005). Accordingly, MMP-7 and IGF-1R gene expression levels were higher in cancer tissue than in adjacent normal mucosa in 205 colorectal specimens (Oshima et al. 2008), and the expression of the IGF-1R correlated with venous invasion and liver metastasis. MMPs can promote apoptotic or anti-apoptotic actions. MMP-7 releases membrane-bound FASL, a transmembrane stimulator of the death receptor FAS (Powell et al. 1999; Mitsiades et al. 2001). Released FASL induces apoptosis of neighboring cells (Powell et al. 1999), or decreases cancer-cell apoptosis (Mitsiades et al. 2001), depending on the experimental system. Likewise, MMP-11 was shown to inhibit apoptosis of cancer cells likely via the release of IGFs (Manes et al. 1997).

In vitro and in vivo studies have demonstrated that IGF-1R regulates the expression of MMP-2. In the Lewis lung carcinoma model of liver metastasis, down or up-modulation of IGF-IR expression was shown to alter MMP-2 expression levels, invasion, and metastasis (Zhang et al. 2004a). Moreover, IGF-1R regulates MMP-14, which is a major proteolytic activator of pro-MMP-2, via PI-3K/Akt/mTOR signaling. In human breast carcinoma cell line MCF-7, IGF-I increased cell surface-associated MMP-9 activity and MMP-9-mediated migration (Mira et al. 1999) and in human nonsmall cell lung carcinoma U-1810 cells, both IGF-I and IGF-II enhanced the expression of MMP-2 and MMP-9, leading to increased cell migration (Bredin et al. 2003). However, there is evidence that IGF-1R overexpression in murine Lewis lung carcinoma cells can reduce MMP-9 levels, which is attributable to decreased PKC-α levels in these cells (Li et al. 2009). In support of this study, it was recently shown that MMP-9-induced ERK signaling in normal Schwann cells was completely ablated by inhibition of the IGF-IR (Chattopadhyay and Shubayev 2009).

The protease system of urokinase plasminogen activator receptor (uPAR)/uPA also plays a major role in ECM proteolysis and tumor invasion, and IGF-IR has been shown to regulate uPA expression or activity in a few tumor cell types. In MDA-MB-231 breast cancer cells, IGF-I induced uPA expression via PI-3K and MAPK-signaling (Dunn et al. 2000, 2001). A reduction in uPA expression and tumorigenesis was also noted in EMT6 murine mammary carcinoma cells expressing antisense IGF-IR (Chernicky et al. 2002). In L3.6pl human pancreatic carcinoma cells, IGF-IR was shown to control cell migration and invasion via regulation of uPA and uPAR expression (Bauer et al. 2005). In addition to direct transcriptional regulation of uPA via MAPK and PI3-K signaling (Dunn et al. 2001), IGF-I and II can also increase the binding of single-chain uPA (scuPA) to cell-surface uPAR, possibly through posttranscriptional modification of uPAR and thereby triggering uPA activation, as was recently shown in a rhabdomyosarcoma cell line (Gallicchio et al. 2003). Other proteases such as the cysteine protease cathepsin L (Navab et al. 2008), or the serine protease Matriptase-2 (TMPRSS6) (Tsai et al. 2006) were implicated in cellular response to IGF and indirectly affect hepatic metastases.

The Role of IGF in Angiogenesis

Angiogenesis is a tightly regulated, multistep process of new blood vessel formation from preexisting vasculature. In the last three decades, the molecular basis for angiogenesis has been resolved and a number of growth factor receptor pathways that activate this process have been identified. Among these receptors are the vascular endothelial growth factor (VEGF) receptors-1 and 2, and neuropilin (NRP) receptors-1 and 2. The VEGFR pathway has been identified as a therapeutic target and to date there are a few humanized anti-VEGFR antibodies as well as small molecule inhibitors in clinical use. VEGFRs and the IGF-1R do not interact directly; however, a few studies have demonstrated some synergy between these two pathways. In thyroid carcinoma cell line SW579, IGF-1 upregulated VEGF mRNA expression and protein secretion, and over-expression of Akt in these cells also stimulated VEGF expression (Poulaki et al. 2003). Another possible link between the IGF-1R and VEGFR pathways is via hypoxia-inducible factor-HIF-1α. HIF-1α is a transcription factor activated under reduced oxygen tension, and is involved in tumor progression/metastasis in various cancers. However, studies have shown that activation of the PI3K/Akt and MAPK pathways by growth factors can activate HIF-1α independently of hypoxia (Zhong et al. 2000; Laughner et al. 2001; Fukuda et al. 2002). This effect appears to depend on the involvement of the molecular chaperone heat-shock protein 90 (HSP90) as the inhibition of HSP90 by SNX-2112 decreased IGF-I-induced Akt and Erk activation in multiple myeloma cells, blocked angiogenesis and overcame the growth advantage conferred by IGF-I (Okawa et al. 2009). Likewise, HSP90 inactivation in a human pancreatic cancer cell by a geldan-amycin derivative impaired IGF-IR signaling and inhibited neovascularization in vivo (Lang et al. 2007). Among the HIF-1α target genes are VEGF, IGF-II, c-Met (a receptor of hepatocyte growth factor) (Pennacchietti et al. 2003; Hayashi et al. 2005) and TGFα (Semenza 2003), all of which are involved in tumor growth and progression. Isolation of preneoplastic lesions from livers of mice injected with diethylnitrosamine revealed that during early stages of hepatocarcinogenesis (before the development of hepatic carcinoma) there was a marked increase in hepatocel-lular HIF-1α protein levels, which was also shown in dysplastic hepatocytes in the three human lesions examined in that study (Tanaka et al. 2006).

Similar to angiogenesis, the growth of lymphatic vessels (lymphangiogenesis) is a complex process orchestrated by many growth factors. VEGF-C and VEGF-D are the most potent lymphangiogenic factors which interact with VEGFR-3, specifi-cally expressed on lymphatic endothelial cells. Accordingly, over-expression of these factors in tumor cells leads to lymphatic metastases (Skobe et al. 2001; Stacker et al. 2001). Lymphatic endothelial cells also express the IGF-1R. In a mouse cornea assay, addition of IGF-1/II stimulated lymphatic endothelial cell proliferation and migration (Bjorndahl et al. 2005). Lymphangiogenesis in the context of hepatic metastasis has not yet been studied. Nonetheless, it has stimulated considerable interest in therapeutic development of potential inhibitors for the treatment or prevention of lymphatic metastasis.

IGF in Animal Models of Cancer

Evidence for the role of the IGF system in cancer has been obtained from studies in animal models. Although the IGF-1R or its ligands (IGF-I, and II) are not tum-origenic by themselves, increased expression of these proteins leads to enhanced tumor incidence and growth in mouse models of cancer. As such, transgenic expres-sion of IGF-1 in basal epithelial cells of the prostate in mice resulted in sponta-neous development of prostate carcinoma (DiGiovanni et al. 2000). Likewise, transgenic expression of IGF-I in epidermal cells under the HK1 promoter increased 12-O-tetradecanoylphorbol-13-acetate (TPA)-induced skin tumors. Furthermore, compared to nontransgenic controls, the number of tumors per mouse was increased and the latent period for tumor development was decreased in mice overexpressing the IGF-1 transgene (Wilker et al. 1999). As mentioned in previous sections, IGFs are bound to the IGFBPs, which regulate their bioactivity. When des-IGF-I, an

IGF-I analogue with low affinity for IGFBP, was expressed under the WAP promoter (WAP-DES), there was a marked increase in the incidence of mammary adenocarcinomas, with 53% of mice developing tumors by 23 months of age. Thus, enhancement of tumor growth and progression appears to be independent of IGFBPs. Interestingly, crossing of WAP-DES with mutant p53 (p53172R-H) mice resulted in increased mammary tumor volume (Hadsell et al. 2000), suggesting that the IGF system accelerated malignant transformation following loss of tumor suppressor expression.

Similarly, IGF-II transgenic expression in the lung epithelium increased the incidence of lung tumors in mice older than 18 months. Molecular characterization of IGF-IR downstream mediators revealed that Erk1/2 were hyperphosphorylated. This model was in accordance with clinical studies showing correlations between high levels of IGF-II and pulmonary adenocarcinoma (Moorehead et al. 2003). The potential role of IGF-II in tumor progression was revealed in transgenic mice expressing the SV40-T antigen under the control of the rat insulin promoter (RIP1-Tag2). These mice exhibited upregulation of IGF-II expression in the pancreatic islet β-cells, leading to the formation of hyperproliferative/dysplastic β-cell lesions. Crossing these mice to IGF-II$^{-/-}$ mice resulted in smaller tumors, likely due to a fivefold increase in β-cell apoptosis (Christofori et al. 1995). Interestingly, when RIP1-Tag2 mice were crossed with RIP7-IGF-IR mice (that overexpress human IGF-IR in β-cells), accelerated β-cell tumor formation, with the rapid development of lymph-node metastases was evident (Lopez and Hanahan 2002). The Igf2 gene is maternally imprinted and controlled by the H19 gene. When the H19 gene was mutated (H19$^{+/-}$ mouse), the Igf2 gene lost its heterozygous expression, and was expressed by both alleles, leading to elevations in IGF-II. Crossing of the H19$^{+/-}$ mouse with the Apc$^{+/Min}$ mouse, which develops colon adenomas, resulted in a twofold increase in the number of colon adenomas (Sakatani et al. 2005).

Ligand-independent, constitutive activation of the IGF-1R in the mouse mammary using the CD8a-IGF-IR fusion protein under the control of the mouse mammary tumor virus (MMTV), led to rapid tumor development. As early as 6 weeks of age, the MMTV-CD8a-IGF-IR transgenic mice developed salivary and mammary adenocarcinomas, with a palpable mammary mass at 8 weeks of age. The salivary gland tumors were associated with scattered lymphatic vessels and invaded the adjacent striated muscle. The mammary adenomas and adenocarcinomas were multifocal and seen within adjacent lobules (Sakatani et al. 2005).

In animal models where the IGF system was downregulated, opposite effects on tumor growth and progression were evident. In lit/lit mice, which have a significant reduction in IGF-I expression in all tissues due to a growth hormone defect, the growth of human MCF-7 xenotransplanted cells was attenuated (Yang et al. 1996). Likewise, dw/dw dwarf mice which are deficient in GH/IGF-I were shown to be resistant to DMBA-induced carcinogenesis (Ramsey et al. 2002). In transgenic mice which express a growth hormone antagonist and have decreased circulating IGF-I levels, the incidence of DMBA-induced mammary tumors was significantly decreased (Pollak et al. 2001). In liver IGF-1 deficient (LID) mice with a 75% decrease in circulating IGF-I levels, DMBA- or SV40-T-induced mammary tumor growth was attenuated (Wu et al. 2003). The growth and development of several tumor types were studied in conjunction with the LID model and revealed similar observations, namely reduced tumor growth and progression. Growth and hepatic metastasis development of colon MC38 adenocarcinoma orthografts were significantly reduced in LID mice as compared to controls (Wu et al. 2002) while colon carcinogenesis induced by AOM was also reduced in LID mice (Olivo-Marston et al. 2009). Likewise, TPA-induced skin carcinoma tumor volume and incidence were significantly reduced in LID mice (Moore et al. 2008). However, in an osteosarcoma model, reductions in serum IGF-1 did not inhibit orthograft tumor growth (Hong et al. 2009), and in TRAMP-induced prostate cancer, reductions in serum IGF-1 were insufficient to inhibit tumor growth (Anzo et al. 2008).

A reduction in serum IGF-I levels can also be achieved through calorie-restriction. When IGF-I was infused into calorie-restricted, p53-deficient mice, the anticarcinogenic effect of calorie restriction was abolished (Dunn et al. 1997). Similar results were obtained when GH or IGF-I were administered to calorie-restricted Fischer rats bearing mononuclear cell leukemia (Hursting et al. 1993). On the other hand, the role of IGF-I in obesity-increased cancer risk is still unclear. Several studies using mice fed a high calorie diet have shown that obese animals have an increased incidence of transplanted tumors (Earl et al. 2009; Van Saun et al. 2009; Park et al. 2010). One of the suggested mechanisms is inhibition of Igfbp-1 gene expression via hyperinsulinemia, resulting in an increase of free IGF-1 and enhanced IGF-IR and/or insulin receptor-A activation. In a study using the LID mice fed a high calorie diet, it was demonstrated that increases in tumor growth during obesity are regulated by serum IGF-1 (Wu et al. 2010). Hepatic metastasis growth was shown to increase in obese mice harboring various tumors (Wu et al. 2010). When a colon MC38 adenocarcinoma model of hepatic metastasis was applied in obese LID mice the number and volume of hepatic metastases were reduced. However, these reductions were observed only in mice with long-term IGF-1 deficiency (from birth), suggesting that other regulatory factors such as the host immune system are implicated in this process. However, it should be emphasized that obesity leads to multiple physiological changes and causes upregulation of numerous serum proteins that may play a role in tumor growth. The interpretation of these findings, particularly the elucidation of the role of IGF-I in tumor promotion in obese mice, will therefore require further analysis.

Epidemiological studies have suggested an association between elevated circulating IGF-I concentrations and an increased risk of cancer, whereas higher IGFBP-3 concentrations have been linked to a decreased risk of cancer (Yu and Rohan 2000; Giovannucci 2001). Although several studies include evaluations of IGF-II and other IGFBPs, the majority of studies focus on IGF-I and IGFBP-3. Therefore, our discussion will highlight the relationship between cancer and IGF-I and IGFBP-3.

High serum concentrations of IGF-I have been associated with an increased risk of premenopausal breast cancer, colorectal cancer, prostate cancer, lung cancer, endometrial cancer, and bladder cancer (Chan et al. 1998; Hankinson et al. 1998; Ma et al. 1999; Yu et al. 1999; Stattin et al. 2000; Toniolo et al. 2000; Palmqvist et al. 2002; Petridou et al. 2003; Zhao et al. 2003). Elevated IGFBP-3 has been linked to a decreased risk of prostate cancer, premenopausal breast cancer, and postmenopausal breast cancer (Bruning et al. 1995). Over-expression of the IGF-IR has been observed in breast cancer, although the clinical significance of this over-expression is not known (Peyrat et al. 1988; Papa et al. 1993; Railo et al. 1994; Shimizu et al. 2004; Ueda et al. 2006). In contrast, studies focused on the expression levels of the IGF-IR in prostate cancer have yielded conflicting results (Tennant et al. 1996; Figueroa et al. 2001; Hellawell et al. 2002).

Breast Cancer

IGF-I plays an essential role in mammary gland development and is able to mediate glandular mammary development in concert with growth hormone (GH) and estro-gen (Ruan and Kleinberg 1999; Kleinberg et al. 2000). In vitro and in vivo studies have demonstrated that IGF-I stimulates breast cancer cell growth (Pollak et al. 1988; Lee et al. 1999) and epidemiological data suggest that circulating IGF-I levels are higher in breast cancer patients compared with normal controls (Bohlke et al. 1998; Bruning et al. 1995; Peyrat et al. 1988; Hankinson et al. 1998) (Table 6.1). In several of these studies, a direct relationship between elevated IGF-I and breast cancer risk was observed in premenopausal women but not postmenopausal women (Bruning et al. 1995; Hankinson et al. 1998). Hankinson et al. (1998) reported a nearly fivefold increase in breast cancer risk in women under the age of 50 with elevated plasma IGF-I levels (odds ratio 4.58) and this risk increased to more than sevenfold when IGF-I was adjusted for IGFBP-3. Bruning and colleagues showed that premenopausal women with breast cancer had elevated serum IGF-I levels, decreased IGFBP-3 levels, and increased IGF-I/IGFBP-3 ratios. This increased ratio remained a significant risk factor for breast cancer even after adjustment for age, family history, height, body-mass index, body-fat distribution, and serum levels of C-peptide. However, these associations were not observed in postmenopausal women (Bruning et al. 1995). In a prospective case control study nested within a cohort of the New York University Women's Health Study, the authors observed an elevated risk of breast cancer in premenopausal women with increased levels of circulating IGF-I that was not seen in postmenopausal women. When analysis was limited to premenopausal women who were diagnosed before age 50, the risk increased further. In this study, levels of IGFBP-3 and the IGF-I/IGFBP-3 ratio did not appear to affect breast cancer risk (Toniolo et al. 2000). However, some more recent studies have challenged these findings when they have failed to demonstrate an increased breast cancer risk in premenopausal women with elevated IGF-I (Rinaldi et al. 2006; Schernhammer et al. 2006; Baglietto et al. 2007). In two of these studies, an association was seen in postmenopausal but not premenopausal women (Rinaldi et al. 2006; Baglietto et al. 2007). The European Prospective Investigation into Cancer and Nutrition (EPIC) included more than 1,000 female patients with breast cancer and more than 2,000 controls and found that IGF-I and IGFBP-3 were positively associated with breast cancer risk in postmenopausal but not premenopausal women (Rinaldi et al. 2006). Baglietto and colleagues confirmed

Table 6.1 Case control and cohort studies: association between specific cancers by site and IGF-I and IGFBP-3

Study	Site	Association with IGF-I (measure specified) (95% CI)	Association with IGFBP-3 (measure specified) (95% CI)	P value for trend
Bohlke et al. (1998)	Breast	OR: 1.8 (0.7–4.6)	OR: 0.7 (0.3–1.7)	P value not provided
Hankinson et al. (1998)	Breast (overall)	RR: 1.06 (0.66–1.70)	NA	IGF-I 0.86
Hankinson et al. (1998)	Breast (postmenopausal)	RR: 0.85 (0.53–1.39)	NA	IGF-I 0.63
Hankinson et al. (1998)	Breast (premenopausal)	RR: 2.33 (1.06–5.16)	NA	IGF-I 0.08
Del Giudice et al. (1998)	Breast (premenopausal)	OR: 1.47 (0.66–3.27)	OR: 2.05 (0.93–4.53)	IGF-I P value not provided IGFBP-3 0.07
Petridou et al. (2000)	Breast (postmenopausal)	OR: 1.1 (0.7–1.7)	NA	IGF-I 0.59
Petridou et al. (2000)	Breast (premenopausal)	OR: 0.4 (0.1–1.4)	NA	IGF-I 0.16
Toniolo et al. (2000)	Breast (postmenopausal)	RR: 0.95 (0.49–1.86)	RR: 1.08 (0.54–1.16)	IGF-I 0.87 IGFBP-3 0.83
Toniolo et al. (2000)	Breast (premenopausal)	RR: 1.60 (0.91–2.81)	RR: 1.18 (0.66–2.08)	IGF-I 0.09 IGFBP-3 0.63
Rinaldi et al. (2006)	Breast <50 years old	OR: 1.03 (0.60–1.77)	OR: 0.92 (0.50–1.70)	IGF-I 0.81 IGFBP-3 0.69
Rinaldi et al. (2006)	Breast >50 years old	OR: 1 38 (1.02–1.86)	OR: 1.44 (1.04–1.98)	IGF-I 0.01 IGFBP-3 0.01
Baglietto et al. (2007)	Breast	HR: 1.20 (0.87–1.65)	HR: 1.09 (0.78–1.53)	IGF-I 0.38 IGFBP-3 0.50
Gunter et al. (2009)	Breast	OR: Free IGF-I 1.24 (0.72–2.14)	NA	IGF-I 0.47
Manousos et al. (1999)	Colorectal	OR: 2.3 (0.6–9.1)	OR: 0.5 (0.1–1.7)	P values not provided
Ma et al. (1999)	Colorectal (men)	OR: 2.51 (1.15–5.46)	OR: 0.28(0.12–0.66)	IGF-I 0.02 IGFBP-3 0.05
Kaaks et al. (2000)	Colorectal	OR: 1.88 (0.72–4.91)	OR: 2.46 (1.09–5.57)	IGF-I 0.25 IGFBP-3 0.19
Giovannucci et al. (2000)	Colorectal (women)	OR: 2.18 (0.94–5.08)	OR: 0.28 (0.09–0.85)	IGF-I 0.10 IGFBP-3 0.05

Reference	Cancer type	Risk estimate	Risk estimate	p-value
(Palmqvist et al. 2002)	Colon	OR: 1.27 (0.62–2.63)	OR: 1.32 (0.66–2.67)	IGF-1 0.56 / IGFBP-3 0.20
Morris et al. (2006)	Colorectal	OR: 1.10 (0.56–2.18)	OR: 0.72 (0.37–1.37)	IGF-1 0.65 / IGFBP-3 0.46
Yu et al. (1999)	Lung	OR: 2.06 (1.19–3.56)	OR: 0.73 (0.43–1.26)	IGF-1 0.01 / IGFBP-3 0.50
Morris et al. (2006)	Lung	OR: 1.21 (0.62–2.35)	OR: 1.70 (0.87–3.30)	IGF-1 0.45 / IGFBP-3 0.06
Mantzoros et al. (1997)	Prostate	OR: 1.91 (1.00–3.73)	NA	IGF-1 0.05
Wolk et al. (1998)	Prostate	OR: 1.51 (1.0–2.26)	OR: 1.31 (0.95–1.82)	IGF-1 0.04 / IGFBP-3 0.10
Chan et al. (1998)	Prostate	RR: 4.32 (1.76–10.6)	RR: 0.41 (0.17–1.03)	IGF-1 0.001 / IGFBP-3 0.09
Stattin et al. (2000)	Prostate	OR: 1.57 (0.88–2.81)	OR: 1.56 (0.86–2.83)	IGF-1 0.02 / IGFBP-3 0.03
Chen et al. (2005)	Prostate	RR: 0.17 (0.05–0.62)	RR: 0.24 (0.07–0.84)	IGF-1 0.45 / IGFBP-3 0.11
Morris et al. (2006)	Prostate	OR: 1.37 (0.76–2.49)	OR: 1.40 (0.77–2.55)	IGF-1 0.62 / IGFBP-3 0.42
Severi et al. (2006)	Prostate	HR: 1.07 (0.79–1.46)	HR: 1.49 (1.11–2.00)	IGF-1 0.5 / IGFBP-3 0.008
Allen et al. (2007b)	Prostate	OR: 1.35 (0.99–1.82)	OR: 1.01 (0.74–1.37)	IGF-1 0.08 / IGFBP-3 0.38

OR odds ratio, *HR* hazard ratio, *RR* relative risk

the findings of the EPIC when they reported that in their study of more than 400 breast cancer patients and more than 1,900 controls, breast cancer risk was positively associated with IGF-I and IGFBP-3 in postmenopausal women but not premenopausal women (Baglietto et al. 2007). Thus, it is not clear at this time how menopausal status affects the relationship between the risk of breast risk cancer and IGF-I and IGFBP-3. Several other case-control studies failed to demonstrate an association between IGF-I and breast cancer (Del Giudice et al. 1998; Ng et al. 1998; Petridou et al. 2000). A recent prospective study found no statistically significant linear trends in the association between free IGF-I level and risk of breast cancer (Gunter et al. 2009). Taken together, the results of case control and cohort studies exploring the relationship between IGF-I levels and risk of breast cancer have been inconsistent.

Given the conflicting data resulting from case control and cohort studies, meta-analyses have been undertaken to explore the relationship between IGF and IGFBP-3 and breast cancer risk (Renehan et al. 2004; Shi et al. 2004; Sugumar et al. 2004) (Table 6.2). A meta-analysis of six breast cancer studies found that high concentrations of IGF-I and elevated IGFBP-3 levels were associated with premenopausal but not postmenopausal breast cancer (Renehan et al. 2004). In a meta-analysis that included 16 studies, Shi and colleagues reported that higher concentrations of IGF-I were not associated with an increased risk of breast cancer among the women evaluated. However, when only premenopausal women were included in the analysis, there was a positive association between IGF-I and breast cancer risk. This was not observed in postmenopausal women. In addition, the authors report that breast cancer patients (premenopausal, postmenopausal, and overall) had higher levels of IGFBP-3 than control patients (Shi et al. 2004). A meta-analysis of seven studies explored the relationship between premenopausal breast cancer and IGF-I and IGFBP 3. Only a marginally significant association was seen for premenopausal breast cancer and IGF-I. No relationship was observed between premenopausal breast cancer and IGFBP-3. Lastly, "The Endogenous Hormones and Breast Cancer Collaborative Group", established to analyse pooled individual data from 17 prospective studies in 12 countries, found that circulating IGF1 was positively associated with breast-cancer risk and this association was not modified by IGFBP3, and did not differ markedly by menopausal status (Key et al. 2010). However, these relationships seem confined to oestrogen-receptor-positive tumours.

An association between the IGF-IR and breast cancer risk has also been suggested by various studies reporting increased immunostaining of the IGF-IR in breast cancer tissues (Peyrat et al. 1988; Papa et al. 1993; Railo et al. 1994; Shimizu et al. 2004; Ueda et al. 2006). However, these studies have reported conflicting results and the clinical significance of these findings is not clear.

Colorectal Cancer

Colorectal cancer rates have been shown to be higher in patients with acromegaly, who have elevated levels of GH and IGF-I (Cats et al. 1996; Jenkins et al. 1997). In addition, IGF-I has been shown to stimulate colorectal epithelial and cancer cells

Table 6.2 Meta-analyses: association between specific cancers by site and IGF-I and IGFBP-3

Study	Site	# of studies included (IGF-I/IGFBP-3)	IGF-I (odds ratio, 95% CI)	IGFBP-3 (odds ratio, 95% CI)	P value for trend
Shi et al. (2004)	Breast (overall)	16	1.05 (0.94–1.17)	NA	IGF-I>0.40
Renehan et al. (2004)	Breast (postmenopausal)	4/3	0.95 (0.77–1.17)	1.01 (0.74–1.38)	IGF-I 0.63 IGFBP-3 0.93
Shi et al. (2004)	Breast (postmenopausal)	16	0.93 (0.80–1.10)	NA	IGF-I>0.40 IGFBP-3<0.01
Renehan et al. (2004)	Breast (premenopausal)	4/3	1.65 (1.26–2.08)	1.51 (1.01–1.27)	IGF-I<0.01 IGFBP-3 0.05
Shi et al. (2004)	Breast (premenopausal)	16	1.39 (1.16–1.66)	1.42 (1.15–1.74)	IGF-I<0.01 IGFBP-3<0.01
Sugumar et al. (2004)	Breast (premenopausal)	7	1.74 (097–3.13)	1.60 (0.84–3.02)	IGF-I 0.06 IGFBP-3 0.15
Renehan et al. (2004)	Colorectal	4	1.18 (0.92–1.51)	1.16 (0.85–1.57)	IGF-I 0.19 IGFBP-3 0.35
Morris et al. (2006)	Colorectal	7	1.37 (1.05–1.78)	0.98 (0.64–1.51)	IGF-I 0.68 IGFBP-3 0.02
Renehan et al. (2004)	Lung	4	1.01 (0.650–1.58)	0.98 (0.62–1.54)	IGF-I 0.95 IGFBP-3 0.92
Morris et al. (2006)	Lung	5	1.02 (0.80–1.31)	0.98 (0.61–1.58)	IGF-I 0.64 IGFBP-3 0.01
Renehan et al. (2004)	Prostate	3	1.49 (1.14–1.95)	0.95 (0.70–1.28)	IGF-I 0.003 IGFBP-3 0.72
Morris et al. (2006)	Prostate	9	1.31 (1.03–1.67)	1.05 (0.82–1.35)	IGF-I 0.21 IGFBP-3 0.19

in vitro (Pollak et al. 1987; Guo et al. 1992). These findings prompted investigators to explore the relationship between colon cancer risk and IGF-I and IGFBP-3. In a prospective study of almost 15,000 men in the Physician's Health Study, men with the highest level of IGF-I had an increased risk of colorectal cancer as compared to men in the lowest quintile (relative risk 2.51). In addition, men with higher IGFBP-3 values had a lower risk of colorectal cancer (Ma et al. 1999). The Nurses Health Study examined the relationship of colorectal cancer and IGF-I and IGFBP-3 in women and reported that women with elevated IGF-I levels had an elevated risk of intermediate/late stage colorectal neoplasia and adenoma. In addition, women with higher IGFBP-3 levels had a decreased risk of colorectal cancer and adenoma (Giovannucci et al. 2000). A prospective cohort study of more than 14,000 women found a modest but statistically nonsignificant positive association with levels of IGF-I. This study also found an increased risk of colon cancer in patients with increased IGFBP-3 levels (Kaaks et al. 2000) (Table 6.1). As many of the early studies included patients with cancers of both colon and rectum, a subsequent case-control study examined these two groups of patients individually. The authors described a positive association between IGF-I and colon cancer risk and an inverse association between IGFBP-3 and colon cancer risk. However, with regards to rectal cancer, an inverse relationship was observed for cancer risk and both IGF-I and IGFBP-3 (Palmqvist et al. 2002). Meta-analyses have reported an association between elevated levels of IGF-I and increased colorectal cancer risk but no association between IGFBP-3 and colorectal cancer (Renehan et al. 2004; Morris et al. 2006) (Table 6.2). Thus, it appears that IGF-I is positively associated with the risk of colon cancer, although this same statement cannot be made about rectal cancer.

Prostate Cancer

As IGF-I has been shown to stimulate growth of prostate cancer cells in vitro (Iwamura et al. 1993; Culig et al. 1995), epidemiologic studies have been undertaken to determine if there is a relationship between IGF-I and prostate cancer risk. Early epidemiological studies suggested that circulating IGF-I levels were higher in prostate cancer patients compared with normal controls (Mantzoros et al. 1997). A prospective case control study performed on 152 prostate cancer patients and 152 controls as part of the Physicians' Health Study found that men in the highest quartile of IGF-I had an elevated risk of prostate cancer (relative risk 4.3) as compared to men in the lowest quartile. In addition, elevated IGFBP-3 levels were associated with a decreased risk of prostate cancer (Chan et al. 1998). Similar to the earlier studies done on breast cancer, the link between IGF-I and prostate cancer risk was particularly strong in men younger than age 70 (Wolk et al. 1998). Stattin and colleagues also found that prostate cancer and IGF-I were directly related and that this relationship was especially strong in men younger than 59 years of age. The authors suggest that this may occur because elevated IGF-I levels during early adolescence and adulthood favor the development of early preneoplastic lesions that clinically present in later life (Stattin et al. 2000). Some subsequent studies have challenged this positive association, reporting no relationship (Lacey et al. 2001; Woodson et al. 2003; Chen et al. 2005). IGFBP-3 was inversely associated with prostate cancer risk in only one of these studies (Chen et al. 2005), whereas in the other studies, no relationship was observed (Lacey et al. 2001; Woodson et al. 2003). As part of the European Randomized Study of Screening for Prostate Cancer (ERSPC), a cohort of over 4,000 men were studied to evaluate if total IGF-I, free IGF-I, and IGFBP-3 could predict future prostate cancer risk. No relationship was observed between prostate cancer risk and total IGF-I, free IGF-I, or IGFBP3 (Janssen et al. 2004) (Table 6.1). Another study, a case-cohort study that included 524 cases and 1,826 controls as part of the Melbourne Collaborative Cohort Study found no association between IGF-I and prostate cancer risk. Interestingly, this study reported an association between higher levels of IGFBP-3 and increased risk of prostate cancer (Severi et al. 2006). This is in contrast to the aforementioned studies that found either an inverse relationship or no relationship between these two variables. The European Prospective Investigation into Cancer and Nutrition (EPIC), a case control study of 630 prostate cancer patients and 630 controls reported a weakly positive, nonstatistically significant association between IGF-I and prostate cancer risk and no association with IGFBP-3 (Allen et al. 2007b). Case control and cohort studies have yielded conflicting results on the relationship between prostate cancer risk and IGF-I and IGFBP-3.

Meta-analyses have also been undertaken to examine the relationship between IGF-I and IGFBP-3 and prostate cancer risk (Renehan et al. 2004; Morris et al. 2006) (Table 6.2). A meta-analysis by Morris and colleagues performed on nine studies found an increased risk of prostate cancer in patients with elevated IGF-I (OR 1.31) but no association between IGFBP-3 and prostate cancer (Morris et al. 2006). Renehan et al. (2004) examined three studies and reported similar findings. They found an increased risk of prostate cancer in patients with elevated IGF-I (OR 1.49) but no relationship between IGFBP-3 and prostate cancer. Given the conflicting data, further work is necessary to clarify the association between IGF-I and IGFBP-3 and prostate cancer risk.

In the case of breast and prostate cancer, studies have yielded conflicting results regarding the existence and direction of a relationship between these cancers and the IGF-I system. In addition, studies suggest that reproductive status and age may influence these relationships. In colon cancer, the positive association between cancer risk and the IGF-I system has been more consistently demonstrated. Taken together, further study of the relationship between the IGF-I and cancer risk is needed to clarify our understanding of this complex interaction.

IGF-1 as a Target for Cancer Therapy

The aforementioned experimental data, along with epidemiological evidence, have unequivocally shown that the IGFs and their receptor, IGF-1R, are implicated in all aspects of tumor growth and progression, thus identifying the IGF system as target for cancer therapy (Fig. 6.2). A few strategies have been developed to inhibit the

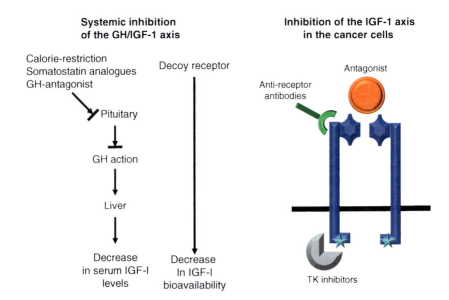

Fig. 6.2 Summary of the therapies currently in use to target the GH/IGF-1 axis for cancer treatment. Strategies involve either systemic inhibition of GH/IGF-1 signaling through caloric restriction and the use of GH antagonists or, alternatively, approaches which challenge the integrity of IGF-1R itself, such as antireceptor antibodies, tyrosine kinase (TK) inhibitors, or IGFI/II antagonists (the figure included in this review is original and created by Dr. Yakar)

IGF system, including interference with ligand binding, blocking the IGF-1R kinase activity, reduction of IGF-1R gene expression, reducing IGF-1 bioavailability, and reducing serum IGF-1 levels (Table 6.3). As of summer 2010, anti-IGF anti cancer drugs were tested in preclinical or early phases of clinical trials and so far treatment outcomes have only been anecdotally published.

The two main approaches that are being tested in preclinical and early clinical phases are humanized monoclonal anti-IGF-IR antibodies and small molecule tyrosine kinase inhibitors (TKI). These two approaches require different exposure to the compound and therefore have diverse efficacy and toxicity profiles. While anti-IGF-IR antibodies are more target-specific, TKI generally have a broader target profile and can cause nonspecific toxicity and may therefore not be well tolerated. It is important to note that prolonged use of those drugs may lead to drug-resistance and activating of alternative survival mechanisms by the tumor cells.

It is important to note that targeting the IGF-I system in vivo poses several challenges: (a) Due to the high degree of homology between the IGF-I and insulin receptors, drugs that target the IGF axis may also affect the insulin receptor/insulin axis with undesirable effects on glucose and lipid metabolism. Inhibition of IGF-I signaling may also result in increased serum GH levels leading to insulin insensitivity. (b) The majority of tumor cells studied to date express the IGF-IR. However, no specific mutations in the receptor or its ligands have been identified in cancerous cells, and therefore specific biomarkers for pathway activation that will allow monitoring of the effects of candidate drugs have not been developed.

Table 6.3 IGF axis as a target for cancer therapy

Target	Class of inhibitors	Inhibitor	Status	Study
Serum IGF-1 levels	Calorie restriction	NA	NA	Dirx et al. (2003) Ross and Bras (1971) Dirx et al. (1999) van Noord (2004)
	Somatostatin analogues	AN-238	Preclinical	Szereday et al. (2003) Pollak and Schally (1998)
	GH antagonist	Pegvisomant	Clinical trials	at http://www.clinicaltrials.gov
	GHRH antagonist	JV-1-38	Preclinical	Kiaris et al. (2003)
IGF-1R ligand binding	Anti IGF-1R antibodies	IMC-A12 (Imclone) R1507 (Roche) AMG479 (Amgen) CP751-871 (Pfizer) MK0646 (Merk/Pierre Fabre) SCH717454 (Schering-Plough) AVE1642 (Sanofi-Aventis) BIIB022 (Biogen Idec)	Clinical trials	at http://clinicaltrials.gov
		H7C10	Preclinical	Goetsch et al. (2005)
	IGF-1R antagonist	JB-1	Preclinical	Häyry et al. (1995) Pietrzkowski et al. (1993) Mitsiades et al. (2004)
	Soluble IGF-1R (decoy receptor)	486/STOP	Preclinical	D'Ambrosio et al. (1996)
		$IGF\text{-}1R^{933}$	Preclinical	Bergsland (2004) Lip et al. (2004)
	IGFBPs	IGFBP-3	Preclinical	Lee et al. (2002) Fowler et al. (2000) Granata et al. (2004) Perks et al. (2000)

(continued)

Table 6.3 (continued)

Target	Class of inhibitors	Inhibitor	Status	Study
IGF-1R signaling	Tyrosine Kinase inhibitors	INSM18 (Insmed/UCSF) OSI906 (OSI pharmaceuticals) XL228 (Exelixis)	Clinical trials	at http://www.clinicaltrials.gov
		BMS536924 (Bristol-Myers Squibb)	Preclinical	Wahner Hendrickson et al. (2009) Litzenburger et al. (2009)
		NVP-ADW742 (Novartis Pharma)	Preclinical	Mitsiades et al. (2004) Warshamana-Greene et al. (2004)
		NVP-AEW541 (Novartis Pharma)	Preclinical	Gariboldi et al. (2010) Hägerstrand et al. (2010) Wolf et al. (2010) Mukohara et al. (2009)
		Cyclolignan PPP	Preclinical	Vasilcanu et al. (2004)
		AG1024 (Merck)	Preclinical	Blum et al. (2000) Párrizas et al. (1997)
IGF-1R gene expression	siRNA	Igf-1r siRNA	Preclinical	Baserga et al. (2003) Surmacz (2003)

Concluding Remarks

There is compelling experimental and epidemiological evidence showing that the IGF axis plays a pivotal role in cancer growth and progression. As such, IGF-1 has been identified as a target for cancer therapy. Clinical trials revealed encouraging results; however, several challenges have been identified, including undesirable metabolic consequences. Results thus far suggest that IGF-axis-targeting agents may be most effective when combined with chemotherapeutic drugs. Indeed, initial preclinical studies suggest that inhibition of the IGF-1R enhances response to chemotherapy, radiation, and siRNA therapy. The use of chemotherapeutic agents, such as CCI-779 and RAD001, which are mTOR inhibitors, in combination with h7C10 antibody against the IGF-1R, resulted in synergistic inhibition of cell survival and reduced tumor burden (Wan et al. 2006). Similarly, in the H460 xenograft model, combining radiation and the A12 antibody against the IGF-1R significantly enhanced antitumor efficacy compared with either modality alone (Allen et al. 2007a). Likewise, in five human hepatoma cell lines the use of AVE1642, anti-IGF-1R antibody, in combination with gefitinib, an EGFR inhibitor or rapamycin, significantly blocked the cell cycle and inhibited AKT phosphorylation, (Desbois-Mouthon et al. 2009). It is now clear that tumor cells activate distinct pro-survival and proliferation pathways, and therefore, therapeutic approaches may be most effective when individualized based on molecular profiling of the malignant cells.

References

Abramovitch, S., T. Glaser, et al. (2003). "BRCA1-Sp1 interactions in transcriptional regulation of the IGF-IR gene." FEBS Lett **541**(1–3): 149–54.

Allen, G.W., C. Saba et al. (2007). "Insulin-like growth factor-I receptor signaling blockade combined with radiation." Cancer Res 67(3):1155–62.

Allen, N. E., T. J. Key, et al. (2007). "Serum insulin-like growth factor (IGF)-I and IGF-binding protein-3 concentrations and prostate cancer risk: results from the European Prospective Investigation into Cancer and Nutrition." Cancer Epidemiol Biomarkers Prev **16**(6): 1121–7.

Andre, F., V. Rigot, et al. (1999). "Integrins and E-cadherin cooperate with IGF-I to induce migration of epithelial colonic cells." Int J Cancer **83**(4): 497–505.

Anzo, M., L. J. Cobb, et al. (2008). "Targeted deletion of hepatic Igf1 in TRAMP mice leads to dramatic alterations in the circulating insulin-like growth factor axis but does not reduce tumor progression." Cancer Res **68**(9): 3342–9.

Baglietto, L., D. R. English, et al. (2007). "Circulating insulin-like growth factor-I and binding protein-3 and the risk of breast cancer." Cancer Epidemiol Biomarkers Prev **16**(4): 763–8.

Balaram, S. K., D. K. Agrawal, et al. (1999). "Insulin like growth factor-1 activates nuclear factor-kappaB and increases transcription of the intercellular adhesion molecule-1 gene in endothelial cells." Cardiovasc Surg **7**(1): 91–7.

Barnes, C. J., K. Ohshiro, et al. (2007). "Insulin-like growth factor receptor as a therapeutic target in head and neck cancer." Clin Cancer Res **13**(14): 4291–9.

Baserga R., F. Peruzzi et al (2003) "The IGF-1 receptor in cancer biology." Int J Cancer **107**(6):873–7.

Bauer, T. W., W. Liu, et al. (2005). "Targeting of urokinase plasminogen activator receptor in human pancreatic carcinoma cells inhibits c-Met- and insulin-like growth factor-I receptor-mediated migration and invasion and orthotopic tumor growth in mice." Cancer Res **65**(17): 7775–81.

Baxter, R. C. (1988). "Characterization of the acid-labile subunit of the growth hormone-dependent insulin-like growth factor binding protein complex." J Clin Endocrinol Metab **67**(2): 265–72.

Bentov, I., D. LeRoith, et al. (2003). "The WT1 Wilms' tumor suppressor gene: a novel target for insulin-like growth factor-I action." Endocrinology **144**(10): 4276–9.

Berfield, A. K., D. Spicer, et al. (1997). "Insulin-like growth factor I (IGF-I) induces unique effects in the cytoskeleton of cultured rat glomerular mesangial cells." J Histochem Cytochem **45**(4): 583–93.

Bergsland E.K. (2004). "Update on clinical trials targeting vascular endothelial growth factor in cancer." Am J Health Syst Pharm 61(21 Suppl 5): S12–20.

Bjorndahl, M., R. Cao, et al. (2005). "Insulin-like growth factors 1 and 2 induce lymphangiogenesis in vivo." Proc Natl Acad Sci USA **102**(43): 15593–8.

Blum G., A. Gazit et al. (2000). "Substrate competitive inhibitors of IGF-1 receptor kinase." Biochemistry **39**(51):15705–12.

Bohlke, K., D. W. Cramer, et al. (1998). "Insulin-like growth factor-I in relation to premenopausal ductal carcinoma in situ of the breast." Epidemiology **9**(5): 570–3.

Bredin, C. G., Z. Liu, et al. (2003). "Growth factor-enhanced expression and activity of matrix metalloproteases in human non-small cell lung cancer cell lines." Anticancer Res **23**(6C): 4877–84.

Bruning, P. F., J. Van Doorn, et al. (1995). "Insulin-like growth-factor-binding protein 3 is decreased in early-stage operable pre-menopausal breast cancer." Int J Cancer **62**(3): 266–70.

Burgering, B. M. and R. H. Medema (2003). "Decisions on life and death: FOXO Forkhead transcription factors are in command when PKB/Akt is off duty." J Leukoc Biol **73**(6): 689–701.

Call, K. M., T. Glaser, et al. (1990). "Isolation and characterization of a zinc finger polypeptide gene at the human chromosome 11 Wilms' tumor locus." Cell **60**(3): 509–20.

Cano, A., M. A. Perez-Moreno, et al. (2000). "The transcription factor snail controls epithelial-mesenchymal transitions by repressing E-cadherin expression." Nat Cell Biol **2**(2): 76–83.

Cantley, L. C. and B. G. Neel (1999). "New insights into tumor suppression: PTEN suppresses tumor formation by restraining the phosphoinositide 3-kinase/AKT pathway." Proc Natl Acad Sci USA **96**(8): 4240–5.

Cats, A., R. P. Dullaart, et al. (1996). "Increased epithelial cell proliferation in the colon of patients with acromegaly." Cancer Res **56**(3): 523–6.

Ceacareanu, A. C., B. Ceacareanu, et al. (2006). "Nitric oxide attenuates IGF-I-induced aortic smooth muscle cell motility by decreasing Rac1 activity: essential role of PTP-PEST and p130cas." Am J Physiol Cell Physiol **290**(4): C1263–70.

Chan, J. M., M. J. Stampfer, et al. (1998). "Plasma insulin-like growth factor-I and prostate cancer risk: a prospective study." Science **279**(5350): 563–6.

Chattopadhyay, S. and V. I. Shubayev (2009). "MMP-9 controls Schwann cell proliferation and phenotypic remodeling via IGF-1 and ErbB receptor-mediated activation of MEK/ERK pathway." Glia **57**(12): 1316–25.

Che, W., N. Lerner-Marmarosh, et al. (2002). "Insulin-like growth factor-1 enhances inflammatory responses in endothelial cells: role of Gab1 and MEKK3 in TNF-alpha-induced c-Jun and NF-kappaB activation and adhesion molecule expression." Circ Res **90**(11): 1222–30.

Chen, C., S. K. Lewis, et al. (2005). "Prostate carcinoma incidence in relation to prediagnostic circulating levels of insulin-like growth factor I, insulin-like growth factor binding protein 3, and insulin." Cancer **103**(1): 76–84.

Chen, Y. W., V. Boyartchuk, et al. (2009). "Differential roles of insulin-like growth factor receptor- and insulin receptor-mediated signaling in the phenotypes of hepatocellular carcinoma cells." Neoplasia **11**(9): 835–45.

Cheng, H. L., M. L. Steinway, et al. (2000). "GTPases and phosphatidylinositol 3-kinase are critical for insulin-like growth factor-I-mediated Schwann cell motility." J Biol Chem **275**(35): 27197–204.

Chernicky, C. L., H. Tan, et al. (2002). "Treatment of murine breast cancer cells with antisense RNA to the type I insulin-like growth factor receptor decreases the level of plasminogen activator transcripts, inhibits cell growth in vitro, and reduces tumorigenesis in vivo." Mol Pathol **55**(2): 102–9.

Chinnadurai, G. (2002). "CtBP, an unconventional transcriptional corepressor in development and oncogenesis." Mol Cell **9**(2): 213–24.

Christofori, G., P. Naik, et al. (1995). "Deregulation of both imprinted and expressed alleles of the insulin-like growth factor 2 gene during beta-cell tumorigenesis." Nat Genet **10**(2): 196–201.

Culig, Z., A. Hobisch, et al. (1995). "Androgen receptor activation in prostatic tumor cell lines by insulin-like growth factor-I, keratinocyte growth factor and epidermal growth factor." Eur Urol **27 Suppl 2**: 45–7.

D'Ambrosio C., A.A. Ferber et al. (1996). "Soluble insulin-like growth factor I receptor that induces apoptosis of tumor cells in vivo and inhibits tumorigenesis." Cancer Res **56**(17): 4013–20.

Del Giudice, M. E., I. G. Fantus, et al. (1998). "Insulin and related factors in premenopausal breast cancer risk." Breast Cancer Res Treat **47**(2): 111–20.

Delling, U., J. Tureckova, et al. (2000). "A calcineurin-NFATc3-dependent pathway regulates skeletal muscle differentiation and slow myosin heavy-chain expression." Mol Cell Biol **20**(17): 6600–11.

Desbois-Mouthon C., A. Baron et al. (2009). "Insulin-like growth factor-1 receptor inhibition induces a resistance mechanism via the epidermal growth factor receptor/HER3/AKT signaling pathway: rational basis for cotargeting insulin-like growth factor-1 receptor and epidermal growth factor receptor in hepatocellular carcinoma." Clin Cancer Res **15**(17):5445–56.

Di Cristofano, A. and P. P. Pandolfi (2000). "The multiple roles of PTEN in tumor suppression." Cell **100**(4): 387–90.

DiGiovanni, J., K. Kiguchi, et al. (2000). "Deregulated expression of insulin-like growth factor 1 in prostate epithelium leads to neoplasia in transgenic mice." Proc Natl Acad Sci USA **97**(7): 3455–60.

Dirx, M.J., P.A. van den Brandt et al. (1999). Diet in adolescence and the risk of breast cancer: results of the Netherlands Cohort Study. Cancer Causes Control **10**(3): 189–99.

Dirx, M.J., M.P. Zeegers et al. (2003). "Energy restriction and the risk of spontaneous mammary tumors in mice: a meta-analysis." Int Journal of Cancer **106**(5): 766–70.

Doerr, M. E. and J. I. Jones (1996). "The roles of integrins and extracellular matrix proteins in the insulin-like growth factor I-stimulated chemotaxis of human breast cancer cells." J Biol Chem **271**(5): 2443–7.

Dominici, F. P., D. P. Argentino, et al. (2005). "Influence of the crosstalk between growth hormone and insulin signalling on the modulation of insulin sensitivity." Growth Horm IGF Res **15**(5): 324–36.

Dunn, S. E., F. W. Kari, et al. (1997). "Dietary restriction reduces insulin-like growth factor I levels, which modulates apoptosis, cell proliferation, and tumor progression in p53-deficient mice." Cancer Res **57**(21): 4667–72.

Dunn, S. E., J. V. Torres, et al. (2000). "The insulin-like growth factor-1 elevates urokinase-type plasminogen activator-1 in human breast cancer cells: a new avenue for breast cancer therapy." Mol Carcinog **27**(1): 10–7.

Dunn, S. E., J. V. Torres, et al. (2001). "Up-regulation of urokinase-type plasminogen activator by insulin-like growth factor-I depends upon phosphatidylinositol-3 kinase and mitogen-activated protein kinase kinase." Cancer Res **61**(4): 1367–74.

Dupont, J., M. Karas, et al. (2000). "The potentiation of estrogen on insulin-like growth factor I action in MCF-7 human breast cancer cells includes cell cycle components." J Biol Chem **275**(46): 35893–901.

Dupont, J., A. Pierre, et al. (2003). "The insulin-like growth factor axis in cell cycle progression." Horm Metab Res **35**(11–12): 740–50.

Earl, T.M., I.B. Nicoud et al. (2009). "Silencing of TLR4 decreases liver tumor burden in a murine model of colorectal metastasis and hepatic steatosis." Ann Surg Oncol **4**:1043–50.

Elia, L., R. Contu, et al. (2009). "Reciprocal regulation of microRNA-1 and insulin-like growth factor-1 signal transduction cascade in cardiac and skeletal muscle in physiological and pathological conditions." Circulation **120**(23): 2377–85.

Etienne-Manneville, S. and A. Hall (2002). "Rho GTPases in cell biology." Nature **420**(6916): 629–35.

Figueroa, J. A., S. De Raad, et al. (2001). "Gene expression of insulin-like growth factors and receptors in neoplastic prostate tissues: correlation with clinico-pathological parameters." Cancer Invest **19**(1): 28–34.

Finlay, D. and D. Cantrell (2010). "Phosphoinositide 3-kinase and the mammalian target of rapamycin pathways control T cell migration." Ann N Y Acad Sci **1183**: 149–57.

Fowler, C.A., C.M. Perks et al (2000). "Insulin-like growth factor binding protein-3 (IGFBP-3) potentiates paclitaxel-induced apoptosis in human breast cancer cells." Int J Cancer **88**(3):448–53.

Friedl, P. (2004). "Prespecification and plasticity: shifting mechanisms of cell migration." Curr Opin Cell Biol **16**(1): 14–23.

Friedl, P., Y. Hegerfeldt, et al. (2004). "Collective cell migration in morphogenesis and cancer." Int J Dev Biol **48**(5–6): 441–9.

Fukuda, R., K. Hirota, et al. (2002). "Insulin-like growth factor 1 induces hypoxia-inducible factor 1-mediated vascular endothelial growth factor expression, which is dependent on MAP kinase and phosphatidylinositol 3-kinase signaling in colon cancer cells." J Biol Chem **277**(41): 38205–11.

Furlanetto, R. W., S. E. Harwell, et al. (1994). "Insulin-like growth factor-I induces cyclin-D1 expression in MG63 human osteosarcoma cells in vitro." Mol Endocrinol **8**(4): 510–7.

Furundzija, V., J. Fritzsche, et al. (2010). "IGF-1 increases macrophage motility via PKC/p38-dependent alphavbeta3-integrin inside-out signaling." Biochem Biophys Res Commun **394**(3): 786–91.

Gallicchio, M. A., C. Kaun, et al. (2003). "Urokinase type plasminogen activator receptor is involved in insulin-like growth factor-induced migration of rhabdomyosarcoma cells in vitro." J Cell Physiol **197**(1): 131–8.

Galvan, V., A. Logvinova, et al. (2003). "Type 1 insulin-like growth factor receptor (IGF-IR) signaling inhibits apoptosis signal-regulating kinase 1 (ASK1)." J Biol Chem **278**(15): 13325–32.

Gariboldi, M.B., R. Ravizza et al. (2010). "The IGFR1 inhibitor NVP-AEW541 disrupts a pro-survival and pro-angiogenic IGF-STAT3-HIF1 pathway in human glioblastoma cells." Biochem Pharmacol. In press.

Gerald, W. L., J. Rosai, et al. (1995). "Characterization of the genomic breakpoint and chimeric transcripts in the EWS-WT1 gene fusion of desmoplastic small round cell tumor." Proc Natl Acad Sci USA **92**(4): 1028–32.

Gessler, M., A. Poustka, et al. (1990). "Homozygous deletion in Wilms tumours of a zinc-finger gene identified by chromosome jumping." Nature **343**(6260): 774–8.

Giannelli, G., J. Falk-Marzillier, et al. (1997). "Induction of cell migration by matrix metalloprotease-2 cleavage of laminin-5." Science **277**(5323): 225–8.

Giovannucci, E., M. N. Pollak, et al. (2000). "A prospective study of plasma insulin-like growth factor-1 and binding protein-3 and risk of colorectal neoplasia in women." Cancer Epidemiol Biomarkers Prev **9**(4): 345–9.

Giovannucci, E. (2001). "Insulin, insulin-like growth factors and colon cancer: a review of the evidence." J Nutr **131**(11 Suppl): 3109S-20S.

Girnita, A., C. All-Ericsson, et al. (2006). "The insulin-like growth factor-I receptor inhibitor picropodophyllin causes tumor regression and attenuates mechanisms involved in invasion of uveal melanoma cells." Clin Cancer Res **12**(4): 1383–91.

Goetsch, L., A. Gonzalez et al. (2005). "A recombinant humanized anti-insulin-like growth factor receptor type I antibody (h7C10) enhances the antitumor activity of vinorelbine and anti-epidermal growth factor receptor therapy against human cancer xenografts." Intl J Cancer **113**(2):316–28.

6 IGF-1 Cellular Action and its Relationship to Cancer...

Graham, T. R., H. E. Zhau, et al. (2008). "Insulin-like growth factor-I-dependent up-regulation of ZEB1 drives epithelial-to-mesenchymal transition in human prostate cancer cells." Cancer Res **68**(7): 2479–88.

Granata, R., L. Trovato et al. (2004). "Dual effects of IGFBP-3 on endothelial cell apoptosis and survival: involvement of the sphingolipid signaling pathways." FASEB J **18**(12):1456–8. In press.

Grooteclaes, M. L. and S. M. Frisch (2000). "Evidence for a function of CtBP in epithelial gene regulation and anoikis." Oncogene **19**(33): 3823–8.

Gumbiner, B. M. (2000). "Regulation of cadherin adhesive activity." J Cell Biol **148**(3): 399–404.

Gunter, M. J., D. R. Hoover, et al. (2009). "Insulin, insulin-like growth factor-I, and risk of breast cancer in postmenopausal women." J Natl Cancer Inst **101**(1): 48–60.

Guo, Y. S., S. Narayan, et al. (1992). "Characterization of insulinlike growth factor I receptors in human colon cancer." Gastroenterology **102**(4 Pt 1): 1101–8.

Hadsell, D. L., K. L. Murphy, et al. (2000). "Cooperative interaction between mutant p53 and des(1–3)IGF-I accelerates mammary tumorigenesis." Oncogene **19**(7): 889–98.

Hägerstrand, D., M.B. Lindh et al. (2010). "PI3K/PTEN/Akt pathway status affects the sensitivity of high-grade glioma cell cultures to the insulin-like growth factor-1 receptor inhibitor NVP-AEW541." Neuro Oncol. In press.

Hamelers, I. H., R. F. van Schaik, et al. (2002). "Insulin-like growth factor I triggers nuclear accumulation of cyclin D1 in MCF-7S breast cancer cells." J Biol Chem **277**(49): 47645–52.

Hankinson, S. E., W. C. Willett, et al. (1998). "Circulating concentrations of insulin-like growth factor-I and risk of breast cancer." Lancet **351**(9113): 1393–6.

Harding, H. P. and D. Ron (2002). "Endoplasmic reticulum stress and the development of diabetes: a review." Diabetes **51 Suppl 3**: S455–61.

Harvey, K. F., N. L. Harvey, et al. (1998). "Caspase-mediated cleavage of the ubiquitin-protein ligase Nedd4 during apoptosis." J Biol Chem **273**(22): 13524–30.

Hayashi, M., M. Sakata, et al. (2005). "Up-regulation of c-met protooncogene product expression through hypoxia-inducible factor-1alpha is involved in trophoblast invasion under low-oxygen tension." Endocrinology **146**(11): 4682–9.

Häyry, P., M. Myllärniemi et al. (1995). "Stabile D-peptide analog of insulin-like growth factor-1 inhibits smooth muscle cell proliferation after carotid ballooning injury in the rat." FASEB J **9**(13):1336–44.

Heck, S., F. Lezoualc'h, et al. (1999). "Insulin-like growth factor-1-mediated neuroprotection against oxidative stress is associated with activation of nuclear factor kappaB." J Biol Chem **274**(14): 9828–35.

Hellawell, G. O., G. D. Turner, et al. (2002). "Expression of the type 1 insulin-like growth factor receptor is up-regulated in primary prostate cancer and commonly persists in metastatic disease." Cancer Res **62**(10): 2942–50.

Hemers, E., C. Duval, et al. (2005). "Insulin-like growth factor binding protein-5 is a target of matrix metalloproteinase-7: implications for epithelial-mesenchymal signaling." Cancer Res **65**(16): 7363–9.

Hong, S. H., J. Briggs, et al. (2009). "Murine osteosarcoma primary tumour growth and metastatic progression is maintained after marked suppression of serum insulin-like growth factor I." Int J Cancer **124**(9): 2042–9.

Horiuchi, A., T. Imai, et al. (2003). "Up-regulation of small GTPases, RhoA and RhoC, is associated with tumor progression in ovarian carcinoma." Lab Invest **83**(6): 861–70.

Hotamisligil, G. S. (2006). "Inflammation and metabolic disorders." Nature **444**(7121): 860–7.

Humphries, M. J. (2000). "Integrin structure." Biochem Soc Trans **28**(4): 311–39.

Hursting, S. D., B. R. Switzer, et al. (1993). "The growth hormone: insulin-like growth factor 1 axis is a mediator of diet restriction-induced inhibition of mononuclear cell leukemia in Fischer rats." Cancer Res **53**(12): 2750–7.

Iwamura, M., P. M. Sluss, et al. (1993). "Insulin-like growth factor I: action and receptor characterization in human prostate cancer cell lines." Prostate **22**(3): 243–52.

Janssen, J. A., M. F. Wildhagen, et al. (2004). "Circulating free insulin-like growth factor (IGF)-I, total IGF-I, and IGF binding protein-3 levels do not predict the future risk to develop prostate cancer: results of a case-control study involving 201 patients within a population-based screening with a 4-year interval." J Clin Endocrinol Metab **89**(9): 4391–6.

Jenkins, P. J., P. D. Fairclough, et al. (1997). "Acromegaly, colonic polyps and carcinoma." Clin Endocrinol (Oxf) **47**(1): 17–22.

Kaaks, R., P. Toniolo, et al. (2000). "Serum C-peptide, insulin-like growth factor (IGF)-I, IGF-binding proteins, and colorectal cancer risk in women." J Natl Cancer Inst **92**(19): 1592–600.

Karnieli, E., H. Werner, et al. (1996). "The IGF-I receptor gene promoter is a molecular target for the Ewing's sarcoma-Wilms' tumor 1 fusion protein." J Biol Chem **271**(32): 19304–9.

Key, T. J., P. N. Appleby, A. W. Roddam, (2010). Endogenous Hormones and Breast Cancer Collaborative Group. "Insulin-like growth factor 1 (IGF1), IGF binding protein 3 (IGFBP3), and breast cancer risk: pooled individual data analysis of 17 prospective studies." Lancet Oncol **11**(6): 530–42.

Kiaris, H., M. Koutsilieris et al. (2003). "Growth hormone-releasing hormone and extra- pituitary tumorigenesis: therapeutic and diagnostic applications of growth hormone-releasing hormone antagonists." Expert Opin Investig Drugs **12**(8):1385–94.

Kiely, P. A., D. O'Gorman, et al. (2006). "Insulin-like growth factor I controls a mutually exclusive association of RACK1 with protein phosphatase 2A and beta1 integrin to promote cell migration." Mol Cell Biol **26**(11): 4041–51.

Kim, H. J., B. C. Litzenburger, et al. (2007). "Constitutively active type I insulin-like growth factor receptor causes transformation and xenograft growth of immortalized mammary epithelial cells and is accompanied by an epithelial-to-mesenchymal transition mediated by NF-kappaB and snail." Mol Cell Biol **27**(8): 3165–75.

Kjoller, L. and A. Hall (1999). "Signaling to Rho GTPases." Exp Cell Res **253**(1): 166–79.

Kleer, C. G., K. L. van Golen, et al. (2002). "Characterization of RhoC expression in benign and malignant breast disease: a potential new marker for small breast carcinomas with metastatic ability." Am J Pathol **160**(2): 579–84.

Kleinberg, D. L., M. Feldman, et al. (2000). "IGF-I: an essential factor in terminal end bud formation and ductal morphogenesis." J Mammary Gland Biol Neoplasia **5**(1): 7–17.

Klemke, R. L., M. Yebra, et al. (1994). "Receptor tyrosine kinase signaling required for integrin alpha v beta 5-directed cell motility but not adhesion on vitronectin." J Cell Biol **127**(3): 859–66.

Knudsen, K. A., A. P. Soler, et al. (1995). "Interaction of alpha-actinin with the cadherin/catenin cell-cell adhesion complex via alpha-catenin." J Cell Biol **130**(1): 67–77.

Lacey, J. V., Jr., A. W. Hsing, et al. (2001). "Null association between insulin-like growth factors, insulin-like growth factor-binding proteins, and prostate cancer in a prospective study." Cancer Epidemiol Biomarkers Prev **10**(10): 1101–2.

Lang, S. A., C. Moser, et al. (2007). "Targeting heat shock protein 90 in pancreatic cancer impairs insulin-like growth factor-I receptor signaling, disrupts an interleukin-6/signal-transducer and activator of transcription 3/hypoxia-inducible factor-1alpha autocrine loop, and reduces orthotopic tumor growth." Clin Cancer Res **13**(21): 6459–68.

Laughner, E., P. Taghavi, et al. (2001). "HER2 (neu) signaling increases the rate of hypoxia-inducible factor 1alpha (HIF-1alpha) synthesis: novel mechanism for HIF-1-mediated vascular endothelial growth factor expression." Mol Cell Biol **21**(12): 3995–4004.

Lavoie, J. N., G. L'Allemain, et al. (1996). "Cyclin D1 expression is regulated positively by the p42/p44MAPK and negatively by the p38/HOGMAPK pathway." J Biol Chem **271**(34): 20608–16.

LeRoith, D. (2007). "Insulin glargine and receptor-mediated signalling: clinical implications in treating type 2 diabetes." Diabetes Metab Res Rev **23**(8): 593–9.

Lee, A. V., J. G. Jackson, et al. (1999). "Enhancement of insulin-like growth factor signaling in human breast cancer: estrogen regulation of insulin receptor substrate-1 expression in vitro and in vivo." Mol Endocrinol **13**(5): 787–96.

Lee, D.Y., H.K. Yee et al. (2002). "Enhanced expression of insulin-like growth factor binding protein-3 sensitizes the growth inhibitory effect of anticancer drugs in gastric cancer cells." Biochem Biophys Res Commun **294**(2): 480–6.

Leger, B., R. Cartoni, et al. (2006). "Akt signalling through GSK-3beta, mTOR and Foxo1 is involved in human skeletal muscle hypertrophy and atrophy." J Physiol **576**(Pt 3): 923–33.

Li, S., D. Zhang, et al. (2009). "The IGF-I receptor can alter the matrix metalloproteinase repertoire of tumor cells through transcriptional regulation of PKC-{alpha}." Mol Endocrinol **23**(12): 2013–25.

Lip P.L., S. Chatterjee et al. (2004). "Plasma vascular endothelial growth factor, angiopoietin-2, and soluble angiopoietin receptor tie-2 in diabetic retinopathy: effects of laser photocoagulation and angiotensin receptor blockade." Br J Opthamol **88**(12):1543–6.

Litzenburger, B.C., H.J. Kim et al. (2009). "BMS-536924 reverses IGF-IR-induced transformation of mammary epithelial cells and causes growth inhibition and polarization of MCF7 cells." Clin Cancer Res **15**(1):226–37.

Lopez, T. and D. Hanahan (2002). "Elevated levels of IGF-1 receptor convey invasive and metastatic capability in a mouse model of pancreatic islet tumorigenesis." Cancer Cell **1**(4): 339–53.

Lynch, L., P. I. Vodyanik, et al. (2005). "Insulin-like growth factor I controls adhesion strength mediated by alpha5beta1 integrins in motile carcinoma cells." Mol Biol Cell **16**(1): 51–63.

Ma, J., M. N. Pollak, et al. (1999). "Prospective study of colorectal cancer risk in men and plasma levels of insulin-like growth factor (IGF)-I and IGF-binding protein-3." J Natl Cancer Inst **91**(7): 620–5.

Ma, Y. and L. M. Hendershot (2004). "The role of the unfolded protein response in tumour development: friend or foe?" Nat Rev Cancer **4**(12): 966–77.

Manes, S., M. Llorente, et al. (1999). "The matrix metalloproteinase-9 regulates the insulin-like growth factor-triggered autocrine response in DU-145 carcinoma cells." J Biol Chem **274**(11): 6935–45.

Manes, S., E. Mira, et al. (1997). "Identification of insulin-like growth factor-binding protein-1 as a potential physiological substrate for human stromelysin-3." J Biol Chem **272**(41): 25706–12.

Manousos, O., J. Souglakos, et al. (1999). "IGF-I and IGF-II in relation to colorectal cancer." Int J Cancer **83**(1): 15–7.

Mantzoros, C. S., A. Tzonou, et al. (1997). "Insulin-like growth factor 1 in relation to prostate cancer and benign prostatic hyperplasia." Br J Cancer **76**(9): 1115–8.

Maor, S. B., S. Abramovitch, et al. (2000). "BRCA1 suppresses insulin-like growth factor-I receptor promoter activity: potential interaction between BRCA1 and Sp1." Mol Genet Metab **69**(2): 130–6.

Maor, S., A. Yosepovich et al. (2007). "Elevated insulin-like growth factor −1 receptor (IGF-1R) levels in primary breast tumors associated with BRCA1 mutations". Cancer Lett **257**(2): 236–43.

Marelli, M. M., R. M. Moretti, et al. (2006). "Insulin-like growth factor-I promotes migration in human androgen-independent prostate cancer cells via the alphavbeta3 integrin and PI3-K/Akt signaling." Int J Oncol **28**(3): 723–30.

Metalli, D., F. Lovat, et al. (2010). "The Insulin-Like Growth Factor Receptor I Promotes Motility and Invasion of Bladder Cancer Cells through Akt- and Mitogen-Activated Protein Kinase-Dependent Activation of Paxillin." Am J Pathol.

Meyer, G. E., E. Shelden, et al. (2001). "Insulin-like growth factor I stimulates motility in human neuroblastoma cells." Oncogene **20**(51): 7542–50.

Miki, H. and T. Takenawa (2003). "Regulation of actin dynamics by WASP family proteins." J Biochem **134**(3): 309–13.

Miller, T. W., M. Perez-Torres, et al. (2009). "Loss of Phosphatase and Tensin homologue deleted on chromosome 10 engages ErbB3 and insulin-like growth factor-I receptor signaling to promote antiestrogen resistance in breast cancer." Cancer Res **69**(10): 4192–201.

Mira, E., S. Manes, et al. (1999). "Insulin-like growth factor I-triggered cell migration and invasion are mediated by matrix metalloproteinase-9." Endocrinology **140**(4): 1657–64.

Mitchison, T. J. and L. P. Cramer (1996). "Actin-based cell motility and cell locomotion." Cell **84**(3): 371–9.

Mitsiades, C.S, N.S. Mitsiades et al. (2004). "Inhibition of the insulin-like growth factor receptor-1 tyrosine kinase activity as a therapeutic strategy for multiple myeloma, other hematologic malignancies, and solid tumors." Cancer Cell **5**(3):221–30.

Mitsiades, N., W. H. Yu, et al. (2001). "Matrix metalloproteinase-7-mediated cleavage of Fas ligand protects tumor cells from chemotherapeutic drug cytotoxicity." Cancer Res **61**(2): 577–81.

Miyashita, T., Y. Takeishi, et al. (2001). "Role of calcineurin in insulin-like growth factor-1-induced hypertrophy of cultured adult rat ventricular myocytes." Jpn Circ J **65**(9): 815–9.

Moore, T., S. Carbajal, et al. (2008). "Reduced susceptibility to two-stage skin carcinogenesis in mice with low circulating insulin-like growth factor I levels." Cancer Res **68**(10): 3680–8.

Moorehead, R. A., O. H. Sanchez, et al. (2003). "Transgenic overexpression of IGF-II induces spontaneous lung tumors: a model for human lung adenocarcinoma." Oncogene **22**(6): 853–7.

Morali, O. G., V. Delmas, et al. (2001). "IGF-II induces rapid beta-catenin relocation to the nucleus during epithelium to mesenchyme transition." Oncogene **20**(36): 4942–50.

Morris, J. K., L. M. George, et al. (2006). "Insulin-like growth factors and cancer: no role in screening. Evidence from the BUPA study and meta-analysis of prospective epidemiological studies." Br J Cancer **95**(1): 112–7.

Mukohara, T., H. Shimada et al. (2009). "Sensitivity of breast cancer cell lines to the novel insulin-like growth factor-1 receptor (IGF-1R) inhibitor NVP-AEW541 is dependent on the level of IRS-1 expression Cancer Lett **282**(1):14–24.

Musaro, A., K. J. McCullagh, et al. (1999). "IGF-1 induces skeletal myocyte hypertrophy through calcineurin in association with GATA-2 and NF-ATc1." Nature **400**(6744): 581–5.

Nakamura, M., S. Miyamoto, et al. (2005). "Matrix metalloproteinase-7 degrades all insulin-like growth factor binding proteins and facilitates insulin-like growth factor bioavailability." Biochem Biophys Res Commun **333**(3): 1011–6.

Nanni, P., Nicoletti, G. et al (2010). High metastatic efficiency of human sarcoma cells in Rag2/γc double knockout mice provides a powerful test system for antimetastatic targeted therapy. European Journal of Cardiovascular prevention and rehabilitation **46** (3):659–68.

Navab, R., C. Pedraza, et al. (2008). "Loss of responsiveness to IGF-I in cells with reduced cathepsin L expression levels." Oncogene **27**(37): 4973–85.

Ng, E. H., C. Y. Ji, et al. (1998). "Altered serum levels of insulin-like growth-factor binding proteins in breast cancer patients." Ann Surg Oncol **5**(2): 194–201.

Nishiya, N., W. B. Kiosses, et al. (2005). "An alpha4 integrin-paxillin-Arf-GAP complex restricts Rac activation to the leading edge of migrating cells." Nat Cell Biol **7**(4): 343–52.

Nobes, C. and A. Hall (1994). "Regulation and function of the Rho subfamily of small GTPases." Curr Opin Genet Dev **4**(1): 77–81.

Novosyadlyy, R., N. Kurshan, et al. (2008). "Insulin-like growth factor-I protects cells from ER stress-induced apoptosis via enhancement of the adaptive capacity of endoplasmic reticulum." Cell Death Differ **15**(8): 1304–17.

Nussbaum, T., J. Samarin, et al. (2008). "Autocrine insulin-like growth factor-II stimulation of tumor cell migration is a progression step in human hepatocarcinogenesis." Hepatology **48**(1): 146–56.

Ohira, T., R. M. Gemmill, et al. (2003). "WNT7a induces E-cadherin in lung cancer cells." Proc Natl Acad Sci USA **100**(18): 10429–34.

Ohlsson, C., N. Kley, et al. (1998). "p53 regulates insulin-like growth factor-I (IGF-I) receptor expression and IGF-I-induced tyrosine phosphorylation in an osteosarcoma cell line: interaction between p53 and Sp1." Endocrinology **139**(3): 1101–7.

Okawa, Y., T. Hideshima, et al. (2009). "SNX-2112, a selective Hsp90 inhibitor, potently inhibits tumor cell growth, angiogenesis, and osteoclastogenesis in multiple myeloma and other hematologic tumors by abrogating signaling via Akt and ERK." Blood **113**(4): 846–55.

Olivo-Marston, S. E., S. D. Hursting, et al. (2009). "Genetic reduction of circulating insulin-like growth factor-1 inhibits azoxymethane-induced colon tumorigenesis in mice." Mol Carcinog **48**(12): 1071–6.

Oshima, T., M. Akaike, et al. (2008). "Clinicopathological significance of the gene expression of matrix metalloproteinase-7, insulin-like growth factor-1, insulin-like growth factor-2 and insulin-like growth factor-1 receptor in patients with colorectal cancer: insulin-like growth factor-1 receptor gene expression is a useful predictor of liver metastasis from colorectal cancer." Oncol Rep **20**(2): 359–64.

Oyadomari, S. and M. Mori (2004). "Roles of CHOP/GADD153 in endoplasmic reticulum stress." Cell Death Differ **11**(4): 381–9.

Palmqvist, R., G. Hallmans, et al. (2002). "Plasma insulin-like growth factor 1, insulin-like growth factor binding protein 3, and risk of colorectal cancer: a prospective study in northern Sweden." Gut **50**(5): 642–6.

Pang, Y., B. Zheng, et al. (2007). "IGF-1 protects oligodendrocyte progenitors against TNFalpha-induced damage by activation of PI3K/Akt and interruption of the mitochondrial apoptotic pathway." Glia **55**(11): 1099–107.

Papa, V., B. Gliozzo, et al. (1993). "Insulin-like growth factor-I receptors are overexpressed and predict a low risk in human breast cancer." Cancer Res **53**(16): 3736–40.

Párrizas, M., A Gazit et al. (1997). "Specific inhibition of insulin-like growth factor-1 and insulin receptor tyrosine kinase activity and biological function by tyrphostins." Endocrinology **138**(4):1427–33.

Park, E.J., J.H. Lee et al. (2010). "Dietary and genetic obesity promote liver inflammation and tumorigenesis by enhancing IL-6 and TNF expression." Cell **140**(2):197–208.

Park, I. H., E. Erbay, et al. (2005). "Skeletal myocyte hypertrophy requires mTOR kinase activity and S6K1." Exp Cell Res **309**(1): 211–9.

Parsons, S. A., D. P. Millay, et al. (2004). "Genetic loss of calcineurin blocks mechanical overload-induced skeletal muscle fiber type switching but not hypertrophy." J Biol Chem **279**(25): 26192–200.

Peinado, H., D. Olmeda, et al. (2007). "Snail, Zeb and bHLH factors in tumour progression: an alliance against the epithelial phenotype?" Nat Rev Cancer **7**(6): 415–28.

Pennacchietti, S., P. Michieli, et al. (2003). "Hypoxia promotes invasive growth by transcriptional activation of the met protooncogene." Cancer Cell **3**(4): 347–61.

Perks,C.M, C. McCaig et al. (2000). "Differential insulin-like growth factor (IGF)- independent interactions of IGF binding protein-3 and IGF binding protein-5 on apoptosis in human breast cancer cells. Involvement of the mitochondria." J Cell Biochem **80**(2):248–58.

Peruzzi, F., M. Prisco, et al. (1999). "Multiple signaling pathways of the insulin-like growth factor 1 receptor in protection from apoptosis." Mol Cell Biol **19**(10): 7203–15.

Peruzzi, F., M. Prisco, et al. (2001). "Anti-apoptotic signaling of the insulin-like growth factor-I receptor through mitochondrial translocation of c-Raf and Nedd4." J Biol Chem **276**(28): 25990–6.

Petridou, E., P. Koukoulomatis, et al. (2003). "Endometrial cancer and the IGF system: a case-control study in Greece." Oncology **64**(4): 341–5.

Petridou, E., Y. Papadiamantis, et al. (2000). "Leptin and insulin growth factor I in relation to breast cancer (Greece)." Cancer Causes Control **11**(5): 383–8.

Peyrat, J. P., J. Bonneterre, et al. (1988). "Presence and characterization of insulin-like growth factor 1 receptors in human benign breast disease." Eur J Cancer Clin Oncol **24**(9): 1425–31.

Pietrzkowski Z., G. Mulholland et al. (1993). "Inhibition of growth of prostatic cancer cell lines by peptide analogues of insulin-like growth factor 1." Cancer Res **53**(5):1102–6.

Pollak, M., M. J. Blouin, et al. (2001). "Reduced mammary gland carcinogenesis in transgenic mice expressing a growth hormone antagonist." Br J Cancer **85**(3): 428–30.

Pollak, M. N., J. F. Perdue, et al. (1987). "Presence of somatomedin receptors on primary human breast and colon carcinomas." Cancer Lett **38**(1–2): 223–30.

Pollak, M. N., C. Polychronakos, et al. (1988). "Characterization of insulin-like growth factor I (IGF-I) receptors of human breast cancer cells." Biochem Biophys Res Commun **154**(1): 326–31.

Pollak,M.N. and A.V. Schally (1998). "Mechanisms of antineoplastic action of somatostatin analogs." Proc Soc Exp Biol Med **217**(2):143–52.

Poulaki, V., C. S. Mitsiades, et al. (2003). "Regulation of vascular endothelial growth factor expression by insulin-like growth factor I in thyroid carcinomas." J Clin Endocrinol Metab **88**(11): 5392–8.

Powell, W. C., B. Fingleton, et al. (1999). "The metalloproteinase matrilysin proteolytically generates active soluble Fas ligand and potentiates epithelial cell apoptosis." Curr Biol **9**(24): 1441–7.

Qiang, Y. W., L. Yao, et al. (2004). "Insulin-like growth factor I induces migration and invasion of human multiple myeloma cells." Blood **103**(1): 301–8.

Quinn, L. S., B. G. Anderson, et al. (2007). "Muscle-specific overexpression of the type 1 IGF receptor results in myoblast-independent muscle hypertrophy via PI3K, and not calcineurin, signaling." Am J Physiol Endocrinol Metab **293**(6): E1538-51.

Raftopoulou, M. and A. Hall (2004). "Cell migration: Rho GTPases lead the way." Dev Biol **265**(1): 23–32.

Railo, M. J., K. von Smitten, et al. (1994). "The prognostic value of insulin-like growth factor-I in breast cancer patients. Results of a follow-up study on 126 patients." Eur J Cancer **30A**(3): 307–11.

Ramsey, M. M., R. L. Ingram, et al. (2002). "Growth hormone-deficient dwarf animals are resistant to dimethylbenzanthracine (DMBA)-induced mammary carcinogenesis." Endocrinology **143**(10): 4139–42.

Remacle-Bonnet, M., F. Garrouste, et al. (2005). "Membrane rafts segregate pro- from anti-apoptotic insulin-like growth factor-I receptor signaling in colon carcinoma cells stimulated by members of the tumor necrosis factor superfamily." Am J Pathol **167**(3): 761–73.

Renehan, A. G., M. Zwahlen, et al. (2004). "Insulin-like growth factor (IGF)-I, IGF binding protein-3, and cancer risk: systematic review and meta-regression analysis." Lancet **363**(9418): 1346–53.

Rinaldi, S., P. H. Peeters, et al. (2006). "IGF-I, IGFBP-3 and breast cancer risk in women: The European Prospective Investigation into Cancer and Nutrition (EPIC)." Endocr Relat Cancer **13**(2): 593–605.

Rosenthal, S. M. and Z. Q. Cheng (1995). "Opposing early and late effects of insulin-like growth factor I on differentiation and the cell cycle regulatory retinoblastoma protein in skeletal myoblasts." Proc Natl Acad Sci USA **92**(22): 10307–11.

Ross, M.H. and G. Bras (1971). "Lasting influence of early caloric restriction on prevalence of neoplasms in the rat." J Natl Cancer Inst **47**(5):1095–113.

Ruan, W. and D. L. Kleinberg (1999). "Insulin-like growth factor I is essential for terminal end bud formation and ductal morphogenesis during mammary development." Endocrinology **140**(11): 5075–81.

Sachdev, D., J. S. Hartell, et al. (2004). "A dominant negative type I insulin-like growth factor receptor inhibits metastasis of human cancer cells." J Biol Chem **279**(6): 5017–24.

Sachdev, P., Y. X. Jiang, et al. (2001). "Differential requirement for Rho family GTPases in an oncogenic insulin-like growth factor-I receptor-induced cell transformation." J Biol Chem **276**(28): 26461–71.

Sah, V. P., T. M. Seasholtz, et al. (2000). "The role of Rho in G protein-coupled receptor signal transduction." Annu Rev Pharmacol Toxicol **40**: 459–89.

Sakatani, T., A. Kaneda, et al. (2005). "Loss of imprinting of Igf2 alters intestinal maturation and tumorigenesis in mice." Science **307**(5717): 1976–8.

Salani, B., L. Briatore, et al. (2008). "Caveolin-1 down-regulation inhibits insulin-like growth factor-I receptor signal transduction in H9C2 rat cardiomyoblasts." Endocrinology **149**(2): 461–5.

Schakman, O., S. Kalista, et al. (2008). "Role of Akt/GSK-3beta/beta-catenin transduction pathway in the muscle anti-atrophy action of insulin-like growth factor-I in glucocorticoid-treated rats." Endocrinology **149**(8): 3900–8.

Schernhammer, E. S., J. M. Holly, et al. (2006). "Insulin-like growth factor-I, its binding proteins (IGFBP-1 and IGFBP-3), and growth hormone and breast cancer risk in The Nurses Health Study II." Endocr Relat Cancer **13**(2): 583–92.

Schroder, M. and R. J. Kaufman (2005). "ER stress and the unfolded protein response." Mutat Res **569**(1–2): 29–63.

Semenza, G. L. (2003). "Targeting HIF-1 for cancer therapy." Nat Rev Cancer **3**(10): 721–32.

Semsarian, C., M. J. Wu, et al. (1999). "Skeletal muscle hypertrophy is mediated by a Ca^{2+}–dependent calcineurin signalling pathway." Nature **400**(6744): 576–81.

Severi, G., H. A. Morris, et al. (2006). "Circulating insulin-like growth factor-I and binding protein-3 and risk of prostate cancer." Cancer Epidemiol Biomarkers Prev 15(6): 1137–41.

Shi, R., H. Yu, et al. (2004). "IGF-I and breast cancer: a meta-analysis." Int J Cancer 111(3): 418–23.

Shields, S. K., C. Nicola, et al. (2007). "Rho guanosine 5'-triphosphatases differentially regulate insulin-like growth factor I (IGF-I) receptor-dependent and -independent actions of IGF-II on human trophoblast migration." Endocrinology 148(10): 4906–17.

Shimizu, C., T. Hasegawa, et al. (2004). "Expression of insulin-like growth factor 1 receptor in primary breast cancer: immunohistochemical analysis." Hum Pathol 35(12): 1537–42.

Skobe, M., T. Hawighorst, et al. (2001). "Induction of tumor lymphangiogenesis by VEGF-C promotes breast cancer metastasis." Nat Med 7(2): 192–8.

Srinivasan, S., M. Ohsugi, et al. (2005). "Endoplasmic reticulum stress-induced apoptosis is partly mediated by reduced insulin signaling through phosphatidylinositol 3-kinase/Akt and increased glycogen synthase kinase-3beta in mouse insulinoma cells." Diabetes 54(4): 968–75.

Stacker, S. A., C. Caesar, et al. (2001). "VEGF-D promotes the metastatic spread of tumor cells via the lymphatics." Nat Med 7(2): 186–91.

Stattin, P., A. Bylund, et al. (2000). "Plasma insulin-like growth factor-I, insulin-like growth factor-binding proteins, and prostate cancer risk: a prospective study." J Natl Cancer Inst 92(23): 1910–7.

Stitt, T. N., D. Drujan, et al. (2004). "The IGF-1/PI3K/Akt pathway prevents expression of muscle atrophy-induced ubiquitin ligases by inhibiting FOXO transcription factors." Mol Cell 14(3): 395–403.

Stoeltzing, O., W. Liu, et al. (2007). "Regulation of cyclooxygenase-2 (COX-2) expression in human pancreatic carcinoma cells by the insulin-like growth factor-I receptor (IGF-IR) system." Cancer Lett 258(2): 291–300.

Stracke, M. L., J. D. Engel, et al. (1989). "The type I insulin-like growth factor receptor is a motility receptor in human melanoma cells." J Biol Chem 264(36): 21544–9.

Sugumar, A., Y. C. Liu, et al. (2004). "Insulin-like growth factor (IGF)-I and IGF-binding protein 3 and the risk of premenopausal breast cancer: a meta-analysis of literature." Int J Cancer 111(2): 293–7.

Surmacz, E. (2003) "Growth factor receptors as therapeutic targets: strategies to inhibit the insulin-like growth factor I receptor." Oncogene 22(42): 6589–97.

Suwa, H., G. Ohshio, et al. (1998). "Overexpression of the rhoC gene correlates with progression of ductal adenocarcinoma of the pancreas." Br J Cancer 77(1): 147–52.

Szereday Z., A.V. Schally et al. (2003). "Effective treatment of H838 human non-small cell lung carcinoma with a targeted cytotoxic somatostatin analog, AN-238." Int J Oncol 22(5): 1141–6.

Takeichi, M. (1991). "Cadherin cell adhesion receptors as a morphogenetic regulator." Science 251(5000): 1451–5.

Takenawa, T. and H. Miki (2001). "WASP and WAVE family proteins: key molecules for rapid rearrangement of cortical actin filaments and cell movement." J Cell Sci 114(Pt 10): 1801–9.

Tanaka, H., M. Yamamoto, et al. (2006). "Hypoxia-independent overexpression of hypoxia-inducible factor 1alpha as an early change in mouse hepatocarcinogenesis." Cancer Res 66(23): 11263–70.

Tanno, S., S. Tanno, et al. (2001). "AKT activation up-regulates insulin-like growth factor I receptor expression and promotes invasiveness of human pancreatic cancer cells." Cancer Res 61(2): 589–93.

Taya, S., N. Inagaki, et al. (2001). "Direct interaction of insulin-like growth factor-1 receptor with leukemia-associated RhoGEF." J Cell Biol 155(5): 809–20.

Tennant, M. K., J. B. Thrasher, et al. (1996). "Protein and messenger ribonucleic acid (mRNA) for the type 1 insulin-like growth factor (IGF) receptor is decreased and IGF-II mRNA is increased in human prostate carcinoma compared to benign prostate epithelium." J Clin Endocrinol Metab 81(10): 3774–82.

Thimmaiah, K. N., J. B. Easton, et al. (2010). "Protection from rapamycin-induced apoptosis by insulin-like growth factor-I is partially dependent on protein kinase C signaling." Cancer Res 70(5): 2000–9.

Tomizawa, M., F. Shinozaki, et al.(2010). "Insulin-like growth factor-I receptor in proliferation and motility of pancreatic cancer." World J Gastroenterol 16(15): 1854–8.

Toniolo, P., P. F. Bruning, et al. (2000). "Serum insulin-like growth factor-I and breast cancer." Int J Cancer **88**(5): 828–32.

Toyoshima, K., N. Ito, et al. (1971). "Tissue culture of urinary bladder tumor induced in a rat by N-butyl-N-(−4-hydroxybutyl)nitrosamine: establishment of cell line, Nara Bladder Tumor II." J Natl Cancer Inst **47**(5): 979–85.

Tsai, W. C., Y. C. Chao, et al. (2006). "Increasing EMMPRIN and matriptase expression in hepatocellular carcinoma: tissue microarray analysis of immunohistochemical scores with clinicopathological parameters." Histopathology **49**(4): 388–95.

Tseng, Y. H., K. Ueki, et al. (2002). "Differential roles of insulin receptor substrates in the antiapoptotic function of insulin-like growth factor-1 and insulin." J Biol Chem **277**(35): 31601–11.

Tsukatani, Y., K. Suzuki, et al. (1997). "Loss of density-dependent growth inhibition and dissociation of alpha-catenin from E-cadherin." J Cell Physiol **173**(1): 54–63.

Ueda, S., H. Tsuda, et al. (2006). "Alternative tyrosine phosphorylation of signaling kinases according to hormone receptor status in breast cancer overexpressing the insulin-like growth factor receptor type 1." Cancer Sci **97**(7): 597–604.

van der Kallen, C. J., M. M. van Greevenbroek, et al. (2009). "Endoplasmic reticulum stress-induced apoptosis in the development of diabetes: is there a role for adipose tissue and liver?" Apoptosis **14**(12): 1424–34.

van Golen, C. M., T. S. Schwab, et al. (2006). "Insulin-like growth factor-I receptor expression regulates neuroblastoma metastasis to bone." Cancer Res **66**(13): 6570–8.

van Golen, K. L., L. Bao, et al. (2002). "Reversion of RhoC GTPase-induced inflammatory breast cancer phenotype by treatment with a farnesyl transferase inhibitor." Mol Cancer Ther **1**(8): 575–83.

van Noord P.A. (2004). "Breast cancer and the brain: a neurodevelopmental hypothesis to explain the opposing effects of caloric deprivation during the Dutch famine of 1944–1945 on breast cancer and its risk factors." J Nutr **134**(12 Suppl): 3399S–3406S.

Van Saun M.N., I.K. Lee et al. (2009). "High fat diet induced hepatic steatosis establishes a permissive microenvironment for colorectal metastases and promotes primary dysplasia in a murine model." Am J Pathol **175**(1): 355–64.

Vasilcanu D., A. Girnita et al. (2004). "The cyclolignan PPP induces activation loop- specific inhibition of tyrosine phosphorylation of the insulin-like growth factor-1 receptor. Link to the phosphatidyl inositol-3 kinase/Akt apoptotic pathway." Oncogene **23**(47): 7854–62.

Vasioukhin, V., C. Bauer, et al. (2000). "Directed actin polymerization is the driving force for epithelial cell-cell adhesion." Cell **100**(2): 209–19.

Vousden, K. H. (2000). "p53: death star." Cell **103**(5): 691–4.

Vyas, D. R., E. E. Spangenburg, et al. (2002). "GSK-3beta negatively regulates skeletal myotube hypertrophy." Am J Physiol Cell Physiol **283**(2): C545–51.

Wahner Hendrickson A.E., P. Haluska et al (2009). "Expression of insulin receptor isoform A and insulin-like growth factor-1 receptor in human acute myelogenous leukemia: effect of the dual-receptor inhibitor BMS-536924 in vitro." Cancer Res **69**(19): 7635–43. In press.

Wan X., B. Harkavy et al. (2006). "Rapamycin induces feedback activation of Akt signaling through an IGF-1R-dependent mechanism." Oncogene **26**(13): 1932–40.

Wang, F., P. Herzmark, et al. (2002). "Lipid products of PI(3)Ks maintain persistent cell polarity and directed motility in neutrophils." Nat Cell Biol **4**(7): 513–8.

Wang, L., Y. Y. Shao, et al. (2010). "Thyroid hormone-mediated growth and differentiation of growth plate chondrocytes involves IGF-1 modulation of beta-catenin signaling." J Bone Miner Res.

Warshamana-Greene G.S., J. Litz et al. (2004). "The insulin-like growth factor-I (IGF-I) receptor kinase inhibitor NVP-ADW742, in combination with STI571, delineates a spectrum of dependence of small cell lung cancer on IGF-I and stem cell factor signaling." Mol Cancer Ther **3**(5): 527–35.

Weiner, O. D., P. O. Neilsen, et al. (2002). "A PtdInsP(3)- and Rho GTPase-mediated positive feedback loop regulates neutrophil polarity." Nat Cell Biol **4**(7): 509–13.

Werner, H., G. G. Re, et al. (1993). "Increased expression of the insulin-like growth factor I receptor gene, IGF1R, in Wilms tumor is correlated with modulation of IGF1R promoter activity by the WT1 Wilms tumor gene product." Proc Natl Acad Sci USA **90**(12): 5828–32.

Werner, H., F. J. Rauscher, et al. (1994). "Transcriptional repression of the insulin-like growth factor I receptor (IGF-I-R) gene by the tumor suppressor WT1 involves binding to sequences both upstream and downstream of the IGF-I-R gene transcription start site." J Biol Chem **269**(17): 12577–82.

Werner, H., E. Karnieli, et al. (1996). "Wild-type and mutant p53 differentially regulate transcription of the insulin-like growth factor I receptor gene." Proc Natl Acad Sci USA **93**(16): 8318–23.

Whitelock, J. M., A. D. Murdoch, et al. (1996). "The degradation of human endothelial cell-derived perlecan and release of bound basic fibroblast growth factor by stromelysin, collagenase, plasmin, and heparanases." J Biol Chem **271**(17): 10079–86.

Wilker, E., D. Bol, et al. (1999). "Enhancement of susceptibility to diverse skin tumor promoters by activation of the insulin-like growth factor-1 receptor in the epidermis of transgenic mice." Mol Carcinog **25**(2): 122–31.

Wolf S., J. Lorenz et al. (2010). "Treatment of biliary tract cancer with NVP-AEW541: mechanisms of action and resistance." World J Gastroenterol **16**(2): 156–66.

Wolk, A., C. S. Mantzoros, et al. (1998). "Insulin-like growth factor 1 and prostate cancer risk: a population-based, case-control study." J Natl Cancer Inst **90**(12): 911–5.

Woodson, K., J. A. Tangrea, et al. (2003). "Serum insulin-like growth factor I: tumor marker or etiologic factor? A prospective study of prostate cancer among Finnish men." Cancer Res **63**(14): 3991–4.

Wu, Y., S. Yakar, et al. (2002). "Circulating insulin-like growth factor-I levels regulate colon cancer growth and metastasis." Cancer Res **62**(4): 1030–5.

Wu, Y., K. Cui, et al. (2003). "Reduced circulating insulin-like growth factor I levels delay the onset of chemically and genetically induced mammary tumors." Cancer Res **63**(15): 4384–8.

Wu, Y., P. Brodt, et al. (2010)"Insulin-like growth factor-I regulates the liver microenvironment in obese mice and promotes liver metastasis." Cancer Res **70**(1): 57–67.

Xu, J., D. Rodriguez, et al. (2001). "Proteolytic exposure of a cryptic site within collagen type IV is required for angiogenesis and tumor growth in vivo." J Cell Biol **154**(5): 1069–79.

Yamaguchi, H., M. Shiraishi, et al. (2009). "MARCKS regulates lamellipodia formation induced by IGF-I via association with PIP2 and beta-actin at membrane microdomains." J Cell Physiol **220**(3): 748–55.

Yamazaki, D., S. Kurisu, et al. (2005). "Regulation of cancer cell motility through actin reorganization." Cancer Sci **96**(7): 379–86.

Yang, X. F., W. G. Beamer, et al. (1996). "Reduced growth of human breast cancer xenografts in hosts homozygous for the lit mutation." Cancer Res **56**(7): 1509–11.

Yao, H., E. J. Dashner, et al. (2006). "RhoC GTPase is required for PC-3 prostate cancer cell invasion but not motility." Oncogene **25**(16): 2285–96.

Ye, P., Q. Hu, et al. (2010) "beta-catenin mediates insulin-like growth factor-I actions to promote cyclin D1 mRNA expression, cell proliferation and survival in oligodendroglial cultures." Glia.

Yu, H. and T. Rohan (2000). "Role of the insulin-like growth factor family in cancer development and progression." J Natl Cancer Inst **92**(18): 1472–89.

Yu, H., M. R. Spitz, et al. (1999). "Plasma levels of insulin-like growth factor-I and lung cancer risk: a case-control analysis." J Natl Cancer Inst **91**(2): 151–6.

Yuen, J. S., M. E. Cockman, et al. (2007). "The VHL tumor suppressor inhibits expression of the IGF1R and its loss induces IGF1R upregulation in human clear cell renal carcinoma." Oncogene **26**(45): 6499–508.

Zhang, D., M. Bar-Eli et al (2004). Dual regulation of MMP-2 Expression by the Type 1 insulin-like Growth Factor Receptor. Journal Biol Chem **279**: 19683–19690.

Zhang, X. and D. Yee (2002). "Insulin-like Growth Factor Binding Protein-1 (IGFBP-1) inhibits Breast Cancer Cell Motility". Cancer Res **62**: 4369–75.

Zhang, X., S. Kamaraju, et al. (2004). "Motility response to insulin-like growth factor-I (IGF-I) in MCF-7 cells is associated with IRS-2 activation and integrin expression." Breast Cancer Res Treat **83**(2): 161–70.

Zhang, X., M. Lin, et al. (2005). "Multiple signaling pathways are activated during insulin-like growth factor-I (IGF-I) stimulated breast cancer cell migration." Breast Cancer Res Treat **93**(2): 159–68.

Zhao, H., J. Dupont, et al. (2004). "PTEN inhibits cell proliferation and induces apoptosis by downregulating cell surface IGF-IR expression in prostate cancer cells." Oncogene **23**(3): 786–94.

Zhao, H., H. B. Grossman, et al. (2003). "Plasma levels of insulin-like growth factor-1 and binding protein-3, and their association with bladder cancer risk." J Urol **169**(2): 714–7.

Zhau, H. E., V. Odero-Marah, et al. (2008). "Epithelial to mesenchymal transition (EMT) in human prostate cancer: lessons learned from ARCaP model." Clin Exp Metastasis **25**(6): 601–10.

Zhong, H., K. Chiles, et al. (2000). "Modulation of hypoxia-inducible factor 1alpha expression by the epidermal growth factor/phosphatidylinositol 3-kinase/PTEN/AKT/FRAP pathway in human prostate cancer cells: implications for tumor angiogenesis and therapeutics." Cancer Res **60**(6): 1541–5.

Zou, C. G., X. Z. Cao, et al. (2009). "The molecular mechanism of endoplasmic reticulum stress-induced apoptosis in PC-12 neuronal cells: the protective effect of insulin-like growth factor I." Endocrinology **150**(1): 277–85.

Chapter 7
Insulin-Like Growth Factor Signaling in Pediatric Sarcomas

Xiaolin Wan, Su Young Kim, and Lee J. Helman

Introduction

Members of the insulin-like growth factor (IGF) family include three cognate ligands [insulin, IGF-I, IGF-II], four cell-membrane receptors [IGF-1R, IGF receptor type 2 (IGF-2R), insulin receptor isoform A (IR-A), insulin receptor isoform B (IR-B)], three hybrid receptors [IGF-1R/IR-A, IGF-1R/IR-B, IR-A/IR-B] and at least six IGF-binding proteins [IGF-BP1-6] (Fig. 7.1) (Pollak et al. 2004; Samani et al. 2007). Binding of IGF-1R by ligand leads to activation of the phosphatidylinositol 3-kinase (PI3K)/Akt/mammalian target of rapamycin (mTOR) and of the mitogen-activated protein kinase (MAPK) pathways (Fig. 7.1) (Pollak et al. 2004).

Sarcomas are rare malignancies of mesenchymal origin that can arise anywhere in the body, but most commonly affect bone, muscle, and connective tissue. Whereas sarcomas comprise only 1% of adult cancers, they make up a much larger percentage of pediatric cases, accounting for 10–15% of all newly diagnosed cancers in children and young adults in the USA (Helman and Meltzer 2003; Raney et al. 2001). Several sarcomas, such as alveolar rhabdomyosarcoma (RMS), Ewing's sarcoma, and synovial sarcoma, occur in younger patients and are characterized by tumor-specific chromosomal translocations, whereas other sarcomas, such as leiomyosarcoma and malignant fibrous histiocytoma, occur more frequently in older adults and are characterized by chaotic karyotypes accompanied by frequent chromosome copy number changes (Helman and Meltzer 2003). The topic of this review

---

L.J. Helman (✉)
Pediatric Oncology Branch, Center for Cancer Research,
National Cancer Institute, National Institute of Health,
Bethesda, MD, USA
e-mail: helmanl@nih.gov

D. LeRoith (ed.), *Insulin-like Growth Factors and Cancer: From Basic Biology to Therapeutics*, Cancer Drug Discovery and Development, DOI 10.1007/978-1-4614-0598-6_7, © Springer Science+Business Media, LLC 2012

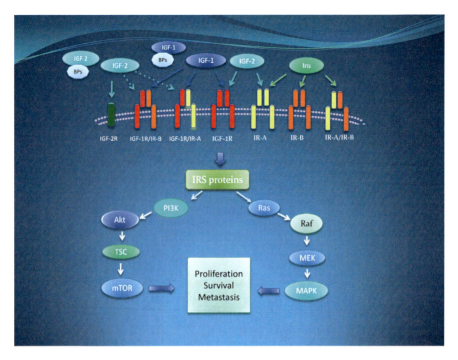

Fig. 7.1 A schematic representation of the key components of the IGF signaling pathway. The ligands IGF-I, IGF-II, and insulin bind to their receptors IGF-1R, IGF-2R, IR-A, and IR-B, as well as a host of hybrid receptors, with varying affinities. The bioavailability of IGF-I and IGF-II are mediated by binding to IGF-BPs. Binding of IGF-II to IGF-2R does not transduce a signal, due to lack of a cytoplasmic signaling domain in the latter. In contrast, binding of IGF-I or IGF-II to IGF-1R leads to autophosphorylation of its tyrosine kinase domain and subsequent activation of downstream signaling pathways, including the PI3K/Akt/mTOR and the Ras/Raf/MAPK signaling pathways, thus promoting cell proliferation, survival, and metastasis

is IGF signaling, which is aberrantly activated in a variety of sarcomas and has a central role in the regulation of cancer cell growth. We discuss the potential for targeting this pathway with a special focus on pediatric sarcomas.

The Role of IGF Signaling in Pediatric Sarcomas

Rhabdomyosarcoma

RMS is the most common pediatric soft tissue sarcoma, accounting for nearly 250 cases of childhood cancer in the USA yearly (Dagher and Helman 1999). Two major subtypes, alveolar (ARMS) and embryonal (ERMS), are associated with distinct clinical characteristics and genetic alterations. ARMS is characterized by nonrandom translocations involving the DNA binding domain of either *PAX3* on the long arm of chromosome 2 or *PAX7* on the short arm of chromosome 1 and the transactivation domain of the *FOXOA1* gene [t(2;13) (PAX3-FOXOA1) or t(1;13) (PAX7-FOXOA1)] (Merlino and Helman 1999).

Loss of heterozygosity (LOH) at chromosome 11p15.5 has been identified in ERMSs (Scrable et al. 1989). Of note, however, this LOH is associated with loss of the maternal allele and duplication of the paternal allele. Since IGF-II maps to 11p15.5 and IGF-II is normally imprinted at the maternal allele, this uniparental isodisomy could lead to a 2× IGF-II gene dosage from LOH. In addition, loss of imprinting (LOI) at the IGF-II locus has been found in ARMS, leading to re-expression of IGF-II from the normally silent (imprinted) maternal allele (Zhan et al. 1994). Thus, LOH or LOI can result in over-expression of IGF-II, which then can function in an autocrine manner to stimulate IGF-1R signaling.

Additional evidence that suggests the involvement of IGF-II in the development of ERMSs comes from mouse models. Mice heterozygous for the patched gene exhibited a high incidence of RMS and overexpressed IGF-II in these tumors (Hahn et al. 1998). Subsequent knockout of IGF-II in these patched-knockout mice resulted in abrogation of tumor formation (Hahn et al. 2000). Furthermore, cotransfection of IGF-II and a PAX3-FOXOA1 construct promoted tumorigenesis in the C2C12 mouse myoblast cell line (Wang et al. 1998). These results suggested that PAX3-FOXOA1 and IGF-II contributed to the oncogenesis of RMS.

Our recent study has shown that IGF-1R expression is detectable in virtually all RMS cell lines, although they differ in abundance by as much as 30-fold based on quantitative protein analysis. Five of nine primary tumor samples also had elevated IGF-1R levels (Cao et al. 2008). Genetic mutations in members of the IGF signaling pathway have not been identified to date, although to our knowledge, there has not yet been a systematic study that has examined every component in this pathway in RMS tumor samples. Taken together, these results suggest that IGF signaling plays an important role in the initiation and progression of RMS.

Ewing's Sarcoma Family of Tumors

Ewing's sarcoma family of tumors (ESFT) is the second most common malignant bone cancer of children and adolescents. The hallmark of ESFT is the characteristic *EWS/ETS* fusion transcription factor. Much of the biology of this tumor can be attributed to this translocation. However, the IGF signaling cascade is of critical importance to ESFT cells, both mediating the activity of the fusion protein and independently contributing to the oncogenic phenotype.

The importance of IGF signaling in ESFT was suggested by the demonstration of high-level expression of both IGF ligand and receptor in tumor samples and cell lines (Yee et al. 1990; Scotlandi et al. 1996). Treatment of these cell lines with a murine anti-IGF-1R antibody severely restricted cell growth, suggesting a role of the IGF cascade in the biology of this tumor (Yee et al. 1990;

Scotlandi et al. 1996). Subsequent studies have demonstrated the contributions of IGF signaling to all aspects of oncogenesis and progression. Toretsky et al. demonstrated the importance of both the EWS-FLI1 translocation and IGF signaling for soft colony agar formation in murine fibroblasts, suggesting a role for the pathway in malignant transformation (1997). More recently, studies on mouse mesenchymal stem cells, which are the presumed cell of origin of ESFT, have shown that the EWS–ETS fusion protein induces the expression of IGF-1 and may explain the permissiveness of these cells for the fusion protein (Cironi et al. 2008). Studies have also shown that continued expression of IGF is required in order to maintain the transformed phenotype, as expression of a dominant negative IGF-1R construct or blockade of the receptor severely impairs proliferation (Yee et al. 1990; Scotlandi et al. 1996). Furthermore, overexpression of the IGF pathway confers a resistant phenotype allowing cells to tolerate various chemotherapeutic agents (Manara et al. 2005).

The dynamic between EWS–ETS and the IGF pathway is likely one of the fundamental mechanisms in ESFT cells. Knockdown of EWS-FLI1 markedly reduced tumorigenicity in immunodeficient mice and downregulated IGF-I expression (Herrero-Martín et al. 2009). In addition, the fusion protein directly inhibits expression of IGF-BP3 leading to increased levels of free IGF ligand (Prieur et al. 2004). Unlike other models, in which silencing of EWS-FLI1 is not tolerated by cells, silencing is tolerated following inactivation of IGF-BP3, all of which is consistent with the permissiveness hypothesis described above (Prieur et al. 2004).

Osteosarcoma

Osteosarcoma is the most common bone tumor in children and young adults. The peak incidence of osteosarcoma occurs during adolescence, corresponding to both the growth spurt and peak concentrations of circulating growth hormone (GH) and IGF-1 (Calle and Kaaks 2004). The involvement of IGF signaling in osteosarcoma is supported by a number of studies that have suggested the role of IGF signaling in the survival, proliferation, invasion, and metastatic capability of osteosarcoma cells (Kappel et al. 1994: Benini et al. 1999; Burrow et al. 1998). High expression of IGF-1R has been observed in some osteosarcoma cell lines. In addition, the majority of osteosarcoma patient samples express IGF ligands and half also have high levels of IGF-1R (Benini et al. 1999; Burrow et al. 1998). Polymorphisms of IGF-2R have also been found in association with an increased risk of developing osteosarcoma (Savage et al. 2007). The mechanism whereby genetic variations in IGF-2R contribute to disease is unclear, since binding of ligand to IGF-2R does not lead to subsequent signaling, due to the lack of an intracellular signaling domain in this receptor.

Gastrointestinal Stromal Tumor

Gastrointestinal stromal tumor (GIST) is a sarcoma of mesenchymal origin that can arise anywhere along the gastrointestinal tract. Typically, these tumors are driven by activating mutations in the cell surface receptors KIT or platelet-derived growth factor receptor alpha (PDGFRA) (Demetri et al. 2007). Pediatric patients also develop GIST, but they rarely have these characteristic mutations and are therefore termed wild-type. Studies have revealed high mRNA levels of IGF-1R and other pathway members in pediatric GIST (Prakash et al. 2005; Agaram et al. 2008). Other studies have confirmed these findings and have also shown that almost all samples from wild-type GIST tumors have a much higher abundance of IGF-1R protein compared to those from KIT-mutated GISTs (Tarn et al. 2008).

Synovial Sarcomas

Synovial sarcoma is a soft tissue tumor with an incidence of approximately 800 new cases yearly. They have characteristic t(X;18) translocations, resulting in the fusion of the genes SYT with SSX1 or SSX2 (Clark et al. 1994). Knock-down and forced expression experiments using the fusion protein have demonstrated that they are essential in the activation of IGF-II (Sun et al. 2006). High expression of IGF-II and IGF-1R were also found in synovial sarcoma samples (Friedrichs et al. 2008). These findings suggest that IGF signaling may play an important role in the underlying biology of synovial sarcoma.

Together, the IGF signaling pathway is abnormally activated, either by loss of genomic imprinting or by abnormal stimulation by endocrine, autocrine, and paracrine mechanisms, in various types of sarcomas. These changes lead to dysregulation of sarcoma cell growth and contribute to the subsequent development of sarcomas and possibly also resistance to chemotherapy. Hence, targeting of IGF signaling, specifically IGF-1R blockade, has emerged in recent years as a promising therapeutic approach in pediatric sarcomas.

Preclinical Highlights on Targeting IGFs Signaling in Pediatric Sarcomas

A number of approaches have been explored to therapeutically target the IGF signaling pathway, from regulation of ligand to blockade of cellular signaling components. But by far, the use of antibodies has been the most widely utilized strategy to block IGF-1R function. The multitude of antibodies directed against IGF-1R share a common mechanism by binding to the extracellular domain of the receptor, resulting in inhibition of their activation, promotion of receptor internalization and downregulation, thus precluding intracellular signaling. The differences lie in their respective affinities for the various receptors and hybrids. The first anti-IGF-1R antibody was αIR3, which has been used for more than 20 years (Flier et al. 1986). Although this murine antibody was remarkably effective in preclinical models, it was the recent development of fully human monoclonal antibodies that has led to a resurgence of this field. Recently, many pharmaceutical companies have developed therapeutic antibodies to specifically target IGF-1R, such as AMG479, AVE1642, BIIB022, CP751,871, IMCA12, MK0646, R1507, and SCH717454 (Gualberto and Pollak 2009). Extensive preclinical studies have demonstrated that antibody-mediated blockade of IGF-1R affects cell proliferation, survival and anchorage-independent growth in vitro, in a wide variety of pediatric sarcoma cell lines derived from ESFT, osteosarcoma, RMS, as well as other rarer sarcomas. They also decrease tumorigenesis, tumor invasion, and metastasis in vivo, and sensitizes cancer cells to chemotherapy, as described elsewhere in recent reviews (Scotlandi and Picci 2008; Kim et al. 2009a, b; Rikhof et al. 2009). One of these, SCH717454 was used to evaluate activity in 35 pediatric tumor xenografts and demonstrated broad antitumor activity when tested in the Pediatric Preclinical Testing Program (PPTP) in vivo (Kolb et al. 2008). Recently, IMC-A12 has shown its greatest activity in RMS xenografts in the PPTP (Houghton et al. 2010). Our studies have demonstrated that MK-0646 inhibited RMS cell growth in vitro (Wan et al. 2007) and RMS xenograft growth in vivo (Cao et al. 2008).

Parallel to the efforts of blocking IGF-1R activity using antibodies, small-molecule inhibitors aimed at modulating IGF-1R tyrosine kinase activity have also been developed. These tyrosine kinase inhibitors (TKIs) include NVP-AWD742, BMS-554417, NVP-AEW541, and OSI-906. These small molecules inhibit ATP binding to the receptor, thereby hindering autophosphorylation and kinase activation. Similarly to the activity profile observed using antibodies, NVP-AEW541, the first of the small molecule IGF-1R kinase inhibitors, has inhibited tumor cell growth in vitro and in vivo in Ewing's sarcoma cells and xenograft models (Scotlandi et al. 2005; Manara et al. 2007). Specificity of these inhibitors remains a major challenge though because the kinase domains of IGF-1R and IR share very high sequence homology (84%) (Ullrich et al. 1986). However, if a dosage that has antitumor activity while minimizing side effects can be identified, the relative lack of specificity may prove to be advantageous. As an example of such, a transgenic mouse model of pancreatic neuroendocrine tumors has been shown to be IGF dependent, but surprisingly, preclinical tests revealed that there was no response to IGF-1R antibody therapy (Ulanet et al. 2010). The finding in this murine model that IR was overexpressed and that disruption of such resulted in decreased tumor burden suggested that IR could also mediate tumorigenic signals. Furthermore, the finding that IR knockout tumors were exquisitely sensitive to the IGF-1R antibody, gives experimental clues that IGF receptors, insulin receptors and hybrid receptors may all participate in tumor formation and progression. Thus, blocking all three using TKIs may be beneficial. Further preclinical work using sarcoma cell lines will help to address this possibility and may have important implications for anti-IGF-1R therapy in pediatric sarcomas.

Two key pathways, Ras/Raf/MAPK and PI3K/Akt/mTOR, are involved in IGF signaling, mediating cell proliferation and survival (Fig. 7.1). The mTOR signaling pathway is aberrantly activated in many human cancers. As a result, it has been an important target for cancer drug development. Data from preclinical studies have shown that rapamycin and its analogues inhibit cell growth in a wide variety of human cancer cell lines. However, a pitfall of these inhibitors is the fact that cancer cells often develop resistance to treatment with mTOR inhibitors, which is associated with feedback activation of Akt through IGF signaling. Our recent study demonstrated that combined treatment using an IGF-1R antibody and an mTOR inhibitor resulted in abrogation of rapamycin-induced feedback activation of Akt, and enhanced the effect of rapamycin on RMS cell growth inhibition (Wan et al. 2007). Our in vivo data also showed that combination treatment with IGF-1R antibody and rapamycin resulted in additive inhibition of RMS tumor growth and murine survival, compared to either alone (Cao et al. 2008). These data suggest that combining therapy with mTOR and IGF-1R inhibitors may overcome the resistance seen with mTOR inhibitors alone. Similarly, the combination of IGF-1R antibodies with Ras/Raf/MAPK pathway inhibitors is conceptually appealing.

Current Clinical Trials

Many preclinical studies have demonstrated that blockade of IGF signaling affects the growth and survival of pediatric sarcoma cell lines in vitro, tumorigenesis in vivo and sensitizes cancer cells to chemotherapy. This has led to the initiation of several phase I and II trials evaluating the efficacy of targeting IGF-1R, alone or in combination with other agents, for patients who have pediatric sarcomas (Table 7.1) (also accessible online at http://clinicaltrials.gov by searching for a specific compound or by using the term IGF-1R antibody). The primary objectives in these studies have been to assess the maximum tolerated dose and the toxicity profile, followed by determination of efficacy in distinct tumor types.

To date, the studies from phase I trials with therapeutic IGF-1R antibodies have not demonstrated serious toxicities in patients with sarcomas, suggesting that these agents have a generally acceptable safety profile as a single agent. Hyperglycemia, when present, has been mild and has been observed in only a few patients and with only some of the antibodies (Rodon et al. 2007; Higano et al. 2007; Tolcher et al. 2007; Atzori et al. 2008). When it has occurred, it has been either transient or readily manageable with medical intervention. In the pediatric settings, the concern of growth retardation following therapy must be considered because of the important role of IGF signaling in normal growth. Growth plate measurement and monitoring has been instituted in almost all protocols that enroll growing children, but it will take many years to determine with any certainty if this hypothetical risk will be a source of practical concern. If a young child responds well to therapy, there would have to be discussions surrounding the potential benefit of continued therapy and the hypothetical but worrisome complication of stunted growth.

Table 7.1 Summary of actively recruiting clinical trials with anti-IGF-IR antibody in pediatric sarcomas

Agent	Tumor type	Patient age (years)	Type	NCT number	Company
IMC-A12	ESFT/RMS/Leio/Syn	≥12	Phase II	NCT00668148	IMClone
IMC-A12	Solid tumors	Up to 30	Phase II	NCT00831844	
A12+CCI-779	Advanced tumors	≥16	Phase I	NCT00678769	
A12+CCI-779	Sarcomas	≥18	Phase II	NCT01016015	
A12+AZD6244	Advanced solid tumors	≥18	Phase I	NCT01061749	
A12+Doxorubicin	Sarcomas	≥16	Phase II	NCT00720174	
A12+Chemotherapy	RMS	Up to 49	Pilot study	NCT01055314	
CP-751,871+sunitinib	Advanced solid tumors	≥18	Phase I	NCT00729833	Pfizer
CP-751+Pegvisomant	Advanced solid tumors	≥10	Phase I	NCT00976508	
CP-751+PF00299804	Advanced tumors	≥18	Phase I	NCT00728390	
AMG479+AMG655	Solid tumors	≥16	Phase I/II	NCT00819169	Amgen
AMG479+RAD001+Panitumumab	Advanced cancer	≥18	Phase I	NCT01061788	
NOT currently recruiting					
AVE1642					ImmunoGen
R1507					Hoffman-LaRoche
BIIB022					Biogen Idec
MK0646					Merck
SCH717454					Schering-Plough

Source: http://clinicaltrials.gov

ESFT Ewing sarcoma family of tumors, *RMS* rhabdomyosarcoma, *Leio leiomyosarcoma*, *Syn* synovial sarcoma

CCI-779: a mTOR inhibitor; AZD6244: a MEK inhibitor; Sunitinib: a tyrosine kinase inhibitor; Pegvisomant: a growth hormone receptor antagonist; PF00299804: a pan-ERBB small-molecule inhibitor; AMG655: a trail recepto-2 agonist; RAD001: an mTOR inhibitor; Panitumumab: an EGF receptor antibody

The cumulative data from clinical trials have shown that responses have varied to treatment with IGF-1R antibodies. The most activity has been seen in patients with ESFT. A few ESFT patients have displayed sustained clinical remission in trials using various IGF-1R antibodies (Tolcher et al. 2007; Atzori et al. 2008; Gualberto 2010). This is somewhat surprising because almost all recurrent ESFT are highly aggressive tumors that are resistant to all known treatment modalities. However, this is also very encouraging, and these complete and partial responses have furthered the initial excitement of utilizing IGF-1R antibody as a therapeutic agent in pediatric sarcomas, particularly ESFT. Other patients have entered clinical trials with a very rapid rate of disease progression. Although few in number, several patients have then gone on to have months of stable disease or very slow progression while on IGF-1R antibody. Unfortunately, the cumulative slow growth eventually pushes them past the threshold for progressive disease and the patient comes off study. It is unclear how the antibody changes the growth kinetics of the tumor in these patients. What is clear is that for the vast majority of patients who are receiving IGF-1R antibody as a single agent, even initial success will be met by a lack of continued efficacy, indicating the presence of an innately resistant tumor mass or the recruitment of compensatory pathways allowing for continued growth. Thus, following the findings that IGF-1R antibody has been well tolerated, and has been efficacious in some tumor types, trials have started to incorporate this compound in combination with salvage chemotherapy, mTOR inhibitors, and other receptor kinase inhibitors.

Conclusion

Dysregulation of IGF signaling plays a fundamental role in oncogenesis in pediatric sarcomas. Although some gaps exist in our knowledge of the role of targeting IGF signaling in pediatric sarcoma, successes in preclinical studies have been borne out in clinical trials. Phase I/II trials with IGF-1R antibodies have demonstrated activity in sarcomas, especially ESFT, for a small number of patients. Work must proceed on how to potentiate these limited successes. This should occur both at the preclinical and clinical levels. Some preclinical questions that need to be addressed include the following. What are the roles of IR and hybrid receptor pathways in IGF-1R mediated tumorigenicity? How can we prospectively identify patients who will respond to therapy? Clinical studies have moved forward from single agent treatment and are beginning to address the combination of IGF blockade with other therapies in sarcoma treatment to alter outcome. It is hoped that the relative lack of toxicity seen with IGF-1R antibodies will allow for its administration in a multiagent regimen. The patient population, the starting doses of the various agents, and unexpected toxicities in particular combinations will be major challenges for future clinical evaluations. Thus far, emerging clinical data for targeting the IGF signaling pathway is very encouraging and requires continued basic, translational, and clinical research to move this field forward and help patients with devastating diseases.

References

Agaram NP, Laquaglia MP, Ustun B, et al (2008) Molecular characterization of pediatric gastrointestinal stromal tumors. Clin Cancer Res 14:3204–3215

Atzori F, Tabernero J, Cervantes A et al (2008) A phase I, pharmacokinetic (PK) and pharmacodynamic (PD) study of weekly (qW) MK-0646, an insulin-like growth factor-1 receptor (IGF1R) monoclonal antibody (MAb) in patients (pts) with advanced solid tumors. J Clin Oncol 26 (suppl):3519

Benini S, Baldini N, Manara MC et al (1999) Redundancy of autocrine loops in human osteosarcoma cells. Int J Cancer 80:581–588

Burrow S, Andrulis IL, Pollak M, Bell RS (1998) Expression of insulin-like growth factor receptor, IGF-1, and IGF-2 in primary and metastatic osteosarcoma. J Surg Oncol 69:21–27

Calle EE, Kaaks R (2004) Overweight, obesity and cancer: epidemiological evidence and proposed mechanisms. Nat Rev Cancer. 4:579–591

Cao L, Yu Y, Darko I, Currier D et al (2008) Addiction to elevated insulin-like growth factor I receptor and initial modulation of the AKT pathway define the responsiveness of rhabdomyosarcoma to the targeting antibody. Cancer Res 68:8039–8048

Clark J, Rocques PJ, Crew AJ et al (1994) Identification of novel genes, SYT and SSX, involved in the t(X;18)(p11.2;q11.2) translocation found in human synovial sarcoma. Nat Genet 7:502–508

Cironi L, Riggi N, Provero P et al (2008) IGF1 is a common target gene of Ewing's sarcoma fusion proteins in mesenchymal progenitor cells. PLoS One 3:e2634

Dagher R Helman L (1999) Rhabdomyosarcoma: an overview. Oncologist 4:34–44.

Demetri GD, Benjamin RS, Blanke CD et al (2007) NCCN Task Force report: management of patients with gastrointestinal stromal tumor (GIST)--update of the NCCN clinical practice guidelines. J Natl Compr Canc Netw 5 Suppl 2:S1–29

Flier JS, Usher P, Moses AC. (1986) Monoclonal antibody to the type I insulin-like growth factor (IGF-I) receptor blocks IGF-I receptor-mediated DNA synthesis: clarification of the mitogenic mechanisms of IGF-I and insulin in human skin fibroblasts. Proc Natl Acad Sci USA 83:664–668

Friedrichs N, Küchler J, Endl E et al (2008) Insulin-like growth factor-1 receptor acts as a growth regulator in synovial sarcoma. J Pathol 216:428–439

Gualberto A, Pollak M (2009) Emerging role of insulin-like growth factor receptor inhibitors in oncology: early clinical trial results and future directions. Oncogene 28:3009–3021

Gualberto A (2010) Figitumumab (CP-751,871) for cancer therapy. Expert Opin Biol Ther 10: 575–585

Hahn H, Wojnowski L, Zimmer AM et al (1998) Rhabdomyosarcomas and radiation hypersensitivity in a mouse model of Gorlin syndrome. Nat Med 4:619–622

Hahn H, Wojnowski L, Specht K et al (2000) Patched target Igf2 is indispensable for the formation of medulloblastoma and rhabdomyosarcoma. J Biol Chem 275:28341–28344

Helman LJ, Meltzer P (2003) Mechanisms of sarcoma development. Nat Rev Cancer 3:685–694

Herrero-Martín D, Osuna D, Ordóñez JL et al (2009) Stable interference of EWS-FLI1 in an Ewing sarcoma cell line impairs IGF-1/IGF-1R signalling and reveals TOPK as a new target. Br J Cancer 101:80–90

Higano CS, Yu EY, Whiting SH et al (2007) A phase I, first in man study of weekly IMC-A12, a fully human insulin like growth factor-1 receptor IgG1 monoclonal antibody, in patients with advanced solid tumors. J Clin Oncol 25 (suppl):3505

Houghton PJ, Morton CL, Gorlick R et al (2010) Initial testing of a monoclonal antibody (IMC-A12) against IGF-1R by the Pediatric Preclinical Testing Program. Pediatr Blood Cancer 54:921–926

Kappel CC, Velez-Yanguas MC, Hirschfeld S, Helman LJ (1994) Human osteosarcoma cell lines are dependent on insulin-like growth factor I for in vitro growth. Cancer Res 54:2803–2807

Kim SY, Toretsky JA, Scher D, Helman LJ (2009a) The role of IGF-1R in pediatric malignancies. Oncologist 14:83–91

Kim SY, Wan X, Helman LJ (2009b) Targeting IGF-1R in the treatment of sarcomas: past, present and future. Bull Cancer 96:E52–60

Kolb EA, Gorlick R, Houghton PJ et al (2008) Initial testing (stage 1) of a monoclonal antibody (SCH 717454) against the IGF-1 receptor by the pediatric preclinical testing program. Pediatr Blood Cancer 50:1190–1197

Manara MC, Perdichizzi S, Serra M et al (2005) The molecular mechanisms responsible for resistance to ET-743 (Trabectidin; Yondelis) in the Ewing's sarcoma cell line, TC-71. Int Oncol 6:1605–1616

Manara MC, Landuzzi L, Nanni P (2007) Preclinical in vivo study of new insulin-like growth factor-I receptor-specific inhibitor in Ewing's sarcoma. Clin Cancer Res. 13:1322–330

Merlino G, Helman L (1999) Rhabdomyosarcoma – working out the pathways. Oncogene 18:5340–5348

Pollak MN, Schernhammer ES, Hankinson SE (2004) Insulin-like growth factors and neoplasia. Nat Rev Cancer 4:505–518

Prakash S, Sarran L, Socci N et al (2005) Gastrointestinal stromal tumors in children and young adults: a clinicopathologic, molecular, and genomic study of 15 cases and review of the literature. J Pediatr Hematol Oncol 27:179–187

Prieur A, Tirode F, Cohen P, Delattre O (2004) EWS/FLI-1 silencing and gene profiling of Ewing cells reveal downstream oncogenic pathways and a crucial role for repression of insulin-like growth factor binding protein 3. Mol Cell Biol 24:7275–7283

Raney RB, Anderson JR, Barr FG et al (2001) Rhabdomyosarcoma and undifferentiated sarcoma in the first two decades of life: a selective review of intergroup rhabdomyosarcoma study group experience and rationale for Intergroup Rhabdomyosarcoma Study V. J Pediatr Hematol Oncol 23:215–220

Rikhof B, de Jong S, Suurmeijer AJ et al (2009) The insulin-like growth factor system and sarcomas. J Pathol 217:469–482

Rodon J, Patnaik A, Stein M et al (2007) A phase I study of q3W R1507, a human monoclonal antibody IGF-1R antagonist in patients with advanced cancer. J Clin Oncol 25 (suppl):3590

Samani AA, Yakar S, LeRoith D, Brodt P (2007) The role of the IGF system in cancer growth and metastasis: overview and recent insights. Endocr Rev 28:20–47

Savage SA, Woodson K, Walk E et al (2007) Analysis of genes critical for growth regulation identifies Insulin-like Growth Factor 2 Receptor variations with possible functional significance as risk factors for osteosarcoma. Cancer Epidemiol Biomarkers Prev 16:1667–1674

Scotlandi K, Benini S, Sarti M et al (1996) Insulin-like growth factor I receptor-mediated circuit in Ewing's sarcoma/peripheral neuroectodermal tumor: a possible therapeutic target. Cancer Res 56:4570–4574

Scotlandi K, Manara MC, Nicoletti G et al (2005) Antitumor activity of the insulin-like growth factor-I receptor kinase inhibitor NVP-AEW541 in musculoskeletal tumors. Cancer Res 65:3868–3876

Scotlandi K, Picci P (2008) Targeting insulin-like growth factor 1 receptor in sarcomas. Curr Opin Oncol 20:419–427

Scrable H, Cavenee W, Ghavimi F et al (1989) A model for embryonal rhabdomyosarcoma tumorigenesis that involves genome imprinting. Proc Natl Acad Sci USA 86:1117–1121

Sun Y, Gao D, Liu Y et al (2006) IGF2 is critical for tumorigenesis by synovial sarcoma oncoprotein SYT-SSX1. Oncogene 25:1118–1124

Tarn C, Rink L, Merkel E, Flieder D et al (2008) Insulin-like growth factor 1 receptor is a potential therapeutic target for gastrointestinal stromal tumors. Proc Natl Acad Sci USA 105:8387–8392

Toretsky JA, Kalebic T, Blakesley V, LeRoith D, Helman LJ (1997) The insulin-like growth factor-I receptor is required for EWS/FLI-1 transformation of fibroblasts. J Biol Chem 272:30822–30827

Tolcher AW, Rothenberg ML, Rodon J et al (2007) A phase I pharmacokinetic and pharmacodynamic study of AMG 479, a fully human monoclonal antibody against insulin-like growth factor type 1 receptor (IGF-1R), in advanced solid tumors. J Clin Oncol 25 (suppl):3002

Ulanet DB, Ludwig DL, Kahn CR, Hanahan D (2010) Inaugural Article: Insulin receptor functionally enhances multistage tumor progression and conveys intrinsic resistance to IGF-1R targeted therapy. Proc Natl Acad Sci USA May 10. [Epub ahead of print]

Ullrich A, Gray A, Tam AW et al (1986) nsulin-like growth factor I receptor primary structure: comparison with insulin receptor suggests structural determinants that define functional specificity. EMBO J 5:2503–2512

Wan X, Harkavy B, Shen N, Grohar P, Helman LJ (2007) Rapamycin induces feedback activation of Akt signaling through an IGF-1R-dependent mechanism. Oncogene 26:1932–40

Wang W, Kumar P, Wang W et al (1998) Insulin-like growth factor II and PAX3-FKHR cooperate in the oncogenesis of rhabdomyosarcoma. Cancer Res 58:4426–4433

Yee D, Favoni RE, Lebovic GS et al (1990) Insulin-like growth factor I expression by tumors of neuroectodermal origin with the t(11;22) chromosomal translocation. A potential autocrine growth factor. J Clin Invest 86:1806–1814

Zhan S, Shapiro DN, Helman LJ (1994) Activation of an imprinted allele of the insulin-like growth factor II gene implicated in rhabdomyosarcoma. J Clin Invest. 94:445–448

Chapter 8
Cancer Genes, Tumor Suppressors, and Regulation of IGF1-R Gene Expression in Cancer

Haim Werner, Zohar Attias-Geva, Itay Bentov, Rive Sarfstein, Hagit Schayek, Doron Weinstein, and Ilan Bruchim

Introduction

The role of insulin-like growth factor-1 (IGF-1) as a progression/survival factor required for normal cell cycle transition has been firmly established. Similarly well characterized are the biochemical and cellular activities of IGF-1 and IGF-2 in the chain of events leading from a phenotypically normal cell to a diseased one harboring neoplastic traits, including growth factor independence, loss of cell–cell contact inhibition, chromosomal abnormalities, accumulation of mutations, activation of oncogenes, etc. In recent years, genomic and proteomic approaches, as well as other high-throughput platforms, have a huge impact on our understanding of both basic and clinical issues. This *gain-of-knowledge* is particularly manifest in the area of IGF research, and "-omic" technologies are allowing us to analyze physiological and pathological processes at a level of integration that was, until recently, unthinkable. Furthermore, and given that the IGF system emerged as a promising interventional target in cancer therapy, the identification of signaling networks linked to IGF-1 action ("IGF-1 signatures") is expected to have a major impact on our ability to optimize therapeutic tools directed against this growth factor axis, as well as on our capacity to predict responsiveness to anti-IGF1-R selective drugs (Bruchim et al. 2009; Rajski et al. 2010; Werner and Bruchim 2010).

The aim of this chapter is to provide an updated review on a number of basic and clinical aspects concerning the role of the IGF system in cancer biology and, in particular, on the interplay between components of the IGF axis and cancer genes (e.g., oncogenes, tumor suppressors). Specifically, our review focuses on the interactions between a series of tumor suppressors, including p53, the breast cancer

H. Werner (✉)
Department of Human Molecular Genetics and Biochemistry,
Sackler School of Medicine, Tel Aviv University, Tel Aviv, Israel
e-mail: hwerner@post.tau.ac.il

D. LeRoith (ed.), *Insulin-like Growth Factors and Cancer: From Basic Biology to Therapeutics*, Cancer Drug Discovery and Development,
DOI 10.1007/978-1-4614-0598-6_8, © Springer Science+Business Media, LLC 2012

gene-1 (BRCA1), the Wilms' tumor protein-1 (WT1), the von-Hippel Lindau gene (VHL), and others, and the IGF-1 receptor (IGF1-R) gene. A novel and, potentially, general paradigm that emanates from these analyses, suggesting that the mechanisms of action of multiple oncogenic agents involve transcriptional modulation of the IGF1-R gene, is presented. In addition, our chapter provides an overview of the interactions between the IGF signaling pathways and nuclear receptor pathways, with particular emphasis on the estrogen (ER) and androgen (AR) receptors in breast and prostate cancers, respectively. In the next section, we discuss controversial data accumulated over the past years regarding the topic of IGF1-R overexpression in tumors.

Controversies on IGF-R Overexpression in Tumors

The level of expression of the IGF1-R gene as a determinant of IGF action and, in particular, the biological significance of IGF1-R overexpression under pathological conditions are still open questions (LeRoith and Helman 2004; Mitsiades et al. 2004; Werner 2009; Werner and LeRoith 1996). Clinical and experimental studies provide evidence that most tumors and transformed cell lines display augmented IGF1-R concentrations (leading to enhanced IGF-1 and IGF-2 binding) and express high IGF1-R mRNA levels. The typical features of the IGF1-R include (1) potent antiapoptotic and mitogenic capacities, (2) important roles in invasion, metastasis, and angiogenesis, and (3) involvement in oncogenic transformation (Baserga 1999; Pollak 2008; Samani et al. 2007). Support in favor of a key role for the IGF1-R in oncogenesis is provided by the fact that IGF1-R-null fibroblasts do not undergo transformation when exposed to cellular and viral oncogenes (Baserga 2000; Sell et al. 1993). The interpretation of the data is consistent with the notion that IGF1-R expression is a fundamental prerequisite for *acquisition* of a malignant phenotype (Bentov and Werner 2004). The apparent universality of this concept and a few important exceptions are described here. The converse paradigm (i.e., that enhanced IGF1-R gene expression in cancer is a *consequence* of the malignant phenotype) is, similarly, a biologically plausible theory that merits consideration.

Given that malignant transformation represents a reversal to a less differentiated ontogenetic stage, it is important to better understand the normal pattern of IGF1-R developmental regulation. During normal ontogenesis, the IGF1-R is expressed at every single period, including the oocyte stage (Bondy et al. 1990, 1992). In preimplantation embryos, the IGF1-R preferentially mediates the effects of IGF-2, since no insulin or IGF-1 transcripts are detectable at these early stages (at least in rodents). Late embryonic and adult stages, in which the percentage of rapidly proliferating cells declines in favor of terminally differentiated postmitotic cells, are usually associated with an overall reduction in IGF1-R levels (Werner et al. 1989). During the neoplastic process, a "primitive" pattern of IGF1-R expression is established, leading to enhanced IGF1-R gene expression. A similar developmental trend is exhibited by IGF-2, which is produced by most cancer cells, whereas IGF-1 is usually produced by stromal cells or reaches the tumor from the circulation.

The appeal of the "dogma" that IGF1-R overexpression is a universal requisite for malignant transformation lies in the fact that elevated IGF1-R levels and enhanced IGF signaling are considered key events, indispensable for the cell to adopt proliferative/oncogenic pathways. It is important, however, to realize that this paradigm is not necessarily valid in *every* type of cancer. Thus, whereas IGF1-R overexpression is a common feature of most pediatric tumors, often associated with recurrent chromosomal translocations, and other solid tumors such as brain and renal cancers, the situation with epithelial tumors, which are more widespread in adults (e.g., breast, prostate), is more complex (Werner and Roberts 2003). Well-controlled immunohistochemical analyses of IGF1-R expression in breast and prostate cancer revealed that both normal epithelium and early stage tumors express high IGF1-R levels, whereas expression is reduced in advanced cancer (Damon et al. 2001; Schnarr et al. 2000; Tennant et al. 1996). The interpretation of the data is consistent with the view that elevated IGF1-R levels, with augmented activation by circulating IGF-1 and/or locally produced IGF-2, is a critical step in early tumor development, whereas the subsequent decrease in IGF1-R values may represent an attempt by established cancer cells to avoid the potential differentiating effects of IGF-1 at sites of metastasis. Of notice, other authors have shown sustained upregulation of IGF1-R expression throughout the various stages of prostate cancer (Hellawell et al. 2002; Liao et al. 2005).

In summary, IGF1-R overexpression, per se, does not necessarily reflect the existence of a cancerous phenotype. Elevated circulating IGF-1 and insulin can downregulate IGF1-R gene expression under physiological conditions. On the contrary, reduced IGF-1 may lead to IGF1-R upregulation without evidence of malignancy. For example, IGF-1 binding and IGF1-R mRNA levels are markedly enhanced in erythrocytes and lymphocytes, respectively, derived from individuals with Laron syndrome, a condition associated with very low IGF-1 levels (Eshet et al. 1993). Together, the relevance and implications of IGF1-R expression in cancer etiology need to be evaluated in a broader context, including analyses of downstream signaling pathways (e.g., IRS-1, *ras-raf*-MAPK, and PKB/Akt), interactions with cancer genes, etc., (Pollak 2004).

Identification of IGF1-R Promoter-Binding Transcription Factors in Cancer Cells

Regulation of IGF1-R gene expression is mainly attained at the transcriptional level. Analysis of the architecture of the IGF1-R gene promoter, as well as identification of *cis*-elements and *trans*-acting factors, helps to define the physical and functional basis for transcriptional control of this gene (Fig. 8.1). Transcription rate of the IGF1-R gene is heavily dependent on a number of stimulatory nuclear proteins, including zinc-finger protein Sp1 (Beitner-Johnson et al. 1995; Werner et al. 1992),

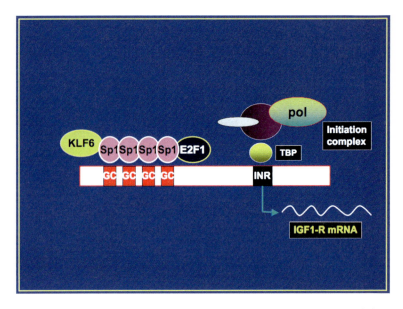

Fig. 8.1 Schematic representation of the IGF1-R promoter. Similar to other growth factor- and growth factor receptor-encoding genes, the regulatory region of the IGF1-R gene lacks canonical TATA and CAAT sequences, two promoter elements that are required for accurate initiation. Transcription of the IGF1-R gene, however, starts from a unique "initiator" (INR) motif, a promoter element able to direct initiation in the absence of a TATA box. Bioinformatic as well as experimental analyses [e.g., DNaseI footprinting, electrophoretic mobility shift assay (EMSA), chromatin immunoprecipitation assay (ChIP)] have identified multiple binding sites (GC-boxes) for members of the Sp/Krüppel-like factor (KLF) family of zinc-finger transcription factors. Sp1, the prototypical paradigm of this family, was shown to bind *cis*-elements in the proximal promoter region with high affinity and to transactivate IGF1-R promoter reporter constructs in coexpression studies. Transcription factor E2F1 was also shown to transactivate the IGF1-R promoter with high potency. The TATA-binding protein (TBP) is responsible for nucleating members of the basal transcription machinery around the "initiator" element. Pol, RNA polymerase II. As described in the text, the IGF1-R promoter is also a target for inhibitory transcription factors, collectively referred to as *tumor suppressors*

E2F1 (Schayek et al. 2010a), Krüppel-like factor-6 (KLF6) (Rubinstein et al. 2004), high-mobility group AT-hook (HMGA1) (Aiello et al. 2010), and others. As described below, IGF1-R gene transcription is also dependent on the presence of negative transcriptional regulators, including p53/p63/p73 (Nahor et al. 2005; Werner et al. 1996), BRCA1 (Abramovitch et al. 2003; Abramovitch and Werner 2003; Maor et al. 2000), WT1 (Idelman et al. 2003; Werner et al. 1994, 1995), and others. The level of expression of the IGF1-R gene is ultimately determined by complex interactions between stimulatory and inhibitory transcription factors. These interactions, therefore, were postulated to have a major impact on the proliferative status of the cell (Werner and Maor 2006). In a recent study we employed a proteomic approach based on DNA affinity chromatography followed either by mass spectroscopy (MS) or Western blot analyses to identify transcription factors

Table 8.1 Functional categories of IGF1-R promoter binding proteins identified by MS

Functional categories	# of proteins identified
Transcription, regulation of nucleobase, nucleoside and nucleic acid metabolism	6
Nuclear stability, chromatin structure, cycle control, and gene expression	2
DNA repair, breaking, replication, and cell death	20
RNA splicing and processing, and translation	24
Other functions, including proliferation, apoptosis, and proteosomal degradation	33
Cytoskeleton-associated proteins	6

MS analysis of DNA affinity chromatography-purified proteins identified a number of previously reported and several novel IGF1-R promoter binding proteins. Most of the proteins were localized in the nucleus, but some of them were found also in the cytoplasm as well as in the plasma membrane. Table 8.1 illustrates the variety of biological processes associated with the identified IGF1-R promoter-binding transcription factors in ER-positive and ER-depleted breast cancer cells

associated with the IGF1-R promoter in ER-positive and ER-depleted breast cancer cells (Sarfstein et al. 2010). To this end, a biotinylated IGF1-R promoter fragment was bound to streptavidin magnetic beads and incubated with nuclear extracts of MCF-7 (ER-positive) and MCF-7-derived C4.12.5 (ER-negative) breast cancer cell lines. IGF1-R promoter-binding proteins were eluted with high salt and analyzed by MS. Out of 91 proteins identified, 6 correspond to cytoskeleton-associated proteins, 6 are involved in transcription, regulation of nucleobase, nucleoside and nucleic acid metabolism, 2 in nuclear stability, chromatin structure, cycle control, and gene expression, 20 in DNA repair, breaking, replication, and cell death, 24 in RNA splicing and processing, and translation, and 33 in other functions, including proliferation, apoptosis, and proteosomal degradation (Table 8.1). Of importance, our analyses identified a number of transcription factors that bind to the IGF1-R promoter *only* in MCF-7 *or* C4.12.5 cell lines, reflecting differences in transcription regulation between hormone-dependent and hormone-independent stages of the disease. Together, the identified proteins may constitute potential biomarkers characteristic of ER-positive or ER-negative tumors. The clinical relevance of these analyses needs to be confirmed by correlations with conventional prognostic factors such as tumor size, lymph nodes status, histological grade, etc.

Regulation of IGF1-R Gene Expression by BRCA1

With about a million new cases annually, breast cancer is the most frequent malignancy in women and represents, after lung cancer, the second leading cause of cancer deaths among women. Systematic reviews and meta-analyses have suggested that high circulating IGF-1 concentrations are associated with an increased risk of premenopausal breast cancer (Renehan et al. 2004; Shi et al. 2004). These epidemiological

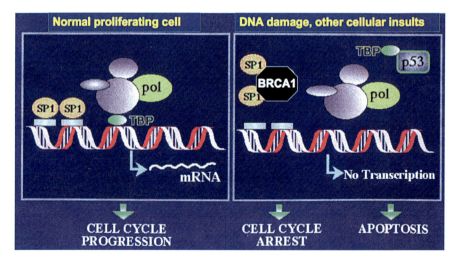

Fig. 8.2 Tumor suppressor control of IGF1-R gene expression. IGF1-R gene expression is dependent on a family of zinc-finger transcription factors, which bind GC boxes in the proximal promoter region and stimulate gene transcription. DNA damage and other cellular insults activate transcription factors BRCA1 and p53. GST-pull down assays have shown that BRCA1 interacts with Sp1, thus preventing it from binding and transactivating the IGF1-R promoter. Likewise, p53 was shown to interact with TBP, leading to disruption of the basal transcription machinery complex. The net result of BRCA1 and p53 induction is a decrease in IGF1-R transcription, with ensuing cell cycle arrest and/or apoptosis

analyses are described in more detail in Chapter 1 of this book. The interactions of the IGF system with several high-penetrance breast cancer susceptibility genes have been explored in recent years. These interactions seem to be of major clinical relevance. BRCA1 is a transcription factor involved in DNA damage repair, cell growth, and apoptosis (Holt et al. 1996; Miki et al. 1994). BRCA1 mutations are detected in a considerable proportion of families with inherited breast and ovarian cancer (Futreal et al. 1994; Wang et al. 2000). BRCA1 mutation carriers have up to 87% estimated cumulative risk of developing breast cancer by age 70.

Consistent with its tumor suppressor role, we have shown that BRCA1 expression in breast cancer cells led to a reduction in endogenous IGF1-R levels and promoter activity (Abramovitch et al. 2003; Abramovitch and Werner 2003; Maor et al. 2000). On the contrary, a mutant BRCA1 gene encoding a truncated version of the molecule (del185AG) had no major effect on IGF1-R expression. These results suggest that the IGF1-R gene is a downstream target for BRCA1 action. Hence, activation of BRCA1 following DNA damage, oxidative stress, or other cellular insults, may lead to a reduction in IGF1-R levels and, subsequently, IGF action (Fig. 8.2). Electrophoretic mobility shift assays (EMSA) performed with the full-length in vitro-translated BRCA1 failed to reveal binding of the protein to IGF1-R promoter sequences. However, BRCA1 was shown to specifically bind zinc-finger protein Sp1, a potent IGF1-R gene transactivator, and to prevent it from binding to the IGF-1R promoter.

8 Cancer Genes, Tumor Suppressors, and Regulation...

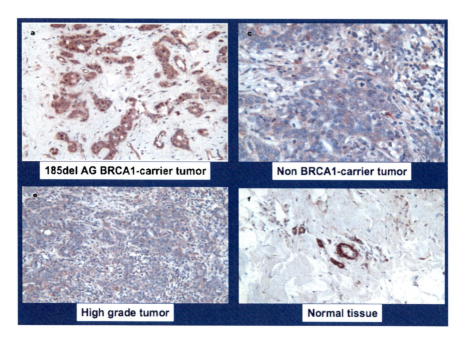

Fig. 8.3 Immunohistochemical analysis of IGF1-R in BRCA1-associated breast cancer. Immunohistochemical analyses with antibodies against both the extracellular (α subunit) and intracellular (β subunit) domains of the IGF1-R revealed that IGF1-R was expressed in all primary tumors and in surrounding normal tissues. Furthermore, IGF1-R immunostaining was predominantly cytoplasmic, although in several of the tumors associated with BRCA1 mutations, IGF1-R was also observed in the plasma membrane. Quantitative evaluation of IGF1-R immunostaining revealed a higher score in mutant BRCA1-associated tumors compared with those from noncarriers (4.64 ± 0.5 vs. 2.64 ± 0.24, mean±SEM, $p < 0.002$) (compare *left* to *right upper panels*). Consistent with previous reports, a large reduction in IGF1-R levels was detected in very high grade tumors (*bottom, left*) compared to normal tissue and tumors

A recent immunohistochemical analysis showed a correlation between somatic IGF1-R expression and germ-line BRCA1 status in breast cancer (Maor et al. 2007b). IGF1-R protein levels were significantly higher in tumors of BRCA1 and BRCA2 mutation carriers compared with those from matched sporadic tumors (Fig. 8.3). Furthermore, infection of breast cancer cells with a wild-type BRCA1-encoding viral vector reduced the endogenous IGF1-R levels. This could be a putative mechanistic explanation for the lower IGF1-R levels observed in tumors derived from non-BRCA1 mutation carriers and for the diminished mitogenic activity in wild-type BRCA1-overexpressing cells (Holt et al. 1996). Furthermore, evidence in support of a complex interplay between the IGF-1 signaling system and tumor suppressor BRCA1 was provided by studies showing that IGF-1 increases BRCA1 protein and mRNA expression and enhances BRCA1 promoter activity (Maor et al. 2007a). In conclusion, inhibitory control of IGF1-R gene expression by BRCA1 may constitute a protection mechanism that prevents from normal breast cells from engaging in mitogenic activity. Lack of IGF1-R inhibition by mutant BRCA1, on the contrary, may lead to enhanced IGF1-R levels, an important prerequisite for malignant transformation (Voskuil et al. 2004).

The role of BRCA1 in prostate cancer is still unclear (Fan et al. 1998; Kirchhoff et al. 2004). We have recently performed an immunohistochemical analysis of BRCA1 on tissue microarrays comprising 203 primary prostate cancer specimens (Schayek et al. 2009). We found significantly elevated BRCA1 levels in prostate cancer in comparison to histologically normal prostate tissue ($p < 0.001$). In addition, an inverse correlation between BRCA1 and IGF1-R levels was observed in the AR-negative P69 and M12 prostate cancer cell lines. Coexpression experiments in M12 cells revealed that BRCA1 was able to suppress IGF1-R promoter activity and endogenous IGF1-R levels. On the contrary, BRCA1 enhanced IGF1-R levels in LnCaP C4-2 cells expressing an endogenous AR, suggesting that BRCA1 regulates IGF1-R expression in prostate cancer cells in an AR-dependent manner. Together, the mechanism of action of BRCA1 involves modulation of IGF1-R gene transcription. In addition, immunohistochemical data is consistent with a potential survival role of BRCA1 in prostate cancer.

Interactions Between the IGF1-R Gene and the p53 Family of Tumor Suppressors

P53 is a transcription factor with tumor suppressor activity which usually accumulates in the cell after DNA damage (Oren 1992). In its hyperphosphorylated state, p53 arrests cell cycle progression at the G_1 phase. Cell cycle arrest enables damaged DNA to be repaired before the replicative phase of the cell cycle (Harris and Hollstein 1993; Kern et al. 1991). Alternatively, p53 can elicit an apoptotic program. p53 is the most frequently mutated molecule in human cancer. Coexpression experiments with p53-encoding vectors and IGF1-R promoter-luciferase reporter vectors have shown that p53 suppresses IGF1-R promoter activity by ~90% as well as endogenous IGF1-R mRNA levels (Werner et al. 1996). By contrast, tumor-derived mutant forms of p53 enhanced IGF1-R gene expression by two- to fourfold. Combined, these results indicate that the mode of action of wild-type p53 involves transcriptional suppression of the strongly antiapoptotic IGF1-R gene. *Gain-of-function* mutation of p53 disrupts its inhibitory activity and generates potentially oncogenic molecules capable of transactivating the IGF1-R gene. In terms of the mechanism of action of p53, EMSA analyses have shown that p53 is not directly involved in DNA binding but appears to exert its effects *via* protein–protein interactions with members of the basal transcription machinery, including the TATA-binding protein (TBP). In addition, p53 was shown to *inhibit* transcription of the antiapoptotic IGF-2 gene and to *enhance* transcription of the proapoptotic IGF-binding protein-3 (IGFBP3) gene (Buckbinder et al. 1995; Zhang et al. 1996). Thus, p53 controls the activity of the entire IGF signaling network by modulating in a coordinated fashion the expression of ligands, receptors, and binding proteins.

To investigate whether the paradigm of p53 suppression of the IGF1-R gene is shared by other members of the p53 family, we addressed the regulation of IGF1-R by p63 and p73 in colon cancer cells (Nahor et al. 2005). Although the structural complexity of the p63/p73 genes and the multiplicity of p63/p73 isoforms preclude any generalization regarding their roles in cancer biology, it is evident that this family of p53 homologues is involved in acquisition and maintenance of the malignant phenotype (Irwin and Kaelin 2001; Yang and McKeon 2000). Results of coexpression studies demonstrated that all p63/p73 isoforms analyzed induced a dose-dependent decrease in endogenous IGF1-R, suggesting that the IGF1-R gene constitutes a physiologically relevant target for p63/p73 action. Moreover, all isoforms assayed suppressed IGF1-R promoter activity. In summary, these studies suggest an antioncogenic role for p53 homologues in colon cancer. Negative regulation of the IGF1-R gene leads to diminished IGF binding, a characteristic feature of terminally differentiated cells. On the contrary, disruption of p63/p73-mediated pathway/s in cancer may result in impaired suppression of IGF1-R transcription, with enhanced binding and receptor activation by endocrine or locally produced IGFs.

Regulation of the IGF1-R Gene by the VHL Protein in Renal Cancer

The VHL gene product has a role in the oxygen-dependent proteolysis of the α-subunits of hypoxia inducible factors (HIF-1 and -2) (Wiesener et al. 2009). pVHL is the substrate recognition component of an E3 ubiquitin ligase complex (Conaway and Conaway 2002). At normal oxygen pressure, HIF-α subunits are hydroxylated on proline residues, targeting them for pVHL-mediated ubiquitylation and proteosomal degradation. In hypoxia, the absence of oxygen-dependent hydroxylation of HIF-α prolines allows HIF-α to accumulate and translocate to the nucleus, triggering transcription of hypoxia-inducible genes. Inactivating VHL mutations occur in ~75% of clear cell renal cell carcinoma (CC-RCC). Inactivation of pVHL allows normoxic accumulation of HIF-α subunits, leading to constitutive expression of hypoxia-inducible genes. IGF1-R levels were found to be unaffected by hypoxia; however, they were higher in CC-RCC cells harboring a mutant inactive VHL than in isogenic cells expressing a wild-type VHL (Yuen et al. 2007). In addition, IGF1-R promoter activity and mRNA levels were lower in CC-RCC cells expressing a wild-type VHL. As described above for BRCA1, IGF1-R promoter activity was dependent on Sp1, and was suppressed by full-length VHL but only partially by truncated VHL lacking an Sp1 binding motif. Finally, the clinical relevance of these findings was confirmed by measurements showing that IGF1-R mRNA levels were higher in CC-RCC biopsies than in benign kidney. Together, these studies have identified a role for tumor suppressor VHL in suppressing IGF1-R transcription and mRNA stability in kidney. VHL inactivation leads to IGF1-R upregulation, contributing to renal tumorigenesis.

Regulation of IGF1-R Gene Expression by Disrupted Transcription Factors

The role of the IGF axis in the biology of Ewing, rhabdomyosarcoma, Wilms' tumor, and other pediatric cancers has been the focus of intensive investigation (Kim et al. 2009; Scotlandi et al. 2005; Scotlandi and Picci 2008). In Wilms' tumor, for example, IGF1-R mRNA levels were almost sixfold higher than in normal adjacent kidney tissue (Werner et al. 1993). In addition, tumor IGF1-R expression was negatively correlated with the expression of WT1, a zinc-finger transcription factor whose mutation is a key event in the etiology of the disease (Werner et al. 1995). WT1 exhibited specific binding to consensus early growth response (EGR)/WT1 sites in the proximal IGF1-R promoter region, whereas WT1 molecules lacking the zinc-finger DNA-binding domain were impaired in their ability to bind and, therefore, to repress the IGF1-R promoter (Werner et al. 1994).

Tumor-specific chromosomal translocations have emerged as a common theme in oncogenesis (Rabbitts 1994). A specific case that provides a valuable general paradigm concerning the involvement and regulation of the IGF1-R gene in tumors displaying disrupted transcription factors is desmoplastic small round cell tumor (DSRCT). DSRCT is a very aggressive primitive tumor afflicting children and young adults which is characterized by a recurrent chromosomal translocation, t(11;22)(p13;q12) (Gerald and Haber 2005; Gerald et al. 1998). This rearrangement fuses the N-terminal (activation) domain of the Ewing sarcoma (EWS) gene, which encodes an RNA-binding protein involved in a number of cancer-related translocation events, to the C-terminal, zinc-finger (DNA-binding) domain of WT1. Fusion of EWS to WT1 in DSRCT abrogates the tumor suppressor role of WT1 and the RNA-binding capacity of EWS, and generates an oncogenic molecule capable of binding and transactivating WT1 target genes, including the IGF1-R promoter (Finkeltov et al. 2002; Karnieli et al. 1996). Hence, whereas wild-type WT1 suppresses IGF1-R gene transcription, mutation or disruption of WT1 leads to enhanced transcription of the IGF1-R gene and augmented activation of cell-surface receptors by IGF-1/2.

Nuclear Receptors

Interactions Between the IGF1-R and Estrogen Receptor Signaling Pathways

Extensive work was aimed at elucidating the association between breast cancer and the activation of the ER signaling pathways. Furthermore, strategies targeting ER activation have become an important tool not only in breast cancer treatment but also in breast cancer prevention in select groups of women. Evidence accumulated in recent years indicates that the biological activity of the IGF system is strongly associated with estrogen status (Lee et al. 1999; Yee and Lee 2000). Estrogens were shown to increase IGF binding and IGF1-R mRNA levels in MCF-7 cells by several fold, suggesting that the mechanism by which estrogens stimulate breast cancer proliferation involves sensitization to the mitogenic effects of IGFs by enhancing IGF1-R concentration (Stewart et al. 1990). In addition, estrogens can modulate IGF signaling by regulating the expression of other members of the IGF family, including ligands, IGFBPs, and IRS-1 (Osborne et al. 1989; Salerno et al. 1999). Using MCF-7-derived sublines that have been selected for loss of ERα by long-term estrogen withdrawal, it was demonstrated that loss of ERα caused reduced expression of IGF-signaling molecules and failure to proliferate in response to IGF-1 or estrogen (Oesterreich et al. 2001). Reexpression of ERα restored the IGF-responsive phenotype, suggesting that ERα is a crucial regulator of the IGF mitogenic loop.

Transient transfection experiments using IGF1-R promoter reporter constructs along with an ERα expression vector showed that the stimulatory effect of estradiol on IGF1-R levels is mediated at the level of transcription (Maor et al. 2006). In addition, deletion analysis showed that the estrogen responsive region in the IGF1-R promoter was mapped to a proximal promoter fragment located between nucleotides -40 and -188. As mentioned above, the IGF1-R promoter includes multiple Sp1 binding sites. Sp1 levels in ER-positive MCF-7 cells were significantly higher than in ER-negative C4 cells. No change in Sp1 levels, however, was seen following estradiol treatment. Expression of Sp1 in conjunction with ERα, but not ERα alone, in C4 cells, induced a strong stimulation of IGF1-R promoter activity. These results are consistent with a crucial role for Sp1 in the ER-induced IGF1-R gene transactivation. The role of Sp1 is further corroborated by experiments showing that mithramycin A (an Sp1 inhibitor) abrogated the estradiol-stimulated increase in IGF1-R promoter activity. In addition, estradiol enhanced both Sp1 and ERα binding to the IGF1-R promoter region in MCF-7 cells whereas no ERα binding was detected in C4 cells. Finally, results of chromatin immunoprecipitation (ChIP) experiments using an ERα antibody indicate that ER binds to the IGF1-R promoter *via* Sp1, and that both proteins can form a DNA-binding high molecular weight complex. Dysregulation of the IGF1-R gene by a defective estrogenic pathway may constitute a key step in breast cancer initiation and progression.

Interactions Between the IGF1-R and Androgen Receptor Signaling Pathways

The involvement of IGF-IR in the initiation and progression of prostate cancer has been the subject of extensive investigation. Contradictory reports, however, have been presented regarding the pattern of IGF1-R expression throughout the various stages of the disease. Acquisition of the malignant phenotype is initially IGF1-R-dependent, however, the progression of prostate cancer from an androgen-dependent to an androgen-independent disease is associated with a decrease in IGF1-R levels (Tennant et al. 1996; Wu et al. 2006). Likewise, IGF1-R expression is extinguished in a majority of human cancer bone marrow metastases (Chott et al. 1999). In addition, Sutherland et al. (2008) showed that prostate epithelial-specific deletion of IGF1-R accelerated the emergence of aggressive prostate cancer. On the contrary, other reports showed a persistent IGF1-R expression in prostate metastases (Hellawell et al. 2002). These seemingly paradoxical results may reflect the ability of IGF1-R to mediate both differentiative and proliferative effects. The molecular mechanisms responsible for regulation of the IGF1-R gene in prostate cancer, however, remain largely unidentified.

Two important features in the progression of prostate cancer from an organ-confined to a metastatic disease are the dysregulation of AR-regulated targets and a change in IGF1-R levels (Kaplan et al. 1999; Tennant et al. 1996). Although these changes could be considered independent epigenetic phenomena, evidence indicates that there is a relationship between IGF1-R signaling and AR action (Lin et al. 2001). Prostate cancer-associated alterations of AR function, including AR gene amplifications, mutations, and altered interaction with coactivators, may contribute to cancer progression. In a recent study we directly examined the effect of wild-type versus mutant AR on IGF1-R gene expression and demonstrated that wild-type AR transfection followed by dihydrotestosterone treatment increased IGF1-R promoter activity in P69 and M12 cells, whereas mutant ARs are impaired in this respect (Schayek et al. 2010c). ChIP analysis showed enhanced AR binding to the IGF1-R promoter in AR-expressing M12 cells. Finally, proliferation assays indicate that wild-type AR-expressing cells consistently displayed an enhanced proliferation rate whereas no enhancement in proliferation was seen in mutant AR-expressing M12 cells. In conclusion, our results suggest that progression from early to advanced stage disease is associated with a decrease in IGF1-R expression which could be the result of impairment in the ability of AR to induce IGF-IR levels. Recently, Pandini et al. (2005) have shown that androgens induced IGF1-R upregulation via a nongenomic AR pathway.

IGF-1 Controls the Expression and Activity of Multiple Tumor Suppressors

The level of expression and activation status of several tumor suppressors has been shown to be regulated by the IGF-1 signaling pathway. For example, IGF-1 was shown to induce exclusion of p53 protein from the nucleus in response to DNA damage in fibroblasts, leading to p53 degradation in the cytoplasm (Heron-Milhavet and LeRoith 2002). Degradation of p53 was associated with an increase in MDM2, an upstream modulator of the half-life and activity of p53. p53 degradation was also associated with downregulation of p21. These results suggest a novel role for IGF-1 in the regulation of the MDM2/p53/p21 pathway during DNA damage.

As mentioned above, IGF-1 was also shown to stimulate BRCA1 mRNA and protein expression in breast cancer-derived cells, and this effect was mediated at the level of transcription of the BRCA1 gene (Maor et al. 2007a). Of interest, the Sp1 zinc finger protein was shown to mediate the IGF-1-induced increase in BRCA1 expression. These studies suggest that dysregulated BRCA1 expression resulting from aberrant IGF signaling may have important consequences relevant to breast cancer pathogenesis. Furthermore, given the role of BRCA1 in regulating IGF1-R expression, our results suggest the possibility of a feedback loop that controls the expression and action of the IGF-1 system and BRCA1 in a coordinated fashion.

An additional tumor suppressor shown to be modulated by IGF-1 is WT1. IGF-1 was shown to reduce WT1 expression in a dose- and time-dependent manner via the MAPK pathway, and this effect was associated with a decrease in WT1 promoter activity (Bentov et al. 2003). Finally, IGF-1 induced KLF6 promoter activity, mRNA, and protein expression (Bentov et al. 2008). KLF6 was originally described as a gene that is rapidly induced in response to several nonspecific insults such as liver damage or hemorrhage. Our results are consistent with combined strong anti-apoptotic signals of KLF6 and IGF-1 to promote proliferation and growth in a tightly regulated fashion. Together, our analyses have identified complex regulatory networks involving the IGFs and cancer associated tumor suppressors.

Studies on Potential Epigenetic Regulation of the IGF1-R Gene

DNA methylation is a major epigenetic alteration affecting gene expression. Methylation involves the addition of methyl groups, catalyzed by DNA methyltransferase, to the 5-carbon of deoxycytosines in the palindromic dinucleotide CpG. Methylation of CpG islands leads to inactivation of gene transcription (Baylin and Herman 2000) and plays a critical role during development. CpG islands are mostly unmethylated in normal tissues and hypermethylated in various cancers (Baylin et al. 1998; Li et al. 2000, 2004). Promoter CpG island hypermethylation of tumor suppressor genes is a common hallmark of all human cancers and affects most cellular pathways. In addition to classical antioncogenes, methylation involves genes in DNA repair pathways, microRNAs, and genes involved in aging.

Bioinformatic analysis of the human IGF1-R promoter region revealed the presence of multiple CpG dinucleotides which constitute potential sites for DNA methylation. To establish whether the decrease in IGF1-R levels in metastatic prostate cancer cells was associated with DNA methylation-induced IGF1-R gene silencing, we evaluated the methylation status of the IGF1-R gene in several prostate cancer cells, representing different stages of the disease, using methylation-specific PCR and sodium bisulfite treatment followed by direct DNA sequencing (Schayek et al. 2010b). No DNA methylation, however, was detected in the IGF1-R promoter region in any prostate cell line, indicating that IGF1-R silencing was not associated with epigenetic control of the gene. Of interest, DNA methylation plays an important role in control of the IGF-2 gene, one of the classical examples of imprinted genes. Loss-of-imprinting leads to biallelic expression of the IGF-2 gene, thus providing a proliferative advantage to transformed cells by elevating the levels of available IGF-2 ligand.

Conclusions

Overexpression of the IGF1-R gene constitutes a common denominator of many human cancers, with some tumors exhibiting a decrease in receptor levels at metastatic stages. The expression of the IGF1-R gene is determined, to a large extent, at the transcriptional level. Evidence has been presented showing that the IGF1-R promoter constitutes a molecular target to a number of stimulatory transcription factors as well as nuclear proteins with tumor suppressor activity. The etiology of cancers associated with *loss-of-function* mutation of tumor suppressors is, in many cases, linked to the inability of mutated tumor suppressors to suppress their downstream targets, including the IGF1-R gene. *Gain-of-function* mutations of oncogenes are associated with increased *trans*activation of the IGF1-R promoter. Interactions between positive and negative transcriptional regulators may ultimately determine the level of expression of this important antiapoptotic gene and, consequently, the proliferative status of the cell. A better understanding of the transcription mechanisms responsible for IGF1-R gene expression as well as identification of the transcription factors associated with the IGF1-R promoter will largely improve our ability to deliver anti-IGF1-R targeted therapies. These analyses will also allow us to predict responsiveness to these therapies.

Acknowledgments Work in the laboratory of H.W. is supported by grants from the Israel Science Foundation, Israel Cancer Association, and Insulin-Dependent Diabetes Trust (IDDT, UK). I.B. wishes to thank the Israel Cancer Research Fund (ICRF, Montreal, Canada) for its generous support.

References

Abramovitch S, Glaser T, Ouchi T, and Werner H (2003) BRCA1-Sp1 interactions in transcriptional regulation of the IGF-IR gene. FEBS Lett 541: 149–154.

Abramovitch S, and Werner H (2003) Functional and physical interactions between BRCA1 and p53 in transcriptional regulation of the IGF-IR gene. Horm Metab Res 35: 758–762.

Aiello A, Pandini G, Sarfstein R, Werner H, Manfioletti G, Vigneri R, and Belfiore A (2010) HMGA1 protein is a positive regulator of the insulin-like growth factor-I receptor gene. Eur J Cancer, in press.

Baserga R (1999) The IGF-I receptor in cancer research. Exp Cell Res 253: 1–6.

Baserga R (2000) The contradictions of the insulin-like growth factor 1 receptor. Oncogene 19: 5574–5581.

Baylin SB, and Herman JG (2000) DNA hypermethylation in tumorigenesis: epigenetics join genetics. Trends Gen 16: 168–174.

8 Cancer Genes, Tumor Suppressors, and Regulation... 173

Baylin SB, Herman JG, Graff JR, Vertino PM, and Issa JP (1998) Alterations in DNA methylation: a fundamental aspect of neoplasia. Adv Cancer Res 72: 141–196.

Beitner-Johnson D, Werner H, Roberts CT, Jr, and LeRoith D (1995) Regulation of insulin-like growth factor I receptor gene expression by Sp1: Physical and functional interactions of Sp1 at GC boxes and at a CT element. Mol Endocrinol 9: 1147–1156.

Bentov I, LeRoith D, and Werner H (2003) Wilms' tumor suppressor gene: a novel target for insulin-like growth factor-I action. Endocrinology 144: 4276–4279.

Bentov I, and Werner H (2004) IGF, IGF receptor and overgrowth syndromes. Ped Endocrinol Rev 1: 352–360.

Bentov I, Narla G, Schayek H, Akita K, Plymate SR, LeRoith D, Friedman SL, and Werner H (2008) Insulin-like growth factor-I regulates Kruppel-like factor-6 gene expression in a p53-dependent manner. Endocrinology 149: 1890–1897.

Bondy CA, Werner H, Roberts CT, Jr, and LeRoith D (1990) Cellular pattern of insulin-like growth factor I (IGF-I) and type I IGF receptor gene expression in early organogenesis: comparison with IGF-II gene expression. Mol Endocrinol 4: 1386–1398.

Bondy CA, Werner H, Roberts CT, Jr, and LeRoith D (1992) Cellular pattern of Type I insulin-like growth factor receptor gene expression during maturation of the rat brain: comparison with insulin-like growth factors I and II. Neuroscience 46: 909–923.

Bruchim I, Attias Z, and Werner H (2009) Targeting the IGF1 axis in cancer proliferation. Exp Opinion Ther Targets 13: 1179–1192.

Buckbinder L, Talbott R, Velasco-Miguel S, Takenaka I, Faha B, Seizinger BR, and Kley N (1995) Induction of the growth inhibitor IGF-binding protein 3 by p53. Nature 377: 1367–1373.

Chott A, Sun Z, Morganstern D, Pan J, Li T, Susani M, Mosberger I, Upton MP, Bubley GJ, and Balk SP (1999) Tyrosine kinases expressed in vivo by human prostate cancer bone marrow metastases and loss of type 1 insulin-like growth factor receptor. Am J Pathol 155: 1271–1279.

Conaway RC, and Conaway JW (2002) The von Hippel-Lindau tumor suppressor complex and regulation of hypoxia-inducible transcription. Adv Cancer Res 85: 1–12.

Damon SE, Plymate SR, Carroll JM, Sprenger CC, Dechsukhum C, Ware JL, and Roberts CT, Jr (2001) Transcriptional regulation of insulin-like growth factor-I receptor gene expression in prostate cancer cells. Endocrinology 142: 21–27.

Eshet R, Werner H, Klinger B, Silbergeld A, Laron Z, LeRoith D, and Roberts CT, Jr (1993) Up-regulation of insulin-like growth factor-I (IGF-I) receptor gene expression in patients with reduced serum IGF-I levels. J Mol Endocrinol 10: 115–120.

Fan S, Wang J, Yuan RQ, Ma Y, Meng Q, Erdos MR, Brody LC, Goldberg ID, and Rosen EM (1998) BRCA1 as a potential human prostate tumor suppressor: modulation of proliferation, damage responses and expression of cell regulatory proteins. Oncogene 16: 3069–3082.

Finkeltov I, Kuhn S, Glaser T, Idelman G, Wright JJ, Roberts CT, Jr, and Werner H (2002) Transcriptional regulation of IGF-I receptor gene expression by novel isoforms of the EWS-WT1 fusion protein. Oncogene 21: 1890–1898.

Futreal PA, Liu Q, Shattuck-Eidens D, Cochran C, Harshman K, Tavtigian S, Bennett LM, Haugen-Strano A, Swensen J, Miki Y, et al (1994) BRCA1 mutations in primary breast and ovarian carcinomas. Science 266: 120–122.

Gerald WL, and Haber DA (2005) The EWS-WT1 gene fusion in desmoplastic small round cell tumor. Sem Cancer Biol 15: 197–205.

Gerald WL, Ladanyi M, de Alava E, Cuatrecasas M, Kushner BH, LaQuaglia MP, and Rosai J (1998) Clinical, pathologic, and molecular spectrum of tumors associated with t(11;22) (p13;q12): desmoplastic small round-cell tumor and its variants. J Clin Oncol 16: 3028–3036.

Harris CC, and Hollstein M (1993) Clinical implications of the p53 tumor suppressor gene. New England J Med 329: 1318–1327.

Hellawell GO, Turner GD, Davies DR, Poulsom R, Brewster SF, and Macaulay VM (2002) Expression of the type 1 insulin-like growth factor receptor is up-regulated in primary prostate cancer and commonly persists in metastatic disease. Cancer Res 62: 2942–2950.

Heron-Milhavet L, and LeRoith D (2002) Insulin-like growth factor-I induces MDM2-dependent degradation of p53 via the p38 MAPK pathway in response to DNA damage. J Biol Chem 277: 15600–15606.

Holt JT, Thompson ME, Szabo C, Robinson-Benion C, Arteaga CL, King MC, and Jensen RA (1996) Growth retardation and tumour inhibition by BRCA1. Nature Gen 12: 298–301.

Idelman G, Glaser T, Roberts CT, Jr, and Werner H (2003) WT1-p53 interactions in IGF-I receptor gene regulation. J Biol Chem 278: 3474–3482.

Irwin MS, and Kaelin WG (2001) p53 family update: p73 and p63 develop their own identities. Cell Growth Diff 12: 337–349.

Kaplan PJ, Mohan S, Cohen P, Foster BA, and Greenberg NM (1999) The insulin-like growth factor axis and prostate cancer: lessons from the transgenic adenocarcinoma of mouse prostate (TRAMP) model. Cancer Res 59: 2203–2209.

Karnieli E, Werner H, Rauscher FJ, III, Benjamin LE, and LeRoith D (1996) The IGF-I receptor gene promoter is a molecular target for the Ewings' sarcoma-Wilms' tumor 1 fusion protein. J Biol Chem 271: 19304–19309.

Kern SE, Kinzler KW, Bruskin A, Jarosz D, Friedman P, Prives C, and Vogelstein B (1991) Identification of p53 as a sequence-specific DNA-binding protein. Science 252: 1708–1711.

Kim SY, Toretsky JA, Scher D, and Helman LJ (2009) The role of IGF-1R in pediatric malignancies. Oncologist 14: 83–91.

Kirchhoff T, Kauff ND, Mitra N, Nafa K, Huang H, Palmer C, Gulati T, Wadsworth E, Donat S, Robson ME, et al (2004) BRCA mutations and risk of prostate cancer in Ashkenazi Jews. Clin Cancer Res 10: 2918–2921.

Lee AV, Jackson JG, Gooch JL, Hilsenbeck SG, Coronado-Heinsohn E, Osborne CK, and Yee D (1999) Enhancement of insulin-like growth factor signaling in human breast cancer: estrogen regulation of insulin receptor substrate-1 expression in vitro and in vivo. Mol Endocrinol 13: 787–796.

LeRoith D, and Helman LJ (2004) The new kid on the block(ade) of the IGF-1 receptor. Cancer Cell 5: 403.

Li L-C, Okino ST, and Dahiya R (2004) DNA methylation in prostate cancer. Biochim et Biophys Acta 1704: 87–102.

Li LC, Chui R, Nakajima K, Oh BR, Au HC, and Dahiya R (2000) Frequent methylation of estrogen receptor in prostate cancer: correlation with tumor progression. Cancer Res 60: 702–706.

Liao Y, Abel U, Grobholz R, Hermani A, Trojan L, Angel P, and Mayer D (2005) Up-regulation of insulin-like growth factor axis components in human primary prostate cancer correlates with tumor grade. Human Pathol 36: 1186–1196.

Lin HK, Yeh S, Kang HY, and Chang C (2001) Akt suppresses androgen-induced apoptosis by phosphorylating and inhibiting androgen receptor. Proc Natl Acad Sci USA 98: 7200–7205.

Maor S, Mayer D, Yarden RI, Lee AV, Sarfstein R, Werner H, and Papa MZ (2006) Estrogen receptor regulates insulin-like growth factor-I receptor gene expression in breast tumor cells: involvement of transcription factor Sp1. J Endocrinol 191: 605–612.

Maor S, Papa MZ, Yarden RI, Friedman E, Lerenthal Y, Lee SW, Mayer D, and Werner H (2007a) Insulin-like growth factor-I controls BRCA1 gene expression through activation of transcription factor Sp1. Horm Metab Res 39: 179–185.

Maor S, Yosepovich A, Papa MZ, Yarden RI, Mayer D, Friedman E, and Werner H (2007b) Elevated insulin-like growth factor-I receptor (IGF-IR) levels in primary breast tumors associated with BRCA1 mutations. Cancer Letters 257: 236–243.

Maor SB, Abramovitch S, Erdos MR, Brody LC, and Werner H (2000) BRCA1 suppresses insulin-like growth factor-I receptor promoter activity: potential interaction between BRCA1 and Sp1. Mol Gen Metab 69: 130–136.

Miki Y, Swensen J, Shattuck-Eidens D, Futreal PA, Harshman K, Tavtigian S, Liu Q, Cochran C, Bennett LM, Ding W, et al (1994) A strong candidate for the breast and ovarian cancer susceptibility gene BRCA1. Science 266: 66–71.

Mitsiades CS, Mitsiades NS, McMullan CJ, Poulaki V, Shringarpure R, Akiyama M, Hideshima T, Chauhan D, Joseph M, Liberman TA, et al (2004) Inhibition of the insulin-like growth factor

8 Cancer Genes, Tumor Suppressors, and Regulation... 175

receptor-1 tyrosine kinase activity as a therapeutic strategy for multiple myeloma, other hematologic malignancies, and solid tumors. Cancer Cell 5: 221–230.

Nahor I, Abramovitch S, Engeland K, and Werner H (2005) The p53-family members p63 and p73 inhibit insulin-like growth factor-I receptor gene expression in colon cancer cells. Growth Hormone IGF Res 15: 388–396.

Oesterreich S, Zhang P, Guler RL, Sun X, Curran EM, Welshons WV, Osborne CK, and Lee AV (2001) Re-expression of estrogen receptor a in estrogen receptor a-negative MCF-7 cells restores both estrogen and insulin-like growth factor-mediated signaling and growth. Cancer Res 61: 5771–5777.

Oren M (1992) p53: The ultimate tumor suppressor gene? FASEB J 6: 3169–3176.

Osborne CK, Coronado EB, Kitten LJ, Arteaga CI, Fuqua SAW, Ramasharma K, Marshall M, and Li CH (1989) Insulin-like growth factor-II (IGF-II): a potential autocrine/paracrine growth factor for human breast cancer acting via the IGF-I receptor. Mol Endocrinol 3: 1701–1709.

Pandini G, Mineo R, Frasca F, Roberts CT, Jr, Marcelli M, Vigneri R, and Belfiore A (2005) Androgens up-regulate the insulin-like growth factor-I receptor in prostate cancer cells. Cancer Res 65: 1849–1857.

Pollak M (2008) Insulin and insulin-like growth factor signalling in neoplasia. Nature Rev Cancer 8: 915–928.

Pollak MN (2004) Insulin-like growth factors and neoplasia. Novartis Found Symp 262: 84–98.

Rabbitts TH (1994) Chromosomal translocations in human cancer. Nature 372: 143–149.

Rajski M, Zanetti-Dallenbach R, Vogel B, Hermann R, Rochlitz C, and Buess M (2010) IGF-I induced genes in stromal fibroblasts predict the clinical outcome of breast and lung cancer patients. BMC Med 8: 1.

Renehan AG, Zwahlen M, C M, O'Dwyer ST, Shalet SM, and Egger M (2004) Insulin-like growth factor-I, IGF binding protein-3, and cancer risk: systematic review and meta-regression analysis. Lancet 363: 1346–1353.

Rubinstein M, Idelman G, Plymate SR, Narla G, Friedman SL, and Werner H (2004) Transcriptional activation of the IGF-I receptor gene by the Kruppel-like factor-6 (KLF6) tumor suppressor protein: potential interactions between KLF6 and p53. Endocrinology 145: 3769–3777.

Salerno M, Sisci D, Mauro L, Guvakova MA, Ando S, and Surmacz E (1999) Insulin receptor substrate 1 is a target for the pure antiestrogen ICI 182,780 in breast cancer cells. Int J Cancer 81: 299–304.

Samani AA, Yakar S, LeRoith D, and Brodt P (2007) The role of the IGF system in cancer growth and metastasis: overview and recent insights. Endocrine Rev 28: 20–47.

Sarfstein R, Belfiore A, and Werner H (2010) Identification of insulin-like growth factor-I receptor gene promoter-binding proteins in estrogen receptor (ER)-positive and ER-depleted breast cancer cells. Cancers 2: 233–261.

Schayek H, Bentov I, Rotem I, Pasmanik-Chor M, Ginsberg D, Plymate SR, and Werner H (2010a) Transcription factor E2F1 is a potent transactivator of the insulin-like growth factor-I receptor gene. Growth Hormone IGF Res 20: 68–72.

Schayek H, Bentov I, Sun S, Plymate SR, and Werner H (2010b) Progression to metastatic stage in a cellular model of prostate cancer is associated with methylation of the androgen receptor gene and transcriptional suppression of the insulin-like growth factor-I receptor gene. Exp Cell Res 316: 1479–1488.

Schayek H, Haugk K, Sun S, True LD, Plymate SR, and Werner H (2009) Tumor suppressor BRCA1 is expressed in prostate cancer and controls IGF1-R gene transcription in an androgen receptor-dependent manner. Clin Cancer Res 15: 1558–1565.

Schayek H, Seti H, Greenberg NM, Werner H, and Plymate SR (2010c) Differential regulation of IGF1-R gene transcription by wild type and mutant androgen receptor in prostate cancer cells. Mol Cell Endocrinol 323: 239–245.

Schnarr B, Strunz K, Ohsam J, Benner A, Wacker J, and Mayer D (2000) Down-regulation of insulin-like growth factor-I receptor and insulin receptor substrate-1 expression in advanced human breast cancer. Int J Cancer 89: 506–513.

Scotlandi K, Manara MC, Nicoletti G, Lollini PL, Lukas S, Benini S, Croci S, Perdichizzi S, Zambelli D, Serra M, et al (2005) Antitumor activity of the insulin-like growth factor-I receptor kinase inhibitor NVP-AEW541 in musculoskeletal tumors. Cancer Res 65: 3868–3876.

Scotlandi K, and Picci P (2008) Targeting insulin-like growth factor 1 receptor in sarcomas. Curr Opinion Oncol 20: 419–427.

Sell C, Rubini M, Rubin R, Liu J-P, Efstratiadis A, and Baserga R (1993) Simian virus 40 large tumor antigen is unable to transform mouse embryonic fibroblasts lacking type 1 insulin-like growth factor receptor. Proc Natl Acad Sci USA 90: 11217–11221.

Shi R, Yu H, McLarty J, and Glass J (2004) IGF-I and breast cancer: a meta analysis. Int J Cancer 111: 418–423.

Stewart AJ, Johnson MD, May FEB, and Westley BR (1990) Role of insulin-like growth factors and the type I insulin-like growth factor receptor in the estrogen stimulated proliferation of human breast cancer cells. J Biol Chem 265: 21172–21178.

Sutherland BW, Knoblaugh SE, Kaplan-Lefko PJ, Wang F, Holzenberger M, and Greenberg NM (2008) Conditional deletion of insulin-like growth factor-I receptor in prostate epithelium. Cancer Res 68: 3495–3504.

Tennant MK, Thrasher JB, Twomey PA, Drivdahl RH, Birnbaum RS, and Plymate SR (1996) Protein and mRNA for the type 1 insulin-like growth factor (IGF) receptor is decreased and IGF-II mRNA is increased in human prostate carcinoma compared to benign prostate epithelium. J Clin Endocrinol Metab 81: 3774–3782.

Voskuil DW, Bosma A, Vrieling A, Rookus MA, and van't Veer LJ (2004) Insulin-like growth factor system mRNA quantities in normal and tumor breast tissue of women with sporadic and familial breast cancer risk. Breast Cancer Res Treat 84: 225–233.

Wang Q, Zhang H, Fishel R, and Greene MI (2000) BRCA1 and cell signaling. Oncogene 19: 6152–6158.

Werner H (2009) The pathophysiological significance of IGF-I receptor overexpression: new insights. Ped Endocrinol Rev 7: 2–5.

Werner H, Bach MA, Stannard B, Roberts CT, Jr, and LeRoith D (1992) Structural and functional analysis of the insulin-like growth factor I receptor gene promoter. Mol Endocrinol 6: 1545–1558.

Werner H, and Bruchim I (2010) Basic and clinical significance of IGF-1-induced signatures in cancer. BMC Med 8: 2.

Werner H, Karnieli E, Rauscher FJ, III, and LeRoith D (1996) Wild type and mutant p53 differentially regulate transcription of the insulin-like growth factor I receptor gene. Proc Natl Acad Sci USA 93: 8318–8323.

Werner H, and LeRoith D (1996) The role of the insulin-like growth factor system in human cancer. Adv Cancer Res 68: 183–223.

Werner H, and Maor S (2006) The insulin-like growth factor-I receptor gene: a downstream target for oncogene and tumor suppressor action. Trends Endocrinol Metab 17: 236–242.

Werner H, Rauscher FJ, III, Sukhatme VP, Drummond IA, Roberts CT, Jr, and LeRoith D (1994) Transcriptional repression of the insulin-like growth factor I receptor (IGF-I-R) gene by the tumor suppressor WT1 involves binding to sequences both upstream and downstream of the IGF-I-R gene transcription start site. J Biol Chem 269: 12577–12582.

Werner H, Re GG, Drummond IA, Sukhatme VP, Rauscher FJ, III, Sens DA, Garvin AJ, LeRoith D, and Roberts CT, Jr (1993) Increased expression of the insulin-like growth factor-I receptor gene, IGFIR, in Wilms' tumor is correlated with modulation of IGFIR promoter activity by the WT1 Wilms' tumor gene product. Proc Natl Acad Sci USA 90: 5828–5832.

Werner H, and Roberts CT, Jr (2003) The IGF-I receptor gene: a molecular target for disrupted transcription factors. Genes, Chromosomes & Cancer 36: 113–120.

Werner H, Shen-Orr Z, Rauscher FJ, III, Morris JF, Roberts CT, Jr, and LeRoith D (1995) Inhibition of cellular proliferation by the Wilms' tumor suppressor WT1 is associated with suppression of insulin-like growth factor I receptor gene expression. Mol Cell Biol 15: 3516–3522.

8 Cancer Genes, Tumor Suppressors, and Regulation...

Werner H, Woloschak M, Adamo M, Shen-Orr Z, Roberts CT, Jr, and LeRoith D (1989) Developmental regulation of the rat insulin-like growth factor I receptor gene. Proc Natl Acad Sci USA 86: 7451–7455.

Wiesener MS, Maxwell PH, and Eckardt KU (2009) New insights into the role of the tumor suppressor von Hippel Lindau in cellular differentiation, ciliary biology, and cyst repression. J Mol Med 87: 871–877.

Wu JD, Haugk K, Woodke L, Nelson P, Coleman I, and Plymate SR (2006) Interaction of IGF signaling and the androgen receptor in prostate cancer progression. J Cell Biochem 99: 392–401.

Yang A, and McKeon F (2000) P63 and p73: p53 mimics, menaces and more. Nature Rev 1: 199–207.

Yee D, and Lee AV (2000) Crosstalk between the insulin-like growth factors and estrogens in breast cancer. J Mamm Gland Biol Neoplasia 5: 107–115.

Yuen JSP, Cockman ME, Sullivan M, Protheroe A, Turner GDH, Roberts IS, Pugh CW, Werner H, and Macaulay VM (2007) The VHL tumor suppressor inhibits expression of the IGF1R and its loss induces IGF1R upregulation in human clear cell renal carcinoma. Oncogene 26: 6499–6508.

Zhang L, Kashanchi F, Zhan Q, Zhan S, Brady JN, Fornace AJ, Seth P, and Helman LJ (1996) Regulation of insulin-like growth factor II P3 promoter by p53: a potential mechanism for tumorigenesis. Cancer Res 56: 1367–1373.

Chapter 9
Mouse Models of IGF-1R and Cancer

Craig I. Campbell, James J. Petrik, and Roger A. Moorehead

A variety of systems have been used to evaluate the role of the insulin-like growth factor (IGF) axis in cancer, including human tissue and serum, cell lines derived from spontaneous tumors from humans and other species, and genetically modified animals. As animal models of the IGF ligands (IGF-I, IGF-II) and IGF-binding proteins have been described elsewhere in this book, this chapter focuses on animal models of altered *Igf1r* gene expression.

The concept of manipulating the mouse genome to study human diseases, such as cancer, started in the early 1980s. In 1984, in one of the early transgenic mouse lines, Brinster et al. established that hereditary acquisition of a viral oncogene encoding the viral SV40 large T-antigen protein consistently induced a specific type of brain tumor (Brinster et al. 1984). At approximately the same time, Stewart et al. demonstrated that overexpression of c-myc in the mammary epithelium induced spontaneous tumor formation (Stewart et al. 1984). Subsequently, the transforming potential of a number of potent oncogenes, such as c-myc, K-ras, and erbB2, has been confirmed through similar rodent models [reviewed in (Maddison and Clarke 2005; Siegel et al. 2000)]; many of these genes encode proteins that are currently targeted clinically or are under investigation for their therapeutic potential.

A number of different strategies have been used to stably manipulate gene expression in mice, including gene disruption throughout the entire organism, tissue-specific gene disruption, constitutive expression of transgenes, and inducible expression of transgenes. Gene disruption frequently involves deleting the entire gene or critical exons within particular genes through targeted homologous recombination in embryonic stem cells. These stem cells can then be transferred into developing embryos to produce mice containing one normal copy of a particular gene and one

---

R.A. Moorehead (✉)
Department of Biomedical Sciences, Ontario Veterinary College,
University of Guelph, Guelph, ON, Canada,
e-mail: rmoorehe@uoguelph.ca

D. LeRoith (ed.), *Insulin-like Growth Factors and Cancer: From Basic Biology to Therapeutics*, Cancer Drug Discovery and Development, DOI 10.1007/978-1-4614-0598-6_9, © Springer Science+Business Media, LLC 2012

179

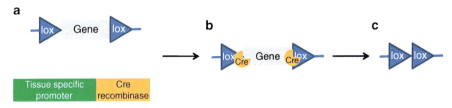

Fig. 9.1 Tissue-specific gene disruption. An endogenous gene of interest or critical exons of an endogenous gene of interest are flanked with loxP (lox) sites using homologous recombination. Homozygous or heterozygous lox-flanked mice are then mated with transgenic mice expressing bacterial Cre recombinase whose expression is driven by a tissue-specific promoter (**a**). The promoter determines which tissue the Cre recombinase is expressed in and, thus, which tissue the gene is disrupted. Cre recombinase cleaves the DNA at the loxP sites (**b**) leading to genomic DNA lacking the gene of interest (**c**)

disrupted copy of that gene; these mice are known as hemizygotes. Mating these hemizygous mice can produce homozygous mice which contain two disrupted copies of the gene and thus are unable to produce a functional protein from the gene of interest. Confirmation of a tumor suppressor role for such gene products as PTEN, p53, and Rb in a number of tissues has been achieved through the generation of such knock-out animals [reviewed in (Frese and Tuveson 2007)].

This approach can be taken one step further by selectively disrupting genes in particular tissues rather than through the entire organism. In this tissue-specific approach, the endogenous gene is flanked with loxP sites. These sites can be cleaved by the bacterial enzyme Cre recombinase. Tissue-specific gene ablation is achieved through tissue-specific expression of the Cre recombinase transgene (Fig. 9.1) [reviewed in (Sauer 1998)]. This strategy is particularly useful for genes that have effects in a variety of different tissues and for genes essential for normal embryonic development, such as the *Igf1r*. Disruption of this gene in the entire organism led to death within minutes of birth (Liu et al. 1993).

Overexpression of a particular gene product is also possible through the use of transgenic animals. An expression construct containing a promoter along with cDNA encoding the gene of interest is microinjected into the pronucleus of a fertilized egg to create a stable germ-line translocation resulting in overexpression of a particular protein [reviewed in (Ristevski 2005)]. Promoters can be selected such that a particular gene can be expressed throughout the entire organism (ubiquitous promoter, such as the β-actin promoter) or in a tissue-specific manner. More recently, transgenic animals have been created such that transgene expression can be regulated by an inducing agent. The most popular approach is the utilization of the Tet-On system. In this system, the cDNA of the gene of interest is cloned downstream of a tetracycline response element and this expression construct is used to create a transgenic mouse. A second transgenic mouse is created using an expression construct containing a tissue-specific promoter upstream of the reverse tetracycline transactivator (rtTA). In mice containing both expression constructs, transgene expression is initiated when a tetracycline derivative, such as doxycycline, is supplied in the animal's food or water.

9 Mouse Models of IGF-1R and Cancer

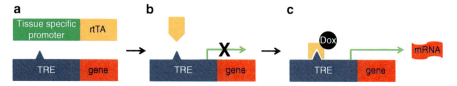

Fig. 9.2 Inducible transgene expression. Two different transgenic mice are created, one containing the reverse tetracycline transactivator (rtTA) downstream of a tissue-specific promoter and one containing the gene of interest downstream of a tetracycline response element (TRE). These two transgenic lines are then mated to produce mice containing both transgenes (**a**). In the absence of doxycycline, the rtTA protein is in a conformation that is unable to bind to the TRE (**b**). In the presence of doxycycline, doxycycline interacts with the rtTA, changing its conformation and allowing it to bind to the TRE and drive transcription of the trangene (**c**)

Doxycycline is required to alter the conformation of the rtTA protein to enable it to bind to the tetracycline response element and, thus, drive expression of the gene of interest (Fig. 9.2). The advantages of the inducible transgenic system are that transgene expression can be initiated and halted as desired by the investigator and the level of transgene expression can be manipulated based on the amount of doxycycline administered [reviewed in (Ristevski 2005)].

Genetic alterations in animals provide an ideal complement to studies utilizing cultured cell lines and those analyzing human tumor tissue samples. Animal models allow genes to be manipulated in a more physiologically relevant environment than cultured cells and provide information on tumor initiation, progression, and metastasis. These properties are difficult to assess in vitro as most of the cells utilized are already transformed and only steps in progression or metastasis, but not the entire cascade, can be evaluated. Similarly, with human tumor samples, transformation has already occurred and the tissue provides information from one time point and thus does not permit the types of longitudinal studies that can be performed in animals. The drawbacks to animal models of altered gene expression are that they are more difficult to generate, time consuming, and expensive compared to cell culture systems.

Although a substantial number of genetically altered animals with alterations in IGF ligands and binding proteins have been created (described elsewhere in this book), only a limited number of animal models manipulating the type I IGF receptor (IGF-1R) have been generated. The most extensively studied tissue in mice with altered IGF-1R expression is the mammary gland (Table 9.1).

Altered IGF-1R Expression in the Mammary Gland

The first transgenic mouse model of IGF-1R overexpression in the mammary gland was the CD8-IGFIR transgenic mice (Carboni et al. 2005). These mice constitutively express a fusion protein containing the extracellular and transmembrane sequences of the human T-cell antigen CD8α fused to the intracellular sequence of

Table 9.1 Summary of IGF-1R animal tumor models

Tissue	Alteration	Tumor phenotype
Mammary	Constitutive overexpression	Mammary tumorigenesis
	Inducible overexpression	Mammary tumorigenesis
	Tissue-specific disruption	Delayed Kras-induced mammary tumorignesis
Lung	Inducible overexpression	Lung tumorigenesis
Pancreas	Tissue-specific disruption	Delayed Tag2-induced pancreatic tumorigenesis
Prostate	Tissue-specific disruption	Increased SV40-induced prostate tumorigenesis
Liver	Tissue-specific disruption	No effect on Myc-induced liver tumorigenesis
Salivary	Constitutive overexpression	Salivary tumorigenesis

human *Igf1r* cDNA. The CD8 portion of this transgene results in homodimerization of the receptor through the formation of disulfide bonds and, thus, constitutive activation of IGF-1R signaling. The expression of this transgene was driven by the mouse mammary tumor virus (MMTV) promoter, and Carboni et al. found high levels of the transgene in the mammary and salivary glands (described below). Expression of the CD8-IGFIR transgene in mammary epithelial cells resulted in hyperplasia accompanied by enhanced proliferation as early as 6 weeks of age and mammary tumors became palpable as early as 8 weeks of age. The mammary tumors consisted of solid sheets of tumor cells with little intervening stroma and displayed histological features of adenomas and adenocarcinomas. A small number of tumors displayed signs of squamous differentiation or spindle cell morphology suggesting that some of the cells acquired a more mesenchymal phenotype and epithelial-to-mesenchymal transition (EMT) may occur in these tumors. Lung metastases were noted in some of the mice, but the percentage of mice harboring metastatic lesions was not reported (Carboni et al. 2005).

Shortly after publication of the CD8-IGFIR transgenic mice, an inducible IGF-1R transgenic model was described. These transgenic mice called MTB-IGFIR expressed high levels of the full-length human *Igf1r* cDNA in mammary epithelial cells in a doxycycline-inducible manner (Jones et al. 2007). When the expression of the IGF-1R transgene was induced at 21 days of age (through the addition of doxycycline to the animal's food or water), mammary epithelial hyperplasia could be detected by 55 days of age and palpable mammary tumors appeared by approximately 70–80 days of age. Tumors were for the most part luminal; however, some tumors contained cells expressing basal markers. Thus, like the CD8-IGFIR transgenic mice, IGF-1R overexpression in MTB-IGFIR transgenic mice produced tumors composed primarily of solid sheets of epithelial cells with some tumor cells acquiring a more mesenchymal phenotype (Jones et al. 2007). The mammary tumors that developed in the MTB-IGFIR transgenics were mainly estrogen receptor and progesterone receptor negative; patients with mammary tumors lacking the estrogen and progesterone receptors typically have a poor prognosis. Lung metastasis has been observed in approximately 40% of the MTB-IGFIR mice, ranging in size from very small microscopic lesions to large macroscopic tumors approaching 7 mm in diameter (Campbell et al. unpublished observations). A cell line maintaining the doxycycline-inducible expression of IGF-1R has been established from these transgenic mice and their characterization is reported in (Jones et al. 2008).

The dependency of the mammary tumors on IGF-1R was also examined using the inducible nature of this model. After removal of doxycycline, 82% of all tumors 10–17 mm in diameter regressed to a nonpalpable state (Jones et al. 2009). Of these regressed tumors, 13% recurred without doxycycline administration, and this process took between 21 and 83 days. Of these recurrent tumors, approximately half were discovered to have reactivated the transgene while the remaining tumors did not express high levels of IGF-1R transgene. Recurrent tumors lacking IGF-1R transgene expression had spindle-shaped cell morphology and markers indicative of an EMT, including high levels of Twist, Zeb, Snail, and Slug and low levels of E-cadherin (Jones et al. 2009).

The inducible nature of the transgene was also exploited to evaluate whether the mammary gland was more susceptible to the oncogenic effects of IGF-1R at different stages of development. Initiating IGF-1R transgene expression in adult mice or in mice that had completed one full pregnancy and lactation cycle delayed tumor development compared to initiating IGF-1R expression prior to puberty (Campbell et al. unpublished observations).

The impact of *Igf1r* loss on mammary tumorigenesis has also been investigated. Klinakis et al. used a model, where mammary tumors were induced by the expression of a constitutively activated Kras allele under the control of the whey acid protein promoter (Klinakis et al. 2009). This promoter is expressed in alveolar and ductal epithelial cells beginning at late pregnancy and continuing through lactation (Robinson et al. 1995). The expression of activated Kras induced mammary tumors as early as 2 days after parturition and 50% of the animals developed palpable mammary tumors 9 days after parturition. Interestingly, one of the modifications observed in these tumors was an approximate threefold increase in endogenous IGF-1R expression (Klinakis et al. 2009). To determine whether IGF-1R expression could regulate Kras-mediated mammary tumorigenesis, the mice containing the activated kras gene were crossed with mice lacking one copy or both copies of *Igf1r* in mammary epithelial cells (whey acidic protein promoter-Cre mice were used to disrupt *Igf1r* expression in mammary epithelial cells). The loss of one copy of the *Igf1r* gene delayed tumor onset approximately fivefold ($T_{50} = 43$ days) while disruption of both copies of the *Igf1r* gene delayed tumor onset approximately 11-fold ($T_{50} = 101$ days) (Klinakis et al. 2009). Moreover, mammary tumors only developed after three pregnancies with both copies of the *Igf1r* gene disrupted while tumors formed after one pregnancy when the mice had one or both copies of the *Igf1r* gene. Klinakis et al. also treated their Kras-induced mammary tumors with the IGF-1R inhibitor cyclolignan picropodophyllin (PPP) and found that PPP inhibited tumor growth rate by increasing tumor cell apoptosis (Klinakis et al. 2009).

Together, these mouse models of altered IGF-1R levels in the mammary gland support the extensive in vitro and in vivo studies demonstrating the importance of

IGF-1R in breast cancer [reviewed in (Surmacz 2000)]. These models have also identified specific properties of IGF-1R during mammary tumorigenesis. (1) Elevated expression of IGF-1R in mammary epithelial cells renders these cells susceptible to transformation and loss of *Igf1r* can suppress transformation induced by other oncogenes (Carboni et al. 2005; Jones et al. 2007; Klinakis et al. 2009). (2) Elevated IGF-1R expression promotes, but is unlikely sufficient to directly induce a metastatic phenotype (Carboni et al. 2005; Jones et al. 2007). (3) Most tumor cells expressing high levels of IGF-1R remain dependent on this oncogene; however, a small percentage of tumor cells can survive independent of their initiating oncogene (Jones et al. 2009). This property will have important implications in future evaluation of agents targeting specific oncogenes. In fact, studies on doxycycline-inducible mammary tumors induced by transgenic expression of ErbB2 are being used to identify how tumors become resistant to the HER2 antibody traztuzumab (Moody et al. 2002; Slamon et al. 2001) and to identify therapeutic strategies to treat traztuzumab-resistant tumors. (4) The developmental stage of the mammary gland influences the susceptibility to oncogene-induced breast cancer. This finding supports the work in rodents that showed pregnancy renders the mammary gland resistant to chemical carcinogens (Medina and Smith 1999; Russo et al. 1991; Sivaraman et al. 1998; Yang et al. 1999) and human epidemiologic data showing that the prepubertal and pubertal females exposed to radiation are more likely to develop breast cancer than females who were adults at the time of exposure (Land et al. 1950).

Elevated IGF-1R Expression in the Lung

As IGF-1R is expressed at high levels in approximately 80% of human nonsmall cell lung tumors and 95% of small cell lung tumors (Reeve et al. 1993; Quinn et al. 1996; Viktorsson et al. 2005), transgenic mice expressing high levels of IGF-1R in the lung were created to further examine the role of IGF-1R in lung tumorigenesis. Transgenic mice were created such that full-length human *Igf1R* cDNA was expressed in either type II alveolar cells (surfactant protein C promoter; SPC-IGFIR) or Clara cells (Clara cell secretory protein promoter; CCSP-IGFIR) in a doxycycline-inducible manner (Linnerth et al. 2009). Overexpression of IGF-1R in either type II alveolar or Clara cells was shown to result in macroscopic tumor formation as early as 90 days post transgene induction; after 9 months, all mice contained lung tumors. Multifocal adenomatous alveolar hyperplasia as well as papillary and solid adenomas were observed in both CCSP-IGFIR and SPC-IGFIR lungs (Linnerth et al. 2009). In addition to overexpression of IGF-1R, these lesions were shown to have high levels of phosphorylated Akt, a well-established downstream effector of IGF-1R, phosphorylated CREB, an important molecule in lung tumorigenesis (Aggarwal et al. 2008; Seo et al. 2008), and KLF5, a transcription factor with a known role in normal lung physiology and other cancers (Kwak et al. 2008; Nandan et al. 2008; Wan et al. 2008; Zhang et al. 2007). Due to the inducible nature of this model, oncogene dependency was also assessed. After doxycycline withdrawal, lungs from some of the mice did not contain any detectable tumors and only regressed lesions were present in lung tissue while in other cases tumors were still present in the lung and contained variable levels of the IGF-1R transgene. Even tumors not expressing the IGF-1R transgene retained high levels of KLF5 and CREB suggesting that these two proteins were important for lung tumor survival in this model (Linnerth et al. 2009).

As most human lung cancers are a result of smoking, the SPC-IGFIR and CCSP-IGFIR transgenic mice were treated with the nicotine derivative nitrosamine 4-(methylnitrosamino)-1-(3-pyridyl)-1-butanone (NNK) to evaluate whether IGF-1R overexpression enhanced nicotine-induced lung tumorigenesis. Although elevated IGF-1R expression was unable to significantly enhance NNK-induced lung tumor formation, it was observed that NNK-induced tumors expressed high levels of the endogenous murine IGF-1R suggesting that one of the effects of NNK during lung transformation is an elevation of endogenous *Igr1r* expression (Siwicky et al. 2011).

Therefore, this transgenic model confirms the importance of IGF-1R expression in lung tumorigenesis and indicates that IGF-1R is likely involved in human lung tumor initiation as well as progression. In addition, the lack of complete tumor regression following IGF-1R transgene downregulation suggests that, like the mammary tumors, some of the lung tumor cells can become independent of IGF-1R signaling and thus the clinical use of IGF-1R targeting agents in lung cancer will likely be limited by the development of resistance to these agents.

Disruption of *Igf1r* in the Pancreas

The implication of the IGF axis in pancreatic tumorigenesis came in part through the examination of RIP-Tag2 transgenic mice, a model in which the SV40 T antigen is targeted to the β cells of the pancreas through the use of the rat insulin promoter (RIP) (Hanahan 1985). Here, IGF-II was found to be upregulated during tumorigenesis in this model and ablation of IGF-II in vivo resulted in a reduction in malignancy and an increase in apoptosis in tumors (Christofori et al. 1994). In addition, it was determined that while islets of the RIP-Tag2 transgenic mice showed a low uniform expression of IGF-1R, carcinomas showed high expression of this protein at the margins and invasive edges (Lopez and Hanahan 2002). These studies have implicated the IGF system in pancreatic cancer.

To address the role of IGF-1R in pancreatic cancer, Lopez and Hanahan created a pancreas β cell-specific model of IGF-1R overexpression using the aforementioned RIP resulting in the generation of the RIP7-Igf-1R model. Life expectancy and glucose homeostasis were unaltered in the RIP-7-Igf-IR mice and there was no histological evidence of transformation of the pancreas in these mice. The only observed phenotype in the RIP-Igf-IR transgenic mice was an increased cytoplasmic-to-nuclear ratio of the β cells (Lopez and Hanahan 2002). When RIP7-Igf-IR transgenic mice were crossed with RIP1-Tag2 mice, an increased expression of

IGF-1R in the β cells was observed compared to single transgenic (RIP1-Tag2) littermates. Consequently, tumor onset occurred significantly faster and progressed faster to invasive carcinomas, essentially skipping a benign islet tumor step characteristic of this model. Life expectancy was also significantly reduced in the RIP7-Igf-IR/RIP1-Tag2 double-transgenic mice compared to RIP1-Tag2 single-transgenic mice (Lopez and Hanahan 2002).

In addition to studying the role of the IGF-1R in primary tumorigenesis, Lopez and Hanahan determined that IGF-1R overexpression resulted in a marked increase in lymph node metastasis. This was thought to occur at least in part due to downregulation of E-cadherin, a process often associated with increased malignancy in a number of different cancers (Behrens 1999). It is of interest to note that while IGF-II overexpression in the RIP-Tag2 model had no effect on tumorigenesis (Lopez and Hanahan 2002), overexpression of its receptor provided a clear advantage for tumor growth. This highlights the importance of transgenic models of the IGF-1R, suggesting that in some cases overexpression of its ligands may not be sufficient to induce tumorigenesis without a parallel increase in the receptor.

Disruption of *Igf1r* in the Prostate

The function of IGF-1R in human prostate cancer is far from clear. Reports from the 1990s found an association between high serum IGF-I levels and an individual's lifetime risk of developing prostate cancer (Mantzoros et al. 1997; Pollak et al. 2001; Tricoli et al. 1999); however, several recent studies found no correlation between serum IGF-I levels and prostate cancer risk (Chen et al. 2005). Similarly, the expression of IGF-1R has been found to be elevated in human prostate tumors by some investigators (Cardillo et al. 2003; Liao et al. 2005; Ryan et al. 2007), but not all (Tennant et al. 1996). The inconsistent findings in clinical samples led to the creation of a mouse model harboring a deletion of *Igf1r* specifically in the prostate epithelium (Sutherland et al. 2008). Deletion of the *Igf1r* was achieved by crossing mice homozygous for a loxP-flanked *Igf1r* sequence with transgenic mice expressing Cre in the prostate epithelium using the androgen-responsive ARR2PBi promoter (Holzenberger et al. 2000; Jin et al. 2003). Offspring harboring both the Cre transgene and homozygous for loxP-IGF-1R (IGF-1R$^{loxP/loxP}$; Cre mice) were found to be deficient for IGF-1R expression in the prostate epithelium at 12 weeks of age. Histological analysis of the prostate revealed that loss of *Igf1r* expression resulted in epithelial proliferation and the formation of epithelial tufts in the ventral prostate, lateral prostate, and dorsolateral prostate (Sutherland et al. 2008). IGF-1R$^{loxP/loxP}$; Cre mice were then crossed with TRAMP mice, a transgenic model in which the prostate-specific probasin promoter drives expression of the viral SV40 large T-antigen oncogene resulting in prostate tumors that initially express elevated levels of *Igf1r* mRNA, but lose IGF-1R expression in metastatic lesions (Greenberg et al. 1995). *Igf1r* deletion in the TRAMP transgenic mice resulted in an increased tumor volume in comparison to control animals at 18 weeks of age as well as an increase in the percentage of tumors classified as high-grade, poorly differentiated adenocarcinomas (Sutherland et al. 2008). Based on these results, the authors suggested that loss of *Igf1r* promoted the more rapid development of aggressive, less well-differentiated prostate tumors in this model. Therefore, this study supports the clinical findings of Plymate et al. and Chott et al. who found that prostate tumor progression was associated with decreased IGF-1R expression (Chott et al. 1999; Plymate et al. 1997).

Disruption of *Igf1r* in the Liver

The use of tissue-specific *Igf1r* disruption has also been examined with respect to hepatocellular carcinoma. In these mice, an Alfp-Cre transgene was used to specifically delete the *Igf-Ir* gene in hepatocytes of *Igf1r* floxed mice (mice were called LIGFREKO) (Desbois-Mouthon et al. 2006). Liver growth and morphology were normal in LIGFREKO mice, but liver regeneration following partial hepatectomy was defective. To examine the impact of *Igf1r* loss on hepatocellular carcinoma, the LIGFREKO mice were crossed with transgenic mice expressing c-myc using a hepatocyte-specific L-type pyruvate kinase promoter (Cadoret et al. 2005). Mice expressing the c-myc transgene and lacking liver *Igf1r* were called LIGFREKO/Myc. The number of liver tumors, range of tumor sizes, tumor histology, and life expectancy were similar in the LIGFREKO/Myc and Myc transgenic. Interestingly, liver tumors from Myc transgenic and LIGFREKO/Myc mice expressed elevated levels of IRS-1 and IRS-2 compared to normal adjacent tissue. Therefore, even in the absence of hepatocyte IGF-1R protein, there appears to be alterations in the signaling molecules downstream of the IGF-1R which may explain why loss of hepatocyte IGF-1R did not significantly decrease myc-induced hepatocellular carcinoma (Cadoret et al. 2005). Clinically, the most strongly implicated IGF family member in hepatocellular carcinoma is IGF-II. Studies have shown that IGF-II is elevated in preneoplastic lesions and in hepatocellular carcinoma and it is presumed that IGF-II mediates its actions through the binding to IGF-1R, insulin receptor, or IGF-1R/insulin receptor hybrids with subsequent activation of insulin receptor substrates within the cell [Reviewed in (Breuhahn and Schirmacher 2008)]. The anti-IGF-1R antibody IMC-A12 is currently being evaluated in a phase II clinical trial for hepatocellular carcinoma; however, results from this study have not yet been released (Tanaka and Arii 2009).

Transgenic Expression of IGF-1R in the Salivary Gland

As mentioned above, the CD8-IGF1R transgene was also expressed in the salivary gland of the CD8-IGFIR mice, and palpable salivary tumors were discovered at 8 weeks of age (Carboni et al. 2005). Histologically, these tumors were observed to be lobular adenocarcinomas with sporadic squamous differentiation. From one tumor, a xenograft model of salivary cancer was generated through serial passage of tissue in immunodeficient mice; subsequently, one such xenograft was explanted giving rise to the IGF1R-Sal cell line, and this cell line was shown to maintain high levels of the hybrid receptor. This cell line was used to assess the efficacy of the small molecule inhibitor of the IGF-1R, BMS-536924. In vitro, these cells were tenfold more susceptible to the growth inhibitory effects of this compound than a human breast cancer cell line known to depend on Her2 signaling. In vivo, this compound was shown to significantly inhibit tumor formation and growth after implantation of IGF1R-Sal tumors (Carboni et al. 2005).

Although salivary tumors in humans are a rare occurrence, this study suggests that human salivary tumors may be mediated by IGF-1R signaling and may respond to IGF-1R-targeted therapies.

Conclusion

The differences in the models described in this chapter emphasize the complexity and tissue-specific nature of the IGF axis and highlight the requirement for genetically altered animal models. While overexpression of the IGF-1R was shown to be sufficient for salivary, mammary, and lung tumorigenesis, the presence of a second oncogene was required in the pancreas. In the prostate, loss, rather than a gain, of IGF-1R expression conferred a more aggressive tumor phenotype. As vast amount of correlative data continues to emerge implicating the IGF axis in cancers of various tissues, one of the most powerful tools to validate these observations comes from the use of genetically altered animal models. IGF-1R transgenics and knock-out models have not only helped clarify the role of the IGF-1R in different cancers, but have also been used for preclinical drug testing, assessing oncogene dependence, examining the potential of tumors to become resistant to IGF-1R targeting agents, and investigating the role of other oncoproteins and processes that interact with the IGF-1R during tumor initiation, progression, and metastasis.

References

Brinster RL, Chen HY, Messing A, van Dyke T, Levine AJ, Palmiter RD: **Transgenic mice harboring SV40 T-antigen genes develop characteristic brain tumors.** *Cell* 1984, **37:** 367–379.

Stewart TA, Pattengale PK, Leder P: **Spontaneous mammary adenocarcinomas in transgenic mice that carry and express MTV/myc fusion genes.** *Cell* 1984, **38:** 627–637.

Maddison K, Clarke AR: **New approaches for modelling cancer mechanisms in the mouse.** *J Pathol* 2005, **205:** 181–193.

Siegel PM, Hardy WR, Muller WJ: **Mammary gland neoplasia: insights from transgenic mouse models.** *Bioessays* 2000, **22:** 554–563.

Frese KK, Tuveson DA: **Maximizing mouse cancer models.** *Nat Rev Cancer* 2007, **7:** 645–658.

Sauer B: **Inducible gene targeting in mice using the Cre/lox system.** *Methods* 1998, **14:** 381–392.

Liu JP, Baker J, Perkins AS, Robertson EJ, Efstratiadis A: **Mice carrying null mutations of the genes encoding insulin-like growth factor I (Igf-1) and type 1 IGF receptor (Igf1r).** *Cell* 1993, **75:** 59–72.

Ristevski S: **Making better transgenic models: conditional, temporal, and spatial approaches.** *Mol Biotechnol* 2005, **29:** 153–163.

Carboni JM, Lee AV, Hadsell DL, Rowley BR, Lee FY, Bol DK *et al.*: **Tumor development by transgenic expression of a constitutively active insulin-like growth factor I receptor.** *Cancer Res* 2005, **65:** 3781–3787.

Jones RA, Campbell CI, Gunther EJ, Chodosh LA, Petrik JJ, Khokha R *et al.*: **Transgenic overexpression of IGF-IR disrupts mammary ductal morphogenesis and induces tumor formation.** *Oncogene* 2007, **26:** 1636–1644.

Jones RA, Campbell CI, Petrik JJ, Moorehead RA: **Characterization of a novel primary mammary tumor cell line reveals that cyclin D1 is regulated by the type I insulin-like growth factor receptor.** *Mol Cancer Res* 2008, **6:** 819–828.

Jones RA, Campbell CI, Wood GA, Petrik JJ, Moorehead RA: **Reversibility and recurrence of IGF-IR-induced mammary tumors.** *Oncogene* 2009, **28:** 2152–2162.

Klinakis A, Szabolcs M, Chen G, Xuan S, Hibshoosh H, Efstratiadis A: **Igf1r as a therapeutic target in a mouse model of basal-like breast cancer.** *Proc Natl Acad Sci USA* 2009, **106:** 2359–2364.

Robinson GW, McKnight RA, Smith GH, Hennighausen L: **Mammary epithelial cells undergo secretory differentiation in cycling virgins but require pregnancy for the establishment of terminal differentiation.** *Development* 1995, **121:** 2079–2090.

Surmacz E: **Function of the IGF-I receptor in breast cancer.** *J Mammary Gland Biol Neoplasia* 2000, **5:** 95–105.

Moody SE, Sarkisian CJ, Hahn KT, Gunther EJ, Pickup S, Dugan KD *et al.*: **Conditional activation of Neu in the mammary epithelium of transgenic mice results in reversible pulmonary metastasis.** *Cancer Cell* 2002, **2:** 451–461.

Slamon DJ, Leyland-Jones B, Shak S, Fuchs H, Paton V, Bajamonde A *et al.*: **Use of chemotherapy plus a monoclonal antibody against HER2 for metastatic breast cancer that overexpresses HER2.** *N Engl J Med* 2001, **344:** 783–792.

Medina D, Smith GH: **Chemical carcinogen-induced tumorigenesis in parous, involuted mouse mammary glands.** *J Natl Cancer Inst* 1999, **91:** 967–969.

Russo IH, Koszalka M, Russo J: **Comparative study of the influence of pregnancy and hormonal treatment on mammary carcinogenesis.** *Br J Cancer* 1991, **64:** 481–484.

Sivaraman L, Stephens LC, Markaverich BM, Clark JA, Krnacik S, Conneely OM *et al.*: **Hormone-induced refractoriness to mammary carcinogenesis in Wistar-Furth rats.** *Carcinogenesis* 1998, **19:** 1573–1581.

Yang J, Yoshizawa K, Nandi S, Tsubura A: **Protective effects of pregnancy and lactation against N-methyl-N-nitrosourea-induced mammary carcinomas in female Lewis rats.** *Carcinogenesis* 1999, **20:** 623–628.

Land CE, Tokunaga M, Koyama K, Soda M, Preston DL, Nishimori I *et al.*: **Incidence of female breast cancer among atomic bomb survivors, Hiroshima and Nagasaki, 1950–1990.** *Radiat Res* 2003, **160:** 707–717.

Reeve JG, Morgan J, Schwander J, Bleehen NM: **Role for membrane and secreted insulin-like growth factor-binding protein-2 in the regulation of insulin-like growth factor action in lung tumors.** *Cancer Res* 1993, **53:** 4680–4685.

Quinn KA, Treston AM, Unsworth EJ, Miller MJ, Vos M, Grimley C *et al.*: **Insulin-like growth factor expression in human cancer cell lines.** *J Biol Chem* 1996, **271:** 11477–11483.

Viktorsson K, De Petris L, Lewensohn R: **The role of p53 in treatment responses of lung cancer.** *Biochem Biophys Res Commun* 2005, **331:** 868–880.

Linnerth NM, Siwicky MD, Campbell CI, Watson KL, Petrik JJ, Whitsett JA *et al.*: **Type I insulin-like growth factor receptor induces pulmonary tumorigenesis.** *Neoplasia* 2009, **11:** 672–682.

Aggarwal S, Kim SW, Ryu SH, Chung WC, Koo JS: **Growth suppression of lung cancer cells by targeting cyclic AMP response element-binding protein.** *Cancer Res* 2008, **68:** 981–988.

Seo HS, Liu DD, Bekele BN, Kim MK, Pisters K, Lippman SM *et al.*: **Cyclic AMP response element-binding protein overexpression: a feature associated with negative prognosis in never smokers with non-small cell lung cancer.** *Cancer Res* 2008, **68:** 6065–6073.

Kwak MK, Lee HJ, Hur K, Park dJ, Lee HS, Kim WH *et al.*: **Expression of Kruppel-like factor 5 in human gastric carcinomas.** *J Cancer Res Clin Oncol* 2008, **134:** 163–167.

Nandan MO, McConnell BB, Ghaleb AM, Bialkowska AB, Sheng H, Shao J *et al.*: **Kruppel-like factor 5 mediates cellular transformation during oncogenic KRAS-induced intestinal tumorigenesis.** *Gastroenterology* 2008, **134:** 120–130.

Wan H, Luo F, Wert SE, Zhang L, Xu Y, Ikegami M *et al.*: **Kruppel-like factor 5 is required for perinatal lung morphogenesis and function.** *Development* 2008, **135:** 2563–2572.

Zhang H, Bialkowska A, Rusovici R, Chanchevalap S, Shim H, Katz JP *et al.*: **Lysophosphatidic acid facilitates proliferation of colon cancer cells via induction of Kruppel-like factor 5.** *J Biol Chem* 2007, **282:** 15541–15549.

Siwicky MD, Petrik JJ, Moorehead RA: **The function of IGF-IR in NNK-mediated lung tumorigenesis.** *Lung Cancer* 2011, **71:** 11–18.

Hanahan D: **Heritable formation of pancreatic beta-cell tumours in transgenic mice expressing recombinant insulin/simian virus 40 oncogenes.** *Nature* 1985, **315:** 115–122.

Christofori G, Naik P, Hanahan D: **A second signal supplied by insulin-like growth factor II in oncogene-induced tumorigenesis.** *Nature* 1994, **369:** 414–418.

Lopez T, Hanahan D: **Elevated levels of IGF-1 receptor convey invasive and metastatic capability in a mouse model of pancreatic islet tumorigenesis.** *Cancer Cell* 2002, **1:** 339–353.

Behrens J: **Cadherins and catenins: role in signal transduction and tumor progression.** *Cancer Metastasis Rev* 1999, **18:** 15–30.

Mantzoros CS, Tzonou A, Signorello LB, Stampfer M, Trichopoulos D, Adami HO: **Insulin-like growth factor 1 in relation to prostate cancer and benign prostatic hyperplasia.** *Br J Cancer* 1997, **76:** 1115–1118.

Pollak M, Blouin MJ, Zhang JC, Kopchick JJ: **Reduced mammary gland carcinogenesis in transgenic mice expressing a growth hormone antagonist.** *Br J Cancer* 2001, **85:** 428–430.

Tricoli JV, Winter DL, Hanlon AL, Raysor SL, Watkins-Bruner D, Pinover WH *et al.*: **Racial differences in insulin-like growth factor binding protein-3 in men at increased risk of prostate cancer.** *Urology* 1999, **54:** 178–182.

Chen C, Lewis SK, Voigt L, Fitzpatrick A, Plymate SR, Weiss NS: **Prostate carcinoma incidence in relation to prediagnostic circulating levels of insulin-like growth factor I, insulin-like growth factor binding protein 3, and insulin.** *Cancer* 2005, **103:** 76–84.

Cardillo MR, Monti S, Di Silverio F, Gentile V, Sciarra F, Toscano V: **Insulin-like growth factor (IGF)-I, IGF-II and IGF type I receptor (IGFR-I) expression in prostatic cancer.** *Anticancer Res* 2003, **23:** 3825–3835.

Liao Y, Abel U, Grobholz R, Hermani A, Trojan L, Angel P *et al.*: **Up-regulation of insulin-like growth factor axis components in human primary prostate cancer correlates with tumor grade.** *Hum Pathol* 2005, **36:** 1186–1196.

Ryan CJ, Haqq CM, Simko J, Nonaka DF, Chan JM, Weinberg V *et al.*: **Expression of insulin-like growth factor-1 receptor in local and metastatic prostate cancer.** *Urol Oncol* 2007, **25:** 134–140.

Tennant MK, Thrasher JB, Twomey PA, Drivdahl RH, Birnbaum RS, Plymate SR: **Protein and messenger ribonucleic acid (mRNA) for the type 1 insulin-like growth factor (IGF) receptor is decreased and IGF-II mRNA is increased in human prostate carcinoma compared to benign prostate epithelium.** *J Clin Endocrinol Metab* 1996, **81:** 3774–3782.

Sutherland BW, Knoblaugh SE, Kaplan-Lefko PJ, Wang F, Holzenberger M, Greenberg NM: **Conditional deletion of insulin-like growth factor-I receptor in prostate epithelium.** *Cancer Res* 2008, **68:** 3495–3504.

Holzenberger M, Leneuve P, Hamard G, Ducos B, Perin L, Binoux M *et al.*: **A targeted partial invalidation of the insulin-like growth factor I receptor gene in mice causes a postnatal growth deficit.** *Endocrinology* 2000, **141:** 2557–2566.

Jin C, McKeehan K, Guo W, Jauma S, Ittmann MM, Foster B *et al.*: **Cooperation between ectopic FGFR1 and depression of FGFR2 in induction of prostatic intraepithelial neoplasia in the mouse prostate.** *Cancer Res* 2003, **63:** 8784–8790.

Greenberg NM, Demayo F, Finegold MJ, Medina D, Tilley WD, Aspinall JO *et al.*: **Prostate cancer in a transgenic mouse.** *Proc Natl Acad Sci USA* 1995, **92:** 3439–3443.

Chott A, Sun Z, Morganstern D, Pan J, Li T, Susani M *et al.*: **Tyrosine kinases expressed in vivo by human prostate cancer bone marrow metastases and loss of the type 1 insulin-like growth factor receptor.** *Am J Pathol* 1999, **155:** 1271–1279.

Plymate SR, Bae VL, Maddison L, Quinn LS, Ware JL: **Reexpression of the type 1 insulin-like growth factor receptor inhibits the malignant phenotype of simian virus 40 T antigen immortalized human prostate epithelial cells.** *Endocrinology* 1997, **138:** 1728–1735.

Desbois-Mouthon C, Wendum D, Cadoret A, Rey C, Leneuve P, Blaise A *et al.*: **Hepatocyte proliferation during liver regeneration is impaired in mice with liver-specific IGF-1R knockout.** *FASEB J* 2006, **20:** 773–775.

Cadoret A, Desbois-Mouthon C, Wendum D, Leneuve P, Perret C, Tronche F *et al.*: **c-myc-induced hepatocarcinogenesis in the absence of IGF-I receptor.** *Int J Cancer* 2005, **114:** 668–672.

Breuhahn K, Schirmacher P: **Reactivation of the insulin-like growth factor-II signaling pathway in human hepatocellular carcinoma.** *World J Gastroenterol* 2008, **14:** 1690–1698.

Tanaka S, Arii S: **Molecularly targeted therapy for hepatocellular carcinoma.** *Cancer Sci* 2009, **100:** 1–8.

Chapter 10
Targeting the Insulin-Like Growth Factor-I Receptor in Cancer Therapy

David R. Clemmons

Introduction

The insulin-like growth factor-I receptor (IGF-IR) is ubiquitously present in normal tissues; therefore, it is not surprising that many types of tumor cells express IGF-IR. Furthermore, even if the IGF-IR number is low in a tumor, the surrounding stromal tissue often produces ligands, either IGF-I or IGF-II, thus making a constant supply of ligands available (Moschos and Mantzoros 2002). Additionally, IGF-I can function to stimulate synthesis of other growth factors, such as vascular endothelial growth factor (VEGF), and this stimulates tumor angiogenesis. Therefore, multiple mechanisms exist for components of the IGF system to initiate and sustain tumor cell propogation as well as metastases. The structure of the receptor lends itself to targeting by monoclonal antibodies. The receptor is a heterotetrameric structure composed of 2 α and β subunits (Clemmons 2010). The α subunit contains the hormone-binding domain. The α subunits are located in the extracellular region and have been subdivided into regions termed leucine-rich repeat 1 (LR1), cysteine-rich (CR) domain, and leucine-rich repeat 2 (LR2) (Fig. 10.1). All three domains are essential for ligand binding. Mutagenesis studies have shown that the residues Asp8, Tyr28 His30, Leu33, Phe58, Tyr90,79, and Phe90 within LR1 are important for binding (Keyhanfar et al. 2007). Four cysteines within the cysteine-rich region are also essential for high-affinity binding. The receptor also contains three fibronectin-like domains between the LR2 and carboxy terminus (CT) domain. Seven amino acids contained between positions 692 and 702 within the CT domain are important for binding. Following binding to the first α subunit, the ligand becomes immobilized and then cross-links through a second binding domain to a distinct site on the second α subunit. This results in high-affinity binding. The affinity for IGF-I is in

---

D.R. Clemmons (✉)
Division of Endocrinology, University of North Carolina, School of Medicine,
Burnett-Womack, Chapel Hill, NC, USA
e-mail: endo@med.unc.edu

D. LeRoith (ed.), *Insulin-like Growth Factors and Cancer: From Basic Biology to Therapeutics*, Cancer Drug Discovery and Development,
DOI 10.1007/978-1-4614-0598-6_10, © Springer Science+Business Media, LLC 2012

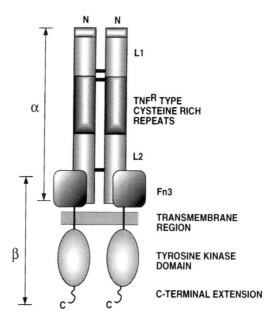

Fig. 10.1 Schematic of IGF-I receptor. The diagram illustrates the location of the ligand binding domains the transmembrane domain and the tyrosine kinase domain. Reprinted with permission Jansson M et al J Biol. Chem 272:8189, 1997

the range of 10^{-9} M, whereas IGF-II binds with a sixfold lower affinity and insulin 1,000-fold lower. Chimeric receptors that are heterodimers containing one insulin and one IGF-IR α/β subunit exist, although their relative abundance in tumors compared to IGF-IR homodimers is not well-defined (Soos et al. 1993). These hybrid receptors have a higher affinity for IGF-I as compared to insulin.

The beta subunit contains intrinsic tyrosine kinase activity. Hormone binding to the α subunits triggers a conformational change resulting in autoactivation of tyrosine kinase activity (Pautsch et al. 2001). The tyrosine kinase then autophosphorylates key tyrosine residues which provide docking sites for SH2 and PTB domain containing proteins, such as insulin receptor substrate-1 and -2 (IRS-1 and 2), that are important docking proteins for the mediators of IGF-I signaling. The signaling components that have been shown to be most relevant for cancer are IRS-1, p85 subunit of PI3 kinase, AKT, mTOR, and p70S6 kinase. This pathway is critical for inhibition of apoptosis and maintenance of tumor cell protein synthesis. IRS-1 activation can also lead to activation of the SHC/MAP kinase pathway which contributes to tumor cell survival and proliferation. Because of the importance of receptor tyrosine activity, several strategies to inhibit the IGFs actions in tumors have focused on inhibiting its enzymatic activity (see Chap. ___) and more recent strategies have focused on inhibiting the activation of downstream signaling elements, such as AKT and mTOR. Receptor number is relatively constant in normal tissues varying between 20 and 35,000 receptors per cell. Although tumors have been described that mutate and markedly overproduce the receptor, this is not common and many tumors have receptor densities that are similar to normal tissues. Therefore, for many types of tumors, IGF-IR-targeting strategies are being directed against a tumor that has a receptor density that is similar to that of normal tissues.

Types of Anti-IGF-IR Antibody-Targeting Strategies

Ligand binding to the receptor activates intrinsic tyrosine kinase activity and this results in major amplification of the growth stimulatory and antiapoptotic signals. Therefore, ligand binding or the conformational changes that occur in response to ligand binding have to be markedly reduced in order to overcome the effect of even small amounts of residual ligand. Four distinct types of blocking antibodies have been described (Doern et al. 2009). These include allosteric IGF-I inhibitors, allosteric IGF-II inhibitors, allosteric IGF-I plus IGF-II inhibitors, and competitive IGF-I and IGF-II blockers. It is presumed that the antibodies that function by allosteric inhibition result in a conformational change in the receptor that reduces ligand binding; however, it is also possible that these antibodies sterically reduce the ability of the receptor to undergo a conformational change that occurs in response to ligand binding that is required to activate the tyrosine kinase activity of the β subunit. Interestingly, some antibodies have been described (including the prototype well-studied murine antibody αIR3) that cause allosteric changes that inhibit IGF-I binding but do not inhibit IGF-II binding (Jacobs et al. 1986). A second class of allosteric inhibitors have been shown to inhibit IGF-II binding but not IGF-I. A third class inhibit both IGF-I and II binding and this inhibition is also allosteric. The fourth class of inhibitors directly bind to the IGF binding site and competitively inhibit both IGF-I and II binding. They are able to reduce binding to extremely low levels when sufficient antibody is utilized. The mechanism of direct ligand competition for this class was proven by demonstrating that increasing concentrations of ligand could competitively block antibody binding to the receptor, whereas this was not possible with the allosteric inhibitors. In analyzing these antibodies further, Doern (2009) demonstrated that at least two separate regions of the receptor can be targeted and that ligand binding is directly inhibited. These include determinants directed against LR1 and the cysteine-rich region or to the fibronectin 3 domain.

Some of the antibodies that have been developed have the additional property of stimulating receptor internalization (Burtrum et al. 2003). This is an extremely important property because internalization markedly favors a greater response and this may be required for inhibition of apoptosis as well as cellular proliferation. However, the duration of the effect and whether tumors respond consistently with IGF-IR downregulation to repetitive doses of antibody are not well-characterized. Whether stimulating internalization favors inhibition of angiogenesis and/or metastasis has not been definitively determined. Since the α subunit of the IGF-IR is less than 60% homologous with the α subunit of the insulin receptor, it has been relatively easy to develop antibodies that have no insulin receptor binding activity. In general, the ability of an antibody to inhibit IGF-I actions is directly related to the IGF-IR number that is expressed by the tumor cells. Increased IGF-IR expression has been shown in breast, lung, thyroid, gastrointestinal tract, and prostate cancers (Samani et al. 2007). Glioblastoma, neuroblastoma, meningioma, and rhabdomyosarcoma can also overexpress IGF-IR. In spite of these results, attempts to correlate tumor prognosis with the degree of IGF-IR expression have led to conflicting results at least for common tumors, such as breast, colon, and prostate cancers (Yuen and Macauley 2008). Other mechanisms can also result in the stimulation of IGF-IR activation. Wilm's tumor and neuroblastoma overexpress IGF-II due to loss of imprinting and Ewing's sarcoma shows an increase in autocrine-secreted IGF-I (Ogawa et al. 1993 and Scotlandi and Picci 2008). Increased IGF-II expression has been shown to occur in Ewing's sarcoma and in neuroectodermal tumors. Other mechanisms that alter sensitivity to IGF-IR activation include constitutive phosphorylation of the IGF-IR beta subunit by other tyrosine kinases and altered glycosylation of the α subunit of the receptor that has also been reported in gliomas and leukemia cells and can alter receptor half-life and degradation (Ota et al. 1988). An alternative form of the insulin receptor (IR-A) that can bind to IGF-II with reasonably high affinity has been shown to be expressed in some breast, colon, and lung carcinomas (Frasca et al. 1999). IGF-binding proteins (IGFBPs) can also regulate ligand occupancy of the receptor by competitively inhibiting IGF binding. Some cancers express very low levels of IGFBPs and this could function to necessitate the use of high concentration of receptor-targeting agents in order to achieve adequate inhibition (Renehan et al. 2004). Additionally, whether compensatory increases that occur in serum GH or IGF-I observations in response to anti-IGF-IR therapy result in changes in IGFBP bioavailability or function has not been determined.

Assessment of Antibody Efficacy in Animal Models

All of the anti-IGF-IR antibodies that have currently entered into clinical testing have been tested in animal models (Table 10.1). Most of these animal model systems have utilized immunocompromised mice and human tumor cell lines to establish xenografts. Occasionally, orthotopic models have been used. Most of the antibodies have been injected intraperitoneally or subcutaneously for several weeks. The parameters that have been analyzed include tumor size, cell growth, apoptosis, metastasis, and mouse survival. Additionally, tumor specimens have been analyzed for evidence of changes in receptor autophosphorylation, downregulation, and degradation and in some cases signaling events, such as IRS-1 phosphorylation. Some investigators have conducted detailed cell cycle analysis. For example, Wu et al. (2005) showed that the same anti-receptor antibody induced apoptosis and G_1 cell cycle arrest in androgen-dependent prostate cancer, whereas it induced G_2 inhibition in androgen-independent tumors. Several tumor cell types have been analyzed, including lung, breast, colon, prostate, biliary tract, pancreatic, and hepatic or head, neck, and thyroid carcinomas (Hofmann and Garcia-Echeverria 2005). A variety of mesenchymal cell tumors, including Ewing's, osteogenic, synovial cell, and rhabdomyosarcoma as well as Wilm's tumor and neuroblastoma, have been studied

10 Targeting the Insulin-Like Growth Factor-I Receptor in Cancer Therapy

Table 10.1 Proof of concept experiments in animal bearing tumor xenografts

Antibody	Tumor cell type	Model	Comment	Reference
CP751/817	Breast cancer	Athymic mice	IGF-IR	Cohen et al. (2005)
			Downregulation	
			Decreased tumor size	
MK0646(h7c10)	NSCLC	Athymic mice	Decreased tumor size Goetsch et al. 2005	
R1507	Osteosarcoma	Athymic mice	Decreased tumor size	Kolb et al. (2010)
			Prolonged survival	
Sch717454(19D12)	Pediatric solid tumors	Athymic mice	Downregulates IGF-IR	Wang et al. (2009b)
			Initiated tumor growth	
			Inhibited angiogenesis	Wang et al. (2005)
AVE1642 (EM164)	Pancreatic cancer	Athymic mice	Decreased tumor growth	Maloney et al. (2003)
AMG479	Pancreatic cancer	Athymic mice	Decreased tumor growth	Beltran et al. (2009)
			Downregulated IGF-IR	
IMC-A12	Breast cancer	Athymic mice	Decreased tumor size	Burtrum et al. (2003)
			Increased apoptosis	Wang et al. (2005)

(Houghton et al. 2010) (Wang et al. 2009b). Hematologic malignancies, such as lymphoma and multiple myeloma, have also been studied (Menu et al. 2009). Each of the antibodies has been tested as a single agent and all have been found to have significant inhibitory activity (Table 10.1). In addition, some antibodies have been tested in combination with chemotherapeutic agents that are known to have activity against a specific tumor type (Geoerger et al. 2010; Cohen et al. 2005; Rowinsky et al. 2007). For example, h7C10 was tested with vinorelbine for activity against nonsmall cell lung carcinoma (NSCLC) (Goetsch et al. 2005). Similarly, CP751,781, and IMCA-12 were tested with docetaxel (Wu et al. 2006 Gridelli et al. 2010). In most cases, the results of these studies have shown a synergistic increase in inhibition of tumor growth. Some antibodies, e.g., IMC-A12 and CP751,871 (Iwasa et al. 2009) (Hewish et al. 2009), have been shown to enhance the effect of radiation on lung carcinoma cells. Additionally, xenograft models have been utilized to test the effect of inhibiting multiple growth factor-signaling pathways. Several studies have analyzed the responses to combined administration of anti-EGF plus anti-IGF-IR antibodies (Carmirand et al. 2005). In general, these studies have shown synergistic inhibition of tumor growth (van der Veeken et al. 2009; Goetsch et al. 2005). One study analyzed a bispecific antibody that was prepared that could bind to both the EGF receptor and IGF-IR. This antibody resulted in inhibition of the growth of the EXPC3 and HD29 tumor cells in mice (Lu et al. 2005). Breast cancer cell growth has been shown to be synergistically inhibited by anti-estrogen receptor blockers, such as Tamoxifen and anti-IGF-IR antibodies (Cohen et al. 2005; Massarweh et al. 2008; Ye et al. 2003). Anti-Her-2 plus IGF-IR antibodies have also been analyzed in combination and have been shown to be effective against Her2 positive tumors (Nahta et al. 2005; Lu et al. 2001). These model systems have also been very useful in determining the development of the mechanisms of action and resistance to antibody therapy. These are discussed in subsequent sections. Additionally, studies have been undertaken that analyzed the effect of antibodies on metastasis and also attempted to define the mechanisms that determine metastatic behavior.

Human Studies

Seven monoclonal antibodies have advanced to the stage of human testing (Table 10.2). All seven have been tested in phase I trials and in some cases the phase I trial has been extended to determine if subjects respond over an extended treatment duration (e.g., 6 months, 1 year). The initial phase I trial was performed using CP751,817 (Figitumumab), a fully human monoclonal antibody. This antibody differs from the others in this class in that it is an IgG_2 antibody. This results in a prolonged half-life, but it also diminishes its ability to trigger a cytotoxic response, that is, there is no antibody-mediated cytotoxicity using this reagent. In the initial phase I trial, 47 patients with refractory myeloma were enrolled (Haluska et al. 2007). Side effects included one case of grade 3 hyperglycemia and one case of anemia. The half-life of a 20 mg/kg dose was estimated to be 20 days. IGF-IR expression was shown to be decreased in granulocytes obtained from these patients and serum IGF-I increased as much as tenfold above baseline with two- to threefold increases in IGFBP-3. A phase I study was also conducted using this drug in patients with refractory solid tumors, including adrenocortical carcinomas and sarcomas (Haluska et al. 2009). This trial had an extension phase which was continued for periods of up to 1 year. Grade 3 toxicities included hepatic enzyme elevation, fatigue, and arthralgias. Serum marker analysis showed that IGF-I and growth hormone levels were increased substantially, e.g., two- to threefold. Two of twenty patients showed stabilization of disease for a 1-year treatment period. Disease stabilization was noted in 8 of 20 sarcomas and 9 of 13 adrenocortical carcinoma patients. Phase I combination studies have also been completed with this antibody. When given in combination with docetaxel to patients with advanced, solid tumors and patients with hormone-resistant prostate cancers, it resulted in significant decreases in circulating tumor cells and serum PSA decreased in 8 of 20 patients (de Bono et al. 2007). The safety and efficacy of this antibody was also investigated and in combination with paclitaxel and carboplatin when administered to patients with NSCLC or ovarian cancer (Karp et al. 2009b). Toxicity was similar to prior studies and increases in IGF-I and IGFBP-3 were similar to prior reports. Complete responses

Table 10.2 Clinical trials reported through May 2010

Antibody name	Tumor cell type	Type of antibody	Comment	References
CP751/817	Ewing's, NSCLC, HRPC, breast, myeloma	IgG2 fully human	Phase I–III trials have been completed	Haluska et al. (2007) Lacy et al. (2008) Kurmasheva et al. (2009) Karp et al. (2009a, b) Jassem et al. (2010) de Bono et al. (2007) Cohen et al. (2005)
MK0646	Colorectal, NSCLC	Humanized mab IgG1	Phase I and II trials have been completed	Hidalgo et al. (2008)
				Javle et al. (2010) Reidy et al. (2010)
R1507	Sarcomas	Fully human IgG1	Phase I and II trials have been completed	Rodon et al. (2007)
	Solid tumors			Pappo et al. (2010) Kurzrock et al. (2010)
Sch717454	Colorectal	Humanized mab IgG1	A phase I trial has been completed	Pollak et al. (2007)
AVE1642	Ewing's, pancreatic cancer	Fully human IgG1 extended	Phase I trials have been completed	Moreau et al. (2007)
				Tolcher et al. (2008)
IMC-A12	Ewing's, pancreatic cancer Fully human IgG1 phase I and II trials have been completed			Higano et al. (2007)
	Head and neck cancer			Busaidy et al. (2010)
AMG 479	Ewing's, pancreatic cancer	Fully human IgG1	Phase I and II trials have been completed	Tolcher et al. (2009)
	Non-Hodgkin's lymphoma NSCLC			Sarantopoulos et al. (2008) Kindler et al. (2010) Tap et al. (2010)
BIIBO22	Various solid tumor types	Fully human IgG4	A phase I trial has been completed	von Mehren et al. (2010)

were noted in two patients with NSCLC and ovarian carcinoma. A phase I extension study of this antibody was also reported in 15 patients with Ewing's sarcoma (Olmos et al. 2010). Two patients had objective responses and eight patients had disease stabilization which lasted 4 months or longer. Grade 3 level side effects e.g., DVT, back pain, vomiting, and hyperglycemia were noted. Elevated liver function tests were noted in eight patients.

A phase II study has also been completed with this monoclonal antibody (Karp et al. 2009a). This was initiated in 156 NSCLC patients. They were randomized to receive either paclitaxel, carboplatin, and the antibody or paclitaxel and carboplatin alone. The antibody was administered at a relatively high dosage, 10–20 mg/kg every 3 weeks. Objective responses were noted in 54% of the antibody-treated group as compared to 42% of the patients who received chemotherapy only. In general, the response rate was higher with the 20 mg/kg dose. Hyperglycemia was noted in 15% of patients. Some patients showed downregulation of IGF-IR abundance on circulating cancer cells in blood. The progression-free survival was also slightly increased with a hazard ratio of 1.181 (Chi et al. 2010). A phase II study has also completed enrollment in patients with localized prostate cancer. These subjects received the 20 mg/kg dose for 3 cycles. PSA levels were shown to decline significantly from baseline and decreased IGF-IR expression was shown in six available tumor specimens. The side effect profile was similar to previous studies. Based on these studies, a phase III trial was initiated using this antibody in patients with NSCLC. Six hundred and eighty-one patients were enrolled (Jassem et al. 2010). The trial was halted when it was determined that survival would not be improved in the antibody-treated patients compared to those who received chemotherapy alone. There was an increase in early deaths in the antibody-treated patients and factors that predicated early death included low body mass and increased creatinine clearance. A second phase III trial was also terminated early in which antibody plus tarceva was compared to tarceva alone in NSCLC patients. This study was also terminated early because it was predicted that survival would not be enhanced in the antibody-treated group.

MK0646

This is an IgG_1 monoclonal antibody. Phase I trials have been conducted in patients with advanced solid tumors. In the first study, 29 patients were given the drug using doses between 1.5 and 20 mg/kg weekly (Hidalgo et al. 2008). The half-life was calculated as 4 days. IGF-IR levels were decreased in circulating mononuclear cells and serum IGF-I levels were increased twofold. In a second study, 28 patients with pancreatic cancer were enrolled (Javle et al. 2010). They were treated with doses of 2.5–15 mg/kg every 2 weeks. Some patients had significant side effects, e.g., grade 3 toxicities including thrombocytopenia, gastrointestinal bleeding, pneumonitis, and increased liver function tests. This study has been extended as a phase II trial in patients with pancreatic cancer, in combination with gemcitabine or gemcitabine plus Erlotinib. Twenty-eight patients have been enrolled. Dose-limiting toxicity was present at 10 mg/kg. Radiographic responses have occurred in ten patients and sustained lack of progression has occurred in five patients treated for intervals between 20 and 44 weeks. A phase II study was completed in 25 patients with neuroendocrine tumors using the drug as monotherapy. No patient had a reduction in tumor size. Five patients had disease stabilization. Hyperglycemia was found in 25% of patients (Reidy et al. 2010).

R1507

This is an IgG1 antibody that has been given in a phase I trial to patients with advanced solid tumors or lymphoma. Twenty-one patients received four escalating doses of 1–16 mg/kg weekly. Two patients had grade 3 level side effects, hyperglycemia and leucopenia (Rodon et al. 2007). Six patients developed an infection and four fatigue. The half-life was estimated to be 8 days. IGF-IR expression on blood cells was reduced by 80%. The trial was extended in patients with Ewing's sarcoma. Two of eight patients had significant reduction in tumor size and stabilization of disease occurred in another two who were treated for a mean duration of 18 weeks. A phase II study enrolled 125 patients with Ewing's sarcoma for a trial of monotherapy (Pappo et al. 2010). Twelve patients had a response that lasted at least 6 weeks with a median duration of 25 weeks. Grade 3–4 toxicities occurred in 16 patients.

SCH717454

This is a human IgG1 antibody. A phase I single-dose study giving doses between 0.3 and 20 mg/kg was conducted in 32 healthy volunteers (Pollak et al. 2007). Two phase II trials are ongoing and the first group of patients with relapsed osteosarcoma are being treated with 1 of 2 dose levels. In the second study, patients with unresectable osteosarcoma or Ewing's sarcoma are receiving a single dose.

AVE1642

This is a fully humanized IgG1 antibody. In the initial phase I study, the drug that was given as monotherapy, 3–12 mg/kg every 3 weeks to patients with refractory multiple myeloma (Moreau et al. 2007). It was well-tolerated in 14 patients for 3 cycles. Worsening hyperglycemia was observed in two patients with diabetes. In a second study, it was administered every 3 weeks with docetaxel to patients with solid tumors (Tolcher et al. 2008). The half-life is estimated as 9 days. Fourteen patients with solid tumors were treated for 4 cycles of therapy and one experienced decreased bone pain and improved proteinuria.

IMC-A12

This antibody has been studied in several phase I trials as well as phase II studies. Additionally, several phase II studies combining this antibody with other forms of treatment are ongoing. In the initial phase I study, the antibody was administered to 21 patients with advanced solid tumors. They received escalating doses between 3 and 12 mg/kg (Higano et al. 2007). The drug was well-tolerated and hyperglycemia was the most common toxicity. Doses of 6 mg/kg had minimal toxicity. There were no objective responses among 15 patients. Nine patients had disease stabilization. In a second phase I trial, the drug was given to 21 patients using doses of 6, 8, or 10 mg/kg with sorafemib to patients with advanced hepatocellular carcinoma (O'Donnell et al. 2010). The purpose of the study was to establish the minimum effective dose when combined with sorafemib, evaluate toxicity, and obtain preliminary efficacy data. No objective responses were observed, but two patients had stabilization for intervals at greater than 12 weeks. Hyperglycemia was observed in 4 of 15 patients. Other adverse events included nausea, fatigue, headache, dermatitis, arthralgias, and nephrotoxicity. Other phase I monotherapy studies have been conducted in patients with Ewing's sarcoma and adrenocortical carcinoma. A phase I trial was completed in 32 patients with solid tumors in combination with temsirolimus, an mTOR inhibitor (Busaidy et al. 2010). The purpose of this study was to evaluate the combined therapy for toxicity. Mild hyperglycemia was noted in 53% of patients. Hypertriglyceridemia was noted in 56% and hypercholesterolemia in 56%. These side effects could be controlled with other medications. The only phase II study to date is a study conducted by NCI in which this antibody is being given with standard platinum chemotherapy to patients with thymoma or thymic carcinoma (Anthony et al. 2010). Thirteen patients have been enrolled; two patients developed hyperuricemia. Other toxicities included elevated liver function tests, neutropenia, and lymphopenia as well as posttreatment pain. Disease stabilization occurred in eight patients and five had disease progression.

AMG479

A phase I study has been completed in patients with advanced solid tumors and non-Hodgkin's lymphoma (Tolcher et al. 2008). The half-life of the drug was determined to be 12 days; therefore, it can be administered at dose of 20 mg/kg every 2 weeks. Grade 3 thrombocytopenia was observed in four patients and transaminitis was observed in 3. One complete response was noted in a patient with Ewing's sarcoma and a partial response was noted in two patients with neuroendocrine tumors.

Hyperglycemia and arthralgias were also reported. Five patients showed stabilization. A phase I study examining the combination of AMG479 and Gemcitabine in patients with NSCLC was reported (Sarantopoulos et al. 2008). Neutropenia was noted in half the patients. Hyperglycemia was noted in 40%. A partial response was noted in one patient and five showed disease stabilization. These were 25 patients with advanced solid tumors. Phase II studies have also been reported. One hundred and twenty-five patients were enrolled in a phase II trial of AMG479 plus Gemcitabine in patients with metastatic pancreatic cancer (Kindler et al. 2010). Survival rate at 6 months was 57% compared to 50% in the Gemcitabine-alone group and 39% vs. 23% at 12 months. The median overall survival was 8.7 months compared to 5.9 months. Toxicities included neutropenia, thrombocytopenia, fatigue, and hyperglycemia. A phase II study has also been reported in patients with Ewing's sarcoma (Tap et al. 2010). Thirty-five patients were enrolled. CT analysis confirmed tumor shrinkage in 29% of patients receiving the antibody. Toxicities included fatigue, nausea, dyspnea, peripheral edema, thrombocytopenia, neutropenia, and hyperglycemia. The drug was used as monotherapy.

BIIB022

This antibody differs in structure from other antibodies since it is an IgG4 monoclonal antibody. Therefore, it is likely to minimally stimulate effector function and cytotoxicity. A single phase I trial has been completed (von Mehren et al. 2010). The drug was administered to 24 patients with advanced solid tumors, 10 were sarcomas. Sixteen patients had treatment-related adverse events, including headache, nausea, fatigue, and hyperglycemia. It was administered using doses between 1.5 and 30 mg/kg. There were no objective responses over 28 days. Three patients showed reduced glucose consumption by PETFGP analysis.

In summary, the phase I trials have all established that these antibodies are reasonably safe when given as monotherapy; however, when administered with combination chemotherapy, the incidence of grade 3 and 4 side effects varied but has been dose limiting in some patients. In general, doses as high as 10–20 mg/kg are tolerated although this has not uniformly been the case when combined with conventional chemotherapy. In the phase II studies reported to date, some subgroups of patients, e.g., with Ewing's sarcoma, have had responses to treatment; however, the incidence of response, e.g., even in sarcomas, has been limited to a relatively small proportion of the patients. Advanced epithelial solid tumors have shown a reasonable incidence of stabilization; however, tumor shrinkage in this group has been less prevalent. Clearly longer trials with more patients enrolled are going to be required to determine whether there are subsets of patients having adequate efficacy to achieve responses that are superior to the results of conventional chemotherapy. The group of patients that has received the most intense focus, those with NSCLC, have had results that have been disappointing. Whether other groups when analyzed this intensively have an improved response rate remains to be determined.

Toxicity

The toxicities that have been noted with this agent are relatively predictable. It is not surprising that hyperglycemia is present in 15–30% of treated patients. IGF-I has insulin-like properties and functions through the IGF-IR to improve insulin sensitivity (Clemmons 2006). Therefore, downregulation of IGF-IRs which occurs frequently with these antibodies is likely to lead to worsening insulin resistance. The hyperglycemia may also be secondary to an elevation of circulating GH levels due to a reduced negative feedback of IGF-1: GH has anti-insulin effects. This has been demonstrated in several subjects by showing elevated plasma insulin concentrations and the presence of hyperglycemia, thus indicating worsening insulin sensitivity. In general, this problem has been able to be managed with oral hypoglycemic agents and therefore it should not represent a major barrier to therapy. Other significant toxicities include bone marrow suppression. Both neutropenia and lymphopenia have been noted as well as thrombocytopenia. To the extent that IGF-I stimulates the proliferation of hematopoetic stem cells, it is not surprising that if it is given with bone marrow-suppressive chemotherapeutic agents it may enhance their suppressive activity. This has clearly been a dose-limiting feature of some studies. The extent to which this problem occurs is likely to be due to the extent of receptor downregulation and the particular chemotherapeutic regimen used as well as individual sensitivity to chemotherapy. Other side effects that are predictable are elevated transaminases, cutaneous reactions, and occasional episodes of an acute allergic reaction to the intravenous infusion. These are not unusual side effects that are noted with many monoclonal antibody therapies. In general, toxicity has not been a major problem with this agent.

Combined Therapy

The combination of this agent with traditional chemotherapy is no doubt the standard in most treatment protocols. The exception to this might be patients who have failed several courses of chemotherapy and have a tumor for which the antibody is being given as a sole treatment. However, to date, only patients with pancreatic cancer and Ewing's sarcoma have shown any significant response to monotherapy; therefore, it is likely that the antibody will be administered in conjunction with traditional chemotherapy (Tolcher et al. 2009; Hidalgo et al. 2008). Since downregulation of the receptor enhances apoptosis, this is certainly a rational use of the drug since many chemotherapeutic agents work by accelerating proapoptotic pathways. Other combined chemotherapeutic approaches are based on known expression of other growth factor receptors by tumors. The hypothesis that has been put forward most frequently is that there is cooperative signaling between the epidermal growth factor receptor (EGFR) and the IGF-IR. Additionally, compensatory increases in EGFR activation have been noted in tumor xenografts following administration of

IGF-IR antibodies. Since very effective monoclonal antibodies that suppress EGFR function are available, several preclinical studies were conducted in mice bearing human tumor xenografts. The results of these studies have shown that suppression of both pathways has an enhanced effect on tumor xenograft growth compared to the effect of either agent alone.

Cooperative Stimulation Through Growth Factor-Signaling Pathways

The estrogen receptor-signaling pathway has received a great deal of attention because of its potential to synergize with the IGF-I-signaling pathway in stimulating breast cancer cell proliferation. IGF-I has been shown to enhance the survival of breast cancer cells that are sensitive to inhibition by tamoxifen (Dunn et al. 1997). AKT activation in response to IGF-I activation has been shown to phosphorylate the estrogen receptor Ser167 which leads to ligand-independent activation of the estrogen receptor (Campbell et al. 2001). A direct interaction between IGF-I and ER has also been demonstrated in cells in culture (Massarweh et al. 2008). Inhibition of IGF-IR tyrosine kinase activity has been shown to enhance the effect of antiestrogens, such as tamoxifen, on breast cancer cells in culture (Knowlden et al. 2005). Treatment of animals bearing ER-positive breast cancer xenografts with CP751,871 enhanced the ability of tamoxifen to inhibit tumor growth in vivo (Cohen et al. 2005). Although these studies have been presumed to be due to antagonism of genomic effects of the estrogen receptor, the ER receptor has also been shown to enhance IGF-I action in breast tumor cells by nongenomic actions. Specifically, Song et al. 2007 showed that sequential activation of the IGF-IR and ER resulted in estradiol stimulation of cell proliferation and that knockdown of the IGF-IR inhibited estradiol-stimulated growth. This pathway was facilitated by activation of matrix metalloproteases and did not require the genomic actions of ER. Cytoplasmic ER also activates Shc and the p85 subunit of PI-3 kinase. Combined targeting of cytoplasmic ER and IGF-IR tyrosine kinase inhibited breast cancer growth in vitro. Currently, one human trial evaluating exemestane with CP751,871 is ongoing and a similar trial is ongoing that is evaluating the effect of AMG479 with exemestane or fulvestamine.

In addition to the estrogen receptor, the EGF receptor pathway is believed to function synergistically with IGF-IR in some tumors. Data from several studies supports the hypothesis that activation of IGF-IR can lead to resistance to anti-EGF receptor therapy. Several mechanisms have been shown to mediate this interaction, including direct association between the two receptors and indirect interactions between common downstream signaling elements. IGF-I has been shown to transactivate the EGF receptor in certain breast cancer cell lines, thus providing another mechanism for cross talk (Saxena et al. 2008). There is evidence of upregulation of the IGF-IR protein and IGF-IR phosphorylation in response to anti-EGFR therapy and this has been proposed to mediate resistance. This has been proposed to be mediated by downregulation of IGFBP-3 expression (Guix et al. 2008). Xenograft studies suggest that targeting both receptors simultaneously with a single bispecific antibody can inhibit breast cancer xenograft growth (Nahta et al. 2005). Similarly, Her2 positive breast cancer patients show upregulation of IGF-IR (Esparis-Ogando et al. 2008). An anti-Her2 inhibitor is being tested in combination with the IMC-A12 antibody in patients in a phase II trial.

Potential interactions between IGF-I and VEGF receptor activation have also been investigated. In certain cancers, overproduction of IGF-I has been shown to induce VEGF synthesis (Kurmasheva et al. 2009). This functions to signal the development of increased vasculature within the tumor bed. Thus, tumor propagation and potential metastasis are facilitated by the ability of IGF-I to induce VEGF synthesis and subsequent VEGF receptor activation. Blocking IGF-I stimulation has been shown to reduce VEGF levels within tumors (Tonra et al. 2006). Recently, this mechanism was shown to predict lymph node metastasis in colorectal cancer (Zhang et al. 2010). Similarly, administration of the CP751,871 antibody downregulated the increase in tumor-derived VEGF. In Ewing's sarcoma and pancreatic cancer xenograft models, blockade to the IGF-IR has been shown to inhibit angiogenesis as well as primary cancer cell growth (Moser et al. 2008; Wang et al. 2010).

Inhibition of intracellular signaling components has also been shown to enhance the cytotoxic effects of IGF-IR antibodies. Prolonged treatment with rapamycin, a potent inhibitor of mTOR which is a key element in mediating the enhanced protein synthesis response of tumors, is associated with the development of tumor resistance. Following its stimulation p70S6 kinase feeds back to suppress AKT activation through serine phosphorylation (O'Reilly et al. 2006). Since rapamycin inhibits mTOR stimulation of p70S6 kinase, it can result in AKT activation and subsequent activation of other downstream signaling components that lead to inhibition of tumor cell apoptosis. Inhibiting IGF-IR activation in tumors that are rapamycin resistant but IGF-I responsive can downregulate this compensatory increase in AKT activation and, thus, inhibit tumor growth (Bertrand et al. 2006). This response has also been observed in tumor xenografts. Specifically, the antitumor antibody R1507 resulted in improved osteosarcoma xenograft responsiveness when administered with rapamycin (Kolb et al. 2010). This approach has also been used in a small number of patients with Ewing's sarcoma with modest success (Naing et al. 2010).

Another pathway which has received recent attention is the LKB/AMP kinase pathway. This pathway is activated by exercise and/or energy deprivation resulting in increased AMP-to-ATP ratios within the cell. The increased kinase activity then functions to utilize fatty acids to increase TCA cycle mobilization providing an alternative of energy source. In order for the cell to conserve energy under these conditions, AMP kinase also acts to inhibit protein synthesis. Specifically functioning through TSC1/TSC-2 phosphorylation, AMP kinase downregulates mTOR and p70S6 kinase induction by growth factors in energy-deprived cells. Induction of AMP kinase has been shown to specifically inhibit IGF-I-stimulated protein synthesis (Ning and Clemmons 2010). This occurs by an interaction between AMP kinase and IRS-1. AMP kinase phosphorylates serine 794 in IRS-1 which inhibits

IRS-1-mediated PI-3 kinase/AKT activation. Based on these observations, investigators have proposed that induction of AMP kinase through stimulation of LKB1 might provide an antiproliferative mechanism which specifically antagonizes the effect of mTOR pathway activation on tumors (Vazquez-Martin et al. 2009). Since AKT can be secondarily activated in response to inhibiting IGF-IR-mediated mTOR activation, stimulation of AMP kinase phosphorylation of AKT might downregulate this compensatory change in AKT, thus inhibiting tumor growth. Metformin combined with anti-IGF-IR antibody has shown to be effective in breast cancer cells (Liu et al. 2009; Alimova et al. 2009).

Mechanisms of Acquired Tumor Resistance to Anti-IGF-IR Therapy

Most human trials have shown that both serum IGF-I and growth hormone concentrations increase following administration of anti-IGF-IR. Preclinical studies have shown that blocking the GH receptor with a GH receptor antagonist reduces growth of xenografts, but this approach has not been tested in combination with anti-IGF-IR in a clinical trial. Additionally, whether the degree of increase that occurs in serum IGF-I overrides the effect of anti-IGF-IR blockade has not been determined. Constitutive phosphorylation occurs in some tumors which may necessitate the use of tyrosine kinase inhibitors (Hendrickson and Haluska 2009). Downregulation of IGF-IR may also occur and this may be associated with a poor prognosis (Chakravarty et al. 2009). Recently, it was demonstrated that resistance to anti-IGF-IR therapy could also be mediated by the insulin receptor using the xenograft model of pancreatic cancer that was IGF-IR-dependent (Ulanet et al. 2010). It was shown that the tumor cells became resistant to an anti-IGF-IR monoclonal antibody through induction of the insulin receptor. Knocking down the insulin receptor restored sensitivity to anti-IGF-IR therapy. The investigators propose that this could be a common mechanism of adaptive resistance.

Novel Therapies in Development

Several novel approaches to targeting the IGF-IR have been developed. SiRNA has been shown to downregulate receptor synthesis and, thereby, inhibit prostate cancer cell growth in vitro and in xenografts.(Furukawa et al. 2009). Colorectal cancers that expressed IGF-IR siRNAs were shown to be more sensitive to radiation or chemotherapy, respectively (Yuen et al. 2009) (Yavari et al. 2010). Dual silencing of the IGF-IR and EGFR has also been shown to be effective (Kalfuss et al. 2009; Niu et al. 2007). Using another approach, autologous bone marrow cells were altered to secrete a soluble form of IGF-IR. When these cells were infused into mice, they were shown to inhibit liver metastases (Wang et al. 2009a).

Recently, a methotrexate/IGF-I conjugate was shown to be delivered effectively to prostate cancer xenografts and to inhibit the cell proliferation (McTavish et al. 2009).

Summary

Since the IGF-IR is ubiquitously expressed, there has been a great deal of interest in its role in propagation and survival of tumor cells. Much remains to be learned regarding how IGF-IR and its associated signaling pathways adapt to the metabolic needs and stresses that are placed upon cancer cells and specifically how IGF-I's potent antiapoptotic effects are propagated over several tumor generations. The ubiquitous presence of this receptor makes an attractive target for cancer chemotherapy. Its ability to synergize with other agents that target growth factor receptors, such as antiHer2 and antiEGFR antibodies, further enhances the likelihood that some patients will respond to this treatment with an improved prognosis. However, the ability to overcome the effects of anti-IGF-I antibodies by the activation of alternative signaling pathways; the induction and heightened sensitivity to other growth factor receptors, i.e., EGFR, or the insulin receptor; as well as receptor-independent mechanisms of tumor resistance remain challenges to this form of therapy. Human trials addressing several of these questions are underway and the results are likely to determine the future success of this treatment.

References

Alimova IN, Liu B, Fan Z, et al (2009) Metformin inhibits breast cancer cell growth colony formation and induces cell cycle arrest in vitro. Cell Cycle 8:909–915.

Anthony LB, Loehrer PJ, Leonog S, et al (2010) Phase II study of cixutumumab (IMC-A12) plus depot octreotide for patients with metastatic carcinoid or islet cell carcinoma. J Clin Oncol 28suppl:220.

Beltran PJ, Mitchell P, Chung YA, et al (2009) AMG 479, a fully human anti-insulin-like growth factor receptor type I monoclonal antibody, inhibits the growth and survival of pancreatic carcinoma cells. Mol Cancer Ther 8:1–11.

Bertrand FE, Steelman LS, Chappell HW, et al (2006) Synergy between an IGF-1R antibody and Raf/MEK/ERK and P13K/Akt/mTOR pathway inhibitors in suppressing IGF-1R-mediated growth in hematopoietic cells. Leukemia 20:1254–1260.

Burtrum D, Zhu Z, Lu D, et al (2003) A fully human monoclonal antibody to the insulin-like growth factor I receptor blocks ligand-dependent signaling and inhibits human tumor growth in vivo. Cancer Res 63:8912–8921.

Busaidy N, Kurzrock R, LoRusso P, et al (2010) Hyperglycemia, hypertriglyceridemia, and hypercholesterolemia in a phase I trial of the combination of an mTOR inhibitor and IGF-1 receptor inhibitor. J Clin Oncol 28 suppl:2597.

Campbell RA, Bhat-Nakshatir P, Patel NM, et al (2001) Phosphatidylinositol 3-kinase/AKT mediated activation of estrogen receptor alpha: a new model for anti-estrogen resistance J Biol Chem 276:9817–9824.

Carmirand A, Zakikhani M, Young F (2005) Inhibition of insulin-like growth factor 1 receptor signaling enhances growth-inhibitory and proapoptotic effects of gefutnib (Iressa) in human breast cancer cells. Breast Cancer Res 7:R570–579.

Chakravarty G, Santillan AA, Galer C, et al (2009) Phosphorylated insulin like growth factor-I receptor expression and its clinico-pathological significance in histologic subtypes of human thyroid cancer. Exp Biol Med 234:372–378.

Chi KN, Gleave ME, Fazil S, et al (2010) A phase II study of preoperative figitumumab (F) in patients (pts) with localized prostate cancer (PCa). J Clin Oncol 28 suppl:4662.

Clemmons DR (2006) Involvement of insulin-like growth factor-I in the control of glucose homeostasis. Curr Opin Pharmacol 6:620–625.

Clemmons DR (2010) Insulin-like growth factor-I and its binding proteins: Jamison JL and DeGroot L (eds) in Endocrinology Adult and Pediatric, Elsevier 6th ed, Philadephia, PA. pp. 454–478.

Cohen BD, Baker DA, Soderstrom C, et al (2005) Combination therapy enhances the inhibition of tumor growth with the fully human antitype I insulin-like growth factor receptor monoclonal antibody CP-751,871. Clin Cancer Res 11:2063–2073.

de Bono JS, Attard G, Adjei A, et al (2007) Potential applications for circulating tumor cells expressing the insulin-like growth factor-I receptor. Clin Cancer Res 13:3611–3616.

Doern A, Cao X, Sereno A, et al (2009) Characterization of inhibitory anti-insulin-like growth factor receptor antibodies with different epitope specificity and ligand-blocking properties: implications for mechanism of action in vivo. J Biol Chem 294:10254–10267.

Dunn SE, Hardman RA, Kari FW, et al (1997) Insulin-like growth factor 1 (IGF-1) alters drug sensitivity of HBL100 human breast cancer cells by inhibition of apoptosis induced by diverse anticancer drugs. Cancer Res 57:2687–2693.

Esparis-Ogando A, Ocana A, Rodriquez-Barrueco R, et al (2008) Synergic antitumoral effect of an IGF-IR inhibitor and trastuzumab on HER2-overexpressing breast cancer cells. Ann Oncol 19:1860–1869.

Frasca F, Pandini G, Scalia P et al (1999) Insulin receptor isoform A, a newly recognized, high-affinity insulin-like growth factor II receptor in fetal and cancer cells. Mol Cell Biol 19:3278–3288.

Furukawa J, Wraight C, Freier SM, et al (2009) Antisense oligonucleotide targeting of insulin-like growth factor-1 receptor (IGF-1R) in prostate cancer. The Prostate 70:206–218.

Geoerger B, Brasme JF, Daudigeos-Dubus E, et al (2010) Anti-insulin-like growth factor 1 receptor antibody EM164 (murine AVE1642) exhibits anti-tumor activity alone and in combination with temozolomide against neuroblastoma. Eur J Cancer epub, June 28.

Goetsch L, Gonzalez A, Leger O, et al (2005) A recombinant humanized anti-insulin-like growth factor receptor type 1 antibody (h7C10) enhances the antitumor activity of vinorelbine and antiepidermal growth factor receptor therapy against human cancers. Int J Cancer 113:316–326.

Gridelli C, Rossi A, Bareschino MA, et al (2010) The potential role of insulin-like growth factor receptor inhibitors in the treatment of advanced non-small cell lung cancer. Expert Opin Investig Drugs 19:631–639.

Guix M, Faber AC, Wang SE, et al (2008) Acquired resistance to EGFR tyrosine kinase inhibitors in cancer cells is mediated by loss of IGF-binding proteins. J Clin Invest 118:2609–2619.

Haluska P, Shaw HM, Batzel GH, et al (2007) Phase I dose escalation study of the anti insulin-like growth factor-I receptor monoclonal antibody (CP-751,871) in patients with refractory solid tumors. Clin Cancer Res 13:5834–5840.

Haluska P, Worden F, Olmos D, et al (2009) Safety, tolerability, and pharmacokinetics of the anti-IGF-1R monoclonal antibody figitumumab in patients with refractory adrenocortical carcinoma. Cancer Chemother Pharmacol 65:765–773.

Hendrickson AW, Haluska P (2009) Resistance pathways relevant to insulin-like growth factor-1 receptor-targeted therapy. Curr Opin Investig Drugs 10:1032–1040.

Hewish M, Chau I, Cunningham D (2009) Insulin-like growth factor 1 receptor targeted therapeutics: novel compounds and novel treatment strategies for cancer medicine. Recent Pat Anticancer Drug Discov 4:54–72.

Hidalgo M, Tirado Gomaz M, Lewis N, et al (2008) A phase I study of MK-0646, a humanized monoclonal antibody against the insulin-like growth factor receptor type 1 (IGF1R) in advanced solid tumor patients in a q2 wk schedule. J Clin Oncol 26 suppl:3520.

Higano CS, Yu EY, Whiting SH, et al (2007) A phase I, first in man study of weekly IMC-A12, a fully human insulin like growth factor-I receptor IgG1 monoclonal antibody, in patients with advanced solid tumors. J Clin Oncol 25 suppl:3505.

Hofmann F, Garcia-Echeverria C (2005) Blocking insulin-like growth factor-I receptor as a strategy for targeting cancer. Drug Discovery Today 10:1041–1047.

Houghton PJ, Morton CL, Gorlick R, et al (2010) Initial testing of a monoclonal antibody (IMC-A12) against IGF-1R by the pediatric preclinical testing program. Pediatr Blood Cancer 54:921–926.

Iwasa T, Okamoto I, Sukuki M, et al (2009) Inhibition of insulin-like growth factor 1 receptor by CP-751,871 radiosensitizes non-small cell lung cancer cells. Clin Cancer Res 15:5117–5125.

Jacobs S, Cook S, Svoboda ME, et al (1986) Interaction of the monoclonal antibodies alpha IR-1 and alpha IR-3 with insulin and somatomedin-C receptors. Endocrinol 118:223–226.

Jassem J, Langer CJ, Karp DD, et al (2010) Randomized, open label, phase III trial of figitmumab in combination with paclitaxel and carboplatin versus paclitaxel and carboplatin in patients with non-small cell lung cancer (NSCLC). J Clin Oncol 28 suppl:15:7500.

Javle MM, Varadhachary RT, Shroff TR, et al (2010) Phase I/II study of MK-0646, the humanized monoclonal IGF-1R antibody in combination with gemcitabine or gemcitabine plus erlontinib (E) for advanced pancreatic cancer. J Clin Onc 28 suppl:4039.

Kalfuss S, Burfeind P, Gaedcke J, et al (2009) Dual silencing of insulin-like growth factor-I receptor and epidermal growth factor receptor in colorectal cancer cells is associated with decreased proliferation and enhanced apoptosis. Mol Cancer Ther 8:821–833.

Karp DD, Paz-Ares LG, Novello S, et al (2009a) Phase II study of the anti-insulin-like growth factor type 1 receptor antibody CP-751,871 in combination with paclitaxel and carboplatin in previously untreated, locally advanced, or metastatic non-small-cell lung cancer. J Clin Onocol 27:2516–2522.

Karp DD, Pollak MN, Cohen RB, et al (2009b) Safety, pharmacokinetics, and pharmacodynamics of the insulin-like growth factor type 1 receptor inhibitor figitumumab (CP-751,871) in combination with paclitaxel and carboplatin. J Thorac Oncol 4:1397–1403.

Keyhanfar M, Booker GW, Whittaker J, et al (2007) Precise mapping of an IGF-I binding site on the IGF-IR. Biochem J 401:269–277.

Kindler HL, Richards DA, Stephenson J, et al (2010) A placebo-controlled, randomized phase II study of conatumumab (C) or AMG 479 (A) or placebo (P) plus gemcitabine (G) in patients (pts) with metastatic pancreatic cancer (mPC). J Clin Oncol 28 suppl:4035.

Knowlden J, Hutchenson IR, Barrow D, et al (2005) Insulin-like growth factor-I receptor signaling in tamoxifen-resistant breast cancer: a supporting role to the epidermal growth factor receptor. Endocrinol 146:4609–4618.

Kolb EW, Kamara D, Zhang W, et al (2010) R1507, a fully human monoclonal antibody targeting IGF-1R, is effective alone and in combination with rapamycin in inhibiting growth of osteosarcoma xenografts. Pediatr Blood Cancer 55:67–75.

Kurmasheva RT, Dudkin L, Billups C, et al (2009) The insulin-like growth factor-1 receptor-targeting antibody, CP-751,871, suppresses tumor-derived VEGF and synergizes with rapamycin in models of childhood sarcoma. Cancer Res 69:7662–7671.

Kurzrock R, Patnaik Am, Aisner J, et al (2010) A Phase I study of weekly R1507, a human monoclonal antibody insulin-like growth factor-I receptor antagonist, in patients with advanced solid tumors. Clin Cancer Res 16:2458–2465.

Lacy MQ, Alsina M, Fonseca R, et al (2008) Phase I, pharmacokinetic and pharmacodynamic study of the anti-insulinlike growth factor ype 1 receptor monoclonal antibody CP-752,871 in patients with multiple myeloma. J Clin Oncol 26:3196–3203.

Liu B, Fan Z, Edgerton SM, et al (2009) Metformin induces unique biological and molecular responses in triple negative breast cancer cells. Cell Cycle 8:2031–2040.

Lu D, Zhang H, Koo H (2005) A fully human recombinant IgG-like bispecific antibody to both the epidermal growth factor receptor and the insulin-like growth factor receptor for enhanced antitumor activity. J Biol Chem 280:19665–19672.

Lu Y, Zi X, Zhao Y, et al (2001) Insulin-like growth factor-I receptor signaling and resistance to trastuzumab (Herceptin) J Natl Cancer Inst 93:1830–1852.

Maloney EK, McLaughlin JL, Dagdigian NE, et al (2003) An anti-insulin-like growth factor I receptor antibody that is a potent inhibitor of cancer cell proliferation. Cancer Res 63:5073–5083.

Massarweh S, Osborne CK, Creighton CJ, et al (2008) Tamoxifen resistance in breast tumors is driven by growth factor receptor signaling with repression of classic estrogen receptor genomic function. Cancer Res 68:826–833.

McTavish H, Griffin RJ, Terai K, et al (2009) Novel insulin-like growth factor-methotrexate covalent conjugate inhibits tumor growth in vivo at lower dosage than methotrexate alone. Transl Res 153:275–282.

Menu E, van Valckenborgh E, van Camp B, et al (2009) The role of the insulin-like growth factor 1 receptor axis in multiple myeloma. Arch Physiol Biochem 115:49–57.

Moreau P, Hulin C, Facon T, et al (2007) Phase I study of AVE1642 and IGF-1R monoclonal antibody in patients with advanced multiple myeloma. Blood 110:1166.

Moschos SJ, Mantzoros (2002) The role of the IGF system in cancer: from basic to clinical studies and clinical applications. Oncology 63:317–332.

Moser C, Schachtschneider P, Lang SA, et al (2008) Inhibition of insulin-like growth factor-I receptor (IGF-IR) using NVP-AEW541, a small molecule kinase inhibitor, reduces orthotopic pancreatic cancer growth and angiogenesis. Eur J Cancer 44:1577–1586.

Nahta R, Yuan LX, Zhang B, et al (2005) Insulin-like growth factor 1 receptor/human epidermal growth factor receptor 2 heterodimerization contributes to trastuzumab resistance of breast cancer cells. Cancer Res 65:11118–111128.

Naing A, LoRusso P, Gupta S, et al (2010) Dual inhibition of IGFR and mTOR pathways. J Clin Oncol 28 suppl:3007.

Niu J, Li XN, Qian N, et al (2007) siRNA mediated the type 1 insulin-like growth factor receptor and epidermal growth factor receptor silencing induces chemosensitization of liver cancer cells. J Cancer Res Clin Oncol 134:503–513.

O'Donnell R, El-Khouriry AB, Lenz H, et al (2010) A phase I trial of escalating doses of the anti-IGF-1R monoclonal antibody (mAb) cixutumumab (IMC-A12) and sorafenib for treatment of advanced hepatocellular carcinoma (HCC). J Clin Oncol 28:173.

O'Reilly KE, Rojo F, She QB, et al (2006) mTOR inhibition induces upstream receptor tyrosine kinase signaling and activates Akt. Cancer Res 66:1500–1508.

Ogawa O, Bercroft DM, Morison IM, et al (1993) Constitutional relaxation of insulin-like growth factor II gene imprinting associated with Wilm's tumour and gigantism. Nat Genet 5:408–412.

Olmos D, Postel-Vinay S, Molife LR, et al (2010) Safety, pharmacokinetics, and preliminary activity of the anti-IGF-1R antibody figitumumab (CP-751,871) in patients with sarcoma and Ewing's sarcoma: a phase 1 expansion cohort study. Lancet Oncol 11:105–106.

Ota, Wilson GL, Leroith D (1988) Insulin-like growth factor I receptors on mouse neuroblastoma cells. Two β subunits are derived from differences in glycosylation. Eur J Biochem 174:521–530.

Pappo AS, Patel S, Crowley J, et al (2010) Activity of R1507, a monoclonal antibody to the insulin-like growth-1 receptor (IGF1R), in patients (pts) with recurrent or refractory Ewing's sarcoma family of tumors (ESFT): Results of a phase II SARC study. J Clin Oncol 28 suppl:1000.

Pautsch A, Zoephel A, Ahorn H et al (2001) Crystal structure of bisphosphorylated IGF-I receptor kinase: insight into domain movements upon kinase activation. Structure 9:955–965.

Pollak LM, Lipton A, Dimers L, et al (2007) Pharmacodynamic properties of the anti-IGF-IR monoclonal antibody CP-751,871 in cancer patients. J Clin Oncol 25 suppl:3587.

Reidy DL, Hollywood E, Segal E, et al (2010) A phase II clinical trial of MK-0646, an insulin-like growth factor-1 receptor inhibitor (IGF-1R), in patients with metastatic well-differentiated neuroendocrine tumor (NETs). J Clin Onc 28 suppl:4163.

Renehan AG, Zwahlen M, Minder C, et al (2004) Insulin-like growth factor (IGF)-I, IGF binding protein-3, and cancer risk: systemic review and meta-regression analysis. Lancet 363:1346–1353

Rodon J, Patnaik A, Stein M, et al (2007) A phase I study of q3W R1507, a human monoclonal antibody IGF-1R antagonist in patients with advanced cancer. J Clin Oncol 25 suppl:3590.

Rowinsky EK, Youssoufian H, Tonra JR, et al (2007) IMC-A12, a human IgG1 monoclonal antibody to the insulin-like growth factor I receptor. Clin Cancer Res 13:5549–5555.

Samani AA, Yakar S, LeRoith D, et al (2007) The role of IGF system in cancer growth and metastasis: overview and recent insights. Endocr Rev 28:20–47.

Sarantopoulos J, Mita AC, Mulay M, et al (2008) A phase 1B study of AMG 479, a type 1 insulin-like growth factor receptor (IGF1R) antibody, in combination with panitumumab (P) or gemcitabine (G). J Clin Oncol 26 suppl:3583.

Saxena NK, Taliaferro-Smith L, Knight BB, et al (2008) Bidirectional crosstalk between leptin and insulin-like growth factor-I signaling promotes invasion and migration of breast cancer cells via transactivation of epidermal growth factor receptor. Cancer Res 68:9712–9722.

Scotlandi K, Picci P (2008) Targeting insulin-like growth factor I receptor in sarcomas. Curr Opin Oncol 20:419–427.

Song RX, Zhang Z, Chen Y, et al (2007) Estrogen signaling via a linear pathway involving insulin-like growth factor I receptor, matrix metalloproteinases, and epidermal growth factor receptor to activate mitogen-activated protein kinase in MCF-7 breast cancer cells. Endocrinol 148:4091–4101.

Soos MA, Field CE, Siddle K (1993) Purified hybrid insulin/insulin-like growth factor-I receptors bind insulin-like growth factor-I but not insulin with high affinity. Biochem J 290:419–426.

Tap WD, Demertri GD, Barnette J, et al (2010) AMG 479 in relapsed or refractory Ewing's family tumors (EFT) or desmoplastic small round cell tumors (DSRCT): Phase II results. J Clin Oncol 28 suppl:10001.

Tolcher AW, Patnaik A, Till E, et al (2008) A phase I study of AVE1642, a humanized monoclonal antibody IGF-IR (insulin-like growth factor 1 receptor) antagonist, in patients (pts) with advanced solid tumor (ST). J Clin Oncol 26 suppl:173.

Tolcher AW, Sarantopoulos J, Patnaik A, et al (2009) Phase I, pharmacokinetic, and pharmacodynamic study of AMG 479, a fully human monoclonal antibody to insulin-like growth factor receptor 1. J Clin Oncol 27:5800–5807.

Tonra JR, Deevi DS, Corcoran E, et al (2006) Combined antibody mediated inhibition of IGF-IR, EGFR, VEGFR2 for more consistent and greater anti-tumor effects. Eur J Cancer 4:2197–2207.

Ulanct DB, Ludwig DL, Kahn CR, et al (2010) Insulin receptor functionally enhances multistage tumor progression and conveys intrinsic resistance to IGF-1R targeted therapy. Proc Natl Acad Sci USA 107:10791–10798.

van der Veeken J, Oliveira S, Schiffelers RM, et al (2009) Crosstalk between epidermal growth factor receptor- and insulin-like growth factor-1 receptor signaling: implications for cancer therapy. Curr Cancer Drug Targets 9:748–760.

Vazquez-Martin A, Oliveras-Ferraros C, Del Barco S, et al (2009) If mammalian target of metformin indirectly is mammalian target of rapamycin, then the insulin-like growth factor-1 receptor axis will audit the efficacy of metformin in cancer clinical trials. J Clin Oncol 27:207–209.

von Mehren M, Britten C, Lear K, et al (2010) Phase I, dose-escalation study of BIIB022 (anti-IGF-1R antibody) in advanced solid tumors. J Clin Onc 28 suppl:2612.

Wang N, Fallavllita L, Nguyen L, et al (2009a) Autologous bone marrow stromal cells genetically engineered to secrete an igf-I receptor decoy prevent the growth of liver metastases. Mol Ther 17:1241–1249.

Wang Y, Hailey J, Williams D, et al (2005) Inhibition of insulin-like growth factor-I receptor (IGF-IR) signaling and tumor cell growth by a fully human neutralizing anti-IGF antibody. Mol Cancer Ther 4:1214–1221.

Wang Y, Lipari P, Wang X, et al (2009b) A fully human insulin-like growth factor-I receptor antibody SCH 717454 (Robatumumab) has antitumor activity as a single agent and in combination with cytotoxics in pediatric tumor xenografts. Mol Cancer Ther 9:410–418.

Wang Y, Lipari P, Wang X, et al (2010) A fully human insulin like growth factor-I receptor antibody SCH 717454 has antitumor activity as a single agent and in combination with cytotoxics in pediatric tumor xenografts. Mol Cancer Ther 9:410–418.

Wu JD, Haugk K, Coleman I (2006) Combined in vivo effect of A12, a type 1 insulin-like growth factor receptor antibody, and docetaxel against prostate cancer tumors. Clin Cancer Res 12:6153–6160.

Wu JD, Odman A, Higgins LM, et al (2005) In vivo effects of the human type 1 insulin-like growth factor receptor antibody A12 on androgen-dependent and androgen-independent human prostate tumors. Clin Cancer Res 11:3065–3074.

Yavari K, Taghikhani M, Maragheh MG, et al (2010) SiRNA-mediated IGF-1R inhibition sensitizes human colon cancer SW480 cells to radiation. Acta Oncol 29:70–75.

Ye JJ, Liang SJ, Guo N, et al (2003) Combined effects of tamoxifen and a chimeric humanized single chain antibody against the type I IGF receptor on breast tumor growth in vivo. Horm Metab Res 35:836–842.

Yuen JS, Akkaya E, Wang Y, et al (2009) Validation of the type 1 insulin-like growth factor receptor as a therapeutic target in renal cancer. Mol Cancer Ther 8:1448–1459.

Yuen JS, Macauley VM (2008) Targeting the type 1 insulin-like growth factor receptor as a treatment for cancer. Expert Opin Ther Targets 12:589–603.

Zhang C, Hao L, Wang L, et al (2010) Elevated IGFIR expression regulating VEGF and VEGF-C predicts lymph node metastasis in human colorectal cancer. BMC Cancer 10:184.

Chapter 11
Targeting Insulin-Like Growth Factor Receptor 1 (IGF-1R) and Insulin Receptor Signaling by Tyrosine Kinase Inhibitors in Cancer

Joan M. Carboni, Mark Wittman, and Fei Huang

Introduction

The insulin-like growth factor receptor 1 (IGF-1R) is an important growth factor receptor in cancer cells and plays an essential role in the establishment and maintenance of the transformed phenotype (LeRoith et al. 1995; Valentinis and Baserga 2001). A significant number of cancers have either overactivated and/or overexpressed IGF-1R and as a result, the IGF-1R signaling pathway has become an attractive target for the development of novel anticancer agents. The convergence of efficacy data for IGF-1R specific antibodies (Gualberto and Pollak 2009) and epidemiological findings (Chan et al. 1998) that correlate higher IGF-1 levels with poor prognosis, has also prominently positioned IGF-1R among the emerging cellular signaling pathways currently being explored for cancer therapy.

IGF-1R is a member of the insulin receptor (IR) family and shares high sequence homology with IR; the role of IR in cancer is just beginning to be explored (Pollak 2008; Hillerman et al. 2010; Ulanet et al. 2010). Two splice variants of IR are expressed in mammalian cells; isoform IR-A, and the classical IR-B. The prevalence of these two IR isoforms varies in different tissues and cell lines (Moller et al. 1989). A variety of human tumors express high levels of IR-A compared with IR-B, which include breast and colon (Frasca et al. 1999; Sciacca et al. 1999), ovarian (Kalli et al. 2002), thyroid (Vella et al. 2002), as well as tumors of smooth and striated muscle (Sciacca et al. 2002). Recent studies show that downregulation of IR alone inhibits cancer cell proliferation, angiogenesis, lymphangiogenesis, and metastasis in tumor models (Zhang et al. 2010). In cells and in tissues, IGF-1R and IR can heterodimerize to form hybrid receptors consisting of a single α and β subunit from IGF-1R and IR (Pandini et al. 2002; Belfiore 2007). As IGF-1R expression levels are also

---

J.M. Carboni (✉)
Oncology Drug Discovery, Bristol Myers Squibb Company, Princeton, NJ, USA
e-mail: joan.carboni@bms.com

D. LeRoith (ed.), *Insulin-like Growth Factors and Cancer: From Basic Biology to Therapeutics*, Cancer Drug Discovery and Development,
DOI 10.1007/978-1-4614-0598-6_11, © Springer Science+Business Media, LLC 2012

Table 11.1 Small-molecule IGF-1R inhibitors

Identifier	Company	Development status	Comments
NVP AEW-541	Novartis AG	Phase I	Multiple Myeloma
			Solid tumors
			Discontinued
NVP ADW-742	Novartis	Preclinical	
PQIP	OSI	Preclinical	
OSI-906	OSI	Phase III	NSCLC, adrenal cortical, ovarian
BMS-536924	BMS	Preclinical	
BMS-754807	BMS	Phase I	All tumor types
XL-228	Exelixis	Phase I	AML, CML, Ph+ ALL leukemia
INSM-18	Insmed/UCSF	Phase II	Prostate
AXL-1717	Axelar AB	Phase I/II	Solid tumors

elevated in primary breast cancer tissues (Pandini et al. 1999), increased levels of hybrid IGF-1R/IR-A receptors likely exist in breast cancer cells. Therefore, dual inhibition of IGF-1R and IR may provide significant advantage in the treatment of cancers dependent on these pathways for survival and growth.

Various strategies have been explored in recent years to modulate the function of IGF-1R. In preclinical models, strategies aimed at reducing receptor number or enzymatic activity have been shown to reverse the malignant phenotype in tumor cells. These strategies include antisense RNA (Long et al. 1995; Andrews et al. 2001), monoclonal antibodies (Arteaga and Osborne 1989), IGF-1 mimetic peptides (Pietrzkowski et al. 1993), dominant negative mutants that lack enzymatic activity (D'Ambrosio et al. 1996), and small-molecule inhibitors of varying specificity (Haluska et al. 2006; Zimmermann et al. 2008; Wittman et al. 2009a).

Tyrosine kinase inhibitors (TKIs) from several different chemotypes have been reported to target IGF-1R (Table 11.1, Fig. 11.1). Small-molecule inhibitors of IGF-1R fall into two subcategories: those that target the ATP-binding pocket of the IGF-1R kinase domain (ATP-competitive) and those that target the substrate-binding site (non-ATP-competitive). This chapter focuses on the IGF-1R compounds that are reported to have entered clinical evaluation as well as selected advanced preclinical leads that have helped define the preclinical profile of small-molecule TKIs. Please refer to the following references for a more thorough treatment of small-molecule inhibitors of IGF-1R (Hubbard and Wilsbacher 2007; Hewish et al. 2009; Li et al. 2009; Wittman et al. 2009b).

IGF-1R ATP-Competitive Inhibitors

Pyrrolopyrimidines

Some of the first IGF-1R "selective" kinase inhibitors were the pyrrolopyrimidines described by Novartis. Among the first of these was *NVP-ADW-742*, a TKI reported to be >16-fold more potent against IGF-1R compared to IR as demonstrated in a capture

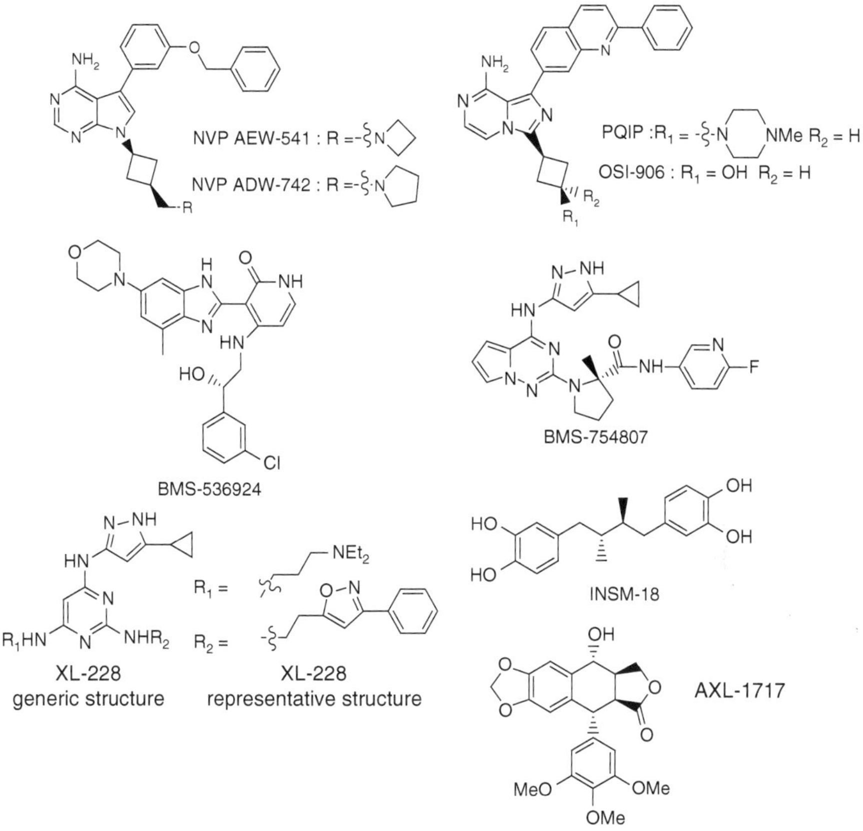

Fig. 11.1 Small-molecule inhibitors of IGF-1R

Elisa assay. NVP-ADW-742 was shown to block IGF-1-induced phosphorylation of IGF-1R and Akt in NIH-3T3 mouse fibroblast-derived fibrosarcoma cells that stably expressed the human IGF-1R (3T3/huIGF1R). This compound was also shown to have activity in vitro against diverse tumor cell types, with particular activity against multiple myeloma, resulting in both antiproliferative and proapoptotic effects as a single agent. Synergy was demonstrated in combination with dexamethasone and/or doxorubicin. In these studies, NVP-ADW-742 was tested in vivo in a clinically relevant mouse model of diffuse multiple myeloma, and was shown to suppress tumor growth, prolong survival, and enhance the antitumor effect of cytotoxic chemotherapy, providing proof of concept for therapeutic use of selective IGF-1R kinase inhibitors in cancer therapy (Mitsiades et al. 2004). A subsequent study also demonstrated that NVP-ADW-742 acted synergistically and enhanced sensitivity of multiple SCLC cell lines to etoposide and carboplatin (Warshamana-Greene et al. 2004).

Tumors express and are capable of activating multiple signaling pathways for survival. Treatment with IGF-1R inhibitors (TKIs or antibodies) may result in their utilization of escape mechanisms given the overlapping spectrum of multiple downstream molecules. To this end, other studies using NVP-ADW-742 showed the importance of SCF/Kit and IGF-1 autocrine loops in SCLC. Two populations of SCLC cells were identified by differential sensitivity to NVP-ADW-742; one that lacked the active SCF/Kit autocrine loop, and a second population which had an active autocrine loop. Due to differences in autocrine loops, a combination study was conducted using NVP-ADW-742 and a Kit kinase inhibitor, STI571; this combination was shown to synergistically inhibit growth and PI3K signaling in SCLC cell lines that have active SCF/Kit autocrine pathways of regulation. These data demonstrate that inhibition of multiple signaling pathways is essential to inhibit activity in SCLC (Warshamana-Greene et al. 2004).

A second pyrrolopyrimidine from Novartis, *NVP-AEW-541*, was found to be orally active and significantly more potent against IGF-1R than NVP-ADW-742, but was equipotent against IR in an in vitro kinase assay (Garcia-Echeverria et al. 2004). However, NVP-AEW-541 was found to be selective for IGF-1R in a cell-based assay using 3T3/huIGF1R. The authors suggest the cellular selectivity arises from conformational differences between the native forms of these receptors that are not recapitulated by the recombinant kinase domains used in the in vitro kinase assays. This compound was able to effectively inhibit IGF-1-mediated survival of MCF-7 cells and to prevent the ability of transformed cells to grow in an anchorage-independent manner at concentrations consistent with its capacity to inhibit IGF-1R autophosphorylation. In vivo studies utilizing the mechanistic 3T3/huIGF1R model, and a pharmacodynamic model (ex vivo murine lung), showed that the compound achieved significant inhibition of tumor growth and inhibition of phosphorylation of downstream signaling molecules in the murine lung model, and was well tolerated when administered orally. Additional studies showed growth inhibition in vitro and in vivo in musculoskeletal tumors (Scotlandi et al. 2005), and in multiple myeloma (Maiso et al. 2008). NVP-AEW-541 did not enter into clinical development.

Imidazopyrazines

Isosteric replacements of the pyrrolopyrimidine core have been investigated by various groups. In general, these isosteric scaffolds possess the same cellular selectivity over IR described for the pyrrolopyrimidines. Included among these scaffolds are the imidazopyrazines (Ji et al. 2007; Mulvihill et al. 2008). [cis-3-[(4-methyl-piper-azin-l-yl)-cyclobutyl]-1-(2-phe-nyl-quinolin-7-yl)-imidazol[1,5-a]pyrazin-8-ylam-ine] (PQIP) is a 1,3-disubstituted-8-amino-imidazopyrazine derivative developed by OSI Pharmaceuticals. PQIP was designed and optimized through structure-based design efforts that built upon co-crystal structures of an earlier imidazopyrazine IGF-1R lead. PQIP was shown to be a highly potent and selective ATP-competitive IGF-1R inhibitor with 14-fold selectivity relative to the human IR in a cell-based assay. It was also highly selective when tested against a panel of 32 other protein kinases. This compound possessed all of the attributes of a robust IGF-1R inhibitor, including inhibition of ligand-stimulated phosphorylation of IGF-1R, AKT, ERK1/2, and p70S6K in serum-starved 3T3/huIGF1R cells. When administered to mice orally, once per day, PQIP inhibited tumor growth in 3T3/huIGF-1R [dose-dependent tumor growth inhibition (TGI; 70–98%) at all doses tested between 25 and 100 mg/kg]. In the human GEO (colon carcinoma) tumor xenograft model using the same dosing regimen for 14 consecutive days, antitumor efficacy was demonstrated with a TGI of 70–97%. In order to assess the drug exposure required for inhibition of tumor IGF-1R in vivo, a pharmacodynamic study was conducted in 3T3/huIGF-1R tumors and the temporal relationship between drug concentration and kinase inhibition indicated that PQIP maintained plasma levels that were sufficient to chronically suppress 90% of IGF-1R phosphorylation in the tumors over a period of 24 h. Efforts to improve the absorption, distribution, metabolism, excretion (ADME) properties of PQIP led to the discovery of *OSI-906* which possessed all of the qualities of PQIP, i.e., potency, selectivity, broad range of tumor growth inhibition, but was orally active without significant effects on glucose (when dosed at 60 mg/kg, BID). OSI-906 also demonstrated synergy when given in combination with Erlotinib in Geo tumor xenograft models (Mulvihill et al. 2008). Results from two phase I clinical studies with dosing of single agent OSI-906 in subjects with cancer have been presented (Carden et al. 2009b; Lindsay et al. 2009).

Additional clinical studies of OSI-906 as single agent or in combination with other cancer agents are underway and include a phase I/II trial in patients with recurrent and/or relapsed ovarian cancer in combination with paclitaxel; a phase III trial in patients with locally advanced or metastatic adrenocortical carcinoma, and a phase I combination study with erlotinib.

Benzimidazoles

BMS-536924, a (1H-benzoimidazol-2-yl)-1H-pyridin-2-one, was identified by Bristol-Myers Squibb as a reversible ATP-competitive inhibitor of IGF-1R, and was among one of the first IGF-1R/IR inhibitors described as "dual" inhibitors with modest activity against Mek, Fak, and Lck.

BMS-536924 was found to be active against a wide range of human tumor cell lines and in vivo against a broad range of human tumor models (breast, rhabdomyosarcoma, colon, multiple myeloma, and IGF-1R Sal). The IGF-1R Sal tumor model was developed as a rapid, 4-day in vivo model, for iterative testing of compounds and is a model that is driven by IGF-1R. This tumor model was developed by fusion of the human CD8α intracellular catalytic domain, making it constitutively activated (CD8-IGF-1R). Overexpression of CD8-IGF-1R in the mammary gland of transgenic mice was sufficient to induce mammary epithelial hyperplasia and tumor formation (Carboni et al. 2005).

Numerous studies have been carried out in various laboratories to examine the efficacy of BMS-536924 in different biological systems. In xenograft studies where CD8-IGF-1R transfected MCF10A cells were implanted into mice, disruption of acini formation and epithelial-to-mesenchymal transition (EMT) was observed and resulted in full transformation. Full transformation of MCF10A cells with a single oncogene is an uncommon finding, underscoring the importance of IGF-1R in oncogenesis (Kim et al. 2007).

Additional studies investigated whether the combination of IGF-1R and HER-2 inhibitors might provide synergistic antiproliferative effects in ovarian cancer cells that were more resistant to HER agents (Haluska et al. 2008). These studies are discussed in section "Cross-Talk Pathways".

The complex interplay between potent CYP3A4 inhibition and CYP3A4 induction via transactivation of the pregnane-X-receptor observed in human hepatocytes for BMS-536924 left questions as to whether this molecule would effectively test the clinical potential of a small-molecule inhibitor of IGF-1R. Work within the pyrrolotriazine chemotype (see below) ultimately provided a clinical candidate with an improved preclinical profile (Velaparthi et al. 2008; Zimmermann et al. 2010). Thus, BMS-536924 was not advanced to the clinic.

Pyrrolotriazines

BMS-754807, a pyrrolotriazine, is a potent and reversible inhibitor of the IGF-1R/IR family kinases (IGF-1R/IR; $K_i < 2$nM) (Wittman et al. 2009a). BMS-754807 effectively inhibits the growth of a broad range of human tumor types in vitro, including: mesenchymal (Ewing's, rhabdomyosarcoma, neuroblastoma, and liposarcoma), epithelial (breast, lung, pancreatic, colon, gastric), and hematopoietic (multiple myeloma and leukemia) tumor cell lines (IC$_{50}$ 5–365 nM). It is also active in xenograft tumor models (epithelial, mesenchymal, and hematopoietic) with TGI ranging from 53 to 115% and a minimum effective dose of as low as 6.25 mg/kg when dosed orally once per day (Carboni et al. 2009). Combination studies with BMS-754807 have been performed with multiple human tumor cell types and in vitro synergies [combination index (CI) < 1.0] have been demonstrated when combined with cytotoxic, hormonal, and targeted agents. In vivo synergy is also observed in the GEO human colon xenograft tumor model when combined with cetuximab (Carboni et al. 2009).

BMS-754807 has activity in triple-negative (TN) breast cancer cell lines. In a tumor xenograft model developed from a primary TN breast tumor, BMS-754807 showed growth inhibition as monotherapy and tumor regressions in combination with docetaxel (Litzenburger et al. 2009). These data provide a biological rationale to test BMS-754807 in combination with chemotherapy in patients with TN breast cancer.

In vivo combination studies were also conducted using BMS-754807 with 4-hydroxy-tamoxifen, and letrozole in the aromatase-expressing estrogen-sensitive postmenopausal breast cancer model, MCF-7/AC-1 (Zhou et al. 1990). BMS-754807 was shown to enhance the activity of both tamoxifen and letrozole in vivo and increased survival, supporting the evaluation of IGF-1R/IR inhibition in combination with hormonal therapy (Haluska et al. 2009).

BMS-754807 is currently studied in phase I/II clinical trials for a variety of human cancers. An initial single-ascending dose study in normal healthy volunteers showed good bioavailability and tolerability (Clemens et al. 2009). Daily administration of BMS-754807 at dose levels that were considered safe led to drug exposures required for efficacy in preclinical models (Desai et al. 2010). Effects on blood glucose were manageable and did not lead to discontinuation of dosing. In both studies, pharmacodynamic effects on insulin and glucose demonstrated pharmacologic activity. Additional clinical studies with BMS-754807 in combination with cetuximab, trastuzumab, and chemotherapeutic agents are ongoing.

2,4,6-Triaminopyrimidine

XL-228, is a multikinase IGF-1R/IR small-molecule inhibitor developed by Exelixis; XL-228 also has activity against Src, Bcr-Abl, mutant BCR-Abl (T315I), Alk, Fak, Aur A/B, and FGFR family members (FGFRs-1,2,3). The specific structure has not been disclosed. Oral administration of XL-228 in vivo demonstrated TGI and regression in Colo205 and MCF7 xenograft models. The half-life of XL-228 is ~40–50 h. Based on favorable preclinical data, an open-label phase I dose-escalation study was conducted evaluating the safety, pharmacokinetics, and pharmacodynamics of XL-228 administered intravenously (1 h infusion) to subjects with either chronic myeloid leukemia (CML) or Philadelphia chromosome-positive acute lymphocytic leukemia (Ph+ ALL) (Cortes et al. 2008). In this study, complete and partial responses were noted in CML and ALL patients, respectively (Gualberto and Pollak 2009). Another trial to evaluate safety, preliminary efficacy, pharmacokinetics, and pharmacodynamic effects in solid tumors or multiple myeloma was conducted and dose limiting toxicity was grade 3 and 4 neutropenia occurring at the 8.0 mg/kg dose level, drug-related adverse events (AEs) in ≥15% of all pts include hyperglycemia (Smith et al. 2010).

IGF-1R Substrate Inhibitors

Catechols

INSM-18 is a naturally occurring bis-catechol, nordihydroguaiaretic acid (NDGA) developed by Insmed/University of California in 2004 for the potential treatment of cancer. INSM-18 is a substrate inhibitor that selectively inhibits both IGF-1R and human epidermal growth factor receptor (Her2/neu). INSM-18 inhibits phosphorylation of a synthetic nonspecific tyrosine kinase substrate by IGF-1R and proliferation of MCF-7 breast cancer cells with an IC_{50} of 0.9 and 24.6 μM, respectively. Two clinical studies have been initiated: A phase I study in 15 patients with recurrent prostate cancer demonstrated some early positive clinical data; 15 patients were treated, and one patient had >50% reduction in PSA, and another had a reduction in PSA doubling time. In a phase II study in patients with hormone-sensitive, nonmetastatic prostate cancer increases in transaminases were reported as an adverse event (Harzstark et al. 2007).

Picropodophyllotoxin

AXL-1717, is an orally active, naturally occurring lignan picropodophyllotoxin (PPP) IGF-1R substrate inhibitor developed by Axelar (Girnita et al. 2004). AXL-1717 demonstrated complete tumor regressions in preclinical models in breast, prostate, melanoma, sarcoma, multiple myeloma, and GBM; AXL-1717 has recently advanced into clinical studies (Harmenberg et al. 2009).

The Role of IGF-1R/IR in Resistance to Cancer Therapies

Cancer treatments utilizing cytotoxic agents, radiation, and specific targeted therapies have provided great value in extending human life. However, resistance is one of the major clinical challenges that impact cancer therapies and drug development. The IGF-1R pathway plays a critical role in drug resistance via its interaction with multiple pathways, including various components of the DNA damage response, estrogen receptor (ER), EGFR, and HER2 pathways (Casa et al. 2008). This section describes the role of the IGF-1R signaling pathway in drug resistance, the benefit of inhibiting this pathway, and the advantage of targeting IGF-1R/IR using TKIs.

Resistance to Chemotherapy

A mechanism of resistance to chemotherapy is the activation of survival pathways that inhibit chemotherapy-induced apoptosis. PI3K and AKT the downstream components of the IGF-1R pathway, are critical to cell survival. Overexpression or activation of IGF-1R has been shown to confer resistance to doxorubicin, 5-fluorouracil, methotrexate, camptothecin, and paclitaxel in various cancer cells (Dunn et al. 1997; Gooch et al. 1999; Lee et al. 2007).

Blocking IGF-1R signaling by either antisense or a dominant-negative mutant can enhance chemosensitivity of cancer cells in vitro and in vivo (Min et al. 2005; D'cunja et al. 2007). Treatment of small cell lung cancer cells with an NVP ADW-742, or breast cancer cells with an anti-IGF-1R antibody, αIR3, also resulted in increased cell death when combined with chemotherapy agents (Beech et al. 2001; Warshamana-Greene et al. 2005). These studies support the notion that IGF-1R targeted therapy in combination with chemotherapy may enhance antitumor activity in certain tumor types and several clinical studies are currently testing this hypothesis (Weroha and Haluska 2008).

Resistance to Radiation Therapy

Several lines of evidence demonstrate that IGF-1R is activated in response to ionizing radiation, and that radiosensitivity is increased when IGF-1R is inhibited using IGF-1R gene deletion, kinase dead IGF-1R mutants, and IGF-1R antisense (Nakamura et al. 1997; Turner et al. 1997; Macaulay et al. 2001). Enhanced cyotoxicity was also observed in a colon cancer model when an IGF-1R antibody was combined with chemotherapy and radiation therapy (Perer et al. 2000). Similar results were obtained when the IGF-1R TKI tyrphostin, AG-1024, was combined with chemoradiation in breast cancer cells (Wen et al. 2001). These data support the premise that IGF-1R plays an important role in preventing radiation-induced cell death (Turner et al. 1997).

IGF-1R modulates radiosensitivity through cell survival and DNA damage response pathways by interaction with ataxia-telangiectasia mutated (ATM) protein kinase and Ku DNA-binding proteins. ATM directly regulates IGF-1R gene expression (Peruzzi et al. 1999; Macaulay et al. 2001; Cosaceanu et al. 2007), and data showed that tumor cells defective in ATM kinase activity expressed low levels of IGF-IR and were highly radiosensitive (Peretz et al. 2001). Downregulation of IGF-1R by antisense resulted in reduction of ATM protein levels and kinase activity, resulting in high sensitivity to radiation (Macaulay et al. 2001). Combination clinical trials (radiation ± IGF-1R TKIs) provide a better understanding of the complex biological processes underlying the response to radiation therapy.

Escape Pathways: Resistance to ErbB Family-Targeted Therapies

Members of the ErbB family of receptor tyrosine kinases, including EGFR, Her2 (ErbB2), ErbB3, and ErbB4 are overexpressed in a variety of human solid tumors (Zhang et al. 2007). Monoclonal antibodies targeting either ErbB2 (trastuzumab and pertuzumab) or EGFR (cetuximab) and small-molecule TKIs directed against the ErbB family (gefitinib, erlotinib, and tykerb) have shown clinical benefit in treating cancers. However, patients initially responsive to ErbB-targeted therapies suffer from recurrence and develop resistance to these treatments via different escape mechanisms (Engelman et al. 2005; Kobayashi et al. 2005; Pao et al. 2005). Because of the cross talk between the ErbB family and IGF-1R pathways, the role of IGF-1R in response to ErbB family-targeted therapies has been investigated both preclinically and clinically (Lu et al. 2001; Nahta et al. 2005; Kostler et al. 2006; Harris et al. 2007).

The role of IGF-1R signaling in resistance to trastuzumab was initially noted in SKBR3 cells that developed acquired resistance to trastuzumab in vitro. Although, the expression of IGF-1R was unchanged between trastuzumab-sensitive and resistant cells, increased IGF-1R signaling as well as heterodimerization of IGF-1R/ErbB2 led to activation of both pathways. Blockade of IGF-1R signaling led to diminished ErbB2 phosphorylation only in the resistant cells (Lu et al. 2001; Nahta et al. 2005). Cross talk between ErbB2 and IGF-1R indicates that targeting both receptors might result in enhanced inhibition of ERK1/2 and AKT activity (Nahta et al. 2007; Chakraborty et al. 2008; Haluska et al. 2008). However, the relevance of IGF-1R in clinical resistance to trastuzumab is still controversial (Kostler et al. 2006; Harris et al. 2007).

EGFR and IGF-1R are coexpressed in multiple tumor types, and data suggest that IGF-1R plays a role in resistance to EGFR inhibitors, gefitinib or erlotinib (Jones et al. 2004; Camirand et al. 2005; Cunningham et al. 2006; Morgillo et al. 2006). Increased levels of IGF-1R/EGFR heterodimers, and activated IGF-1R signaling were observed in NSCLC cells resistant to gefitinib (Morgillo et al. 2007) or erlotinib (Morgillo et al. 2006). Overexpression of IGF-1R in the SKBR3 breast cell line was shown to cause a significant increase in resistance to gefitinib, and the combination of gefitinib and AG-1024 reduced proliferation in a panel of breast cancer cell lines (Camirand et al. 2005). Interestingly, LoVo, a colorectal cancer cell line known to lack functional IGF-1R, preferentially expressed the IR-A isoform as opposed to IR-B, and also generated substantial levels of IGF-2 mRNA. Both pIR and pAkt levels were increased after gefitinib treatment and inhibition of IR-A signaling restored sensitivity to gefitinib, indicating that IR-A may play a role in the resistance to gefitinib (Jones et al. 2006).

In summary, inhibition of IGF-1R/IR signaling can enhance the efficacy of ErbB-targeting therapies to inhibit growth and induce apoptosis in a variety of human cancer cells and reverse the resistance to ErbB-targeting therapies in vitro (Jones et al. 2004; Camirand et al. 2005; Nahta et al. 2007; Huang et al. 2009). These findings need to be validated in clinical studies combining therapies targeting both the ErbB and IGF-1R/IR pathways.

Others: Resistance to Hormonal therapy

ER is expressed in approximately 65–75% of breast cancers (Chu et al. 2001), making it a common therapeutic target. Multiple hormonal therapies have been used to inhibit the different biological effects of ER signaling and provide clinical benefit for the treatment of breast cancer. However, resistance to hormonal therapies is still a clinical problem. Resistance is partially due to cross talk between the ER and various growth factor signaling pathways, including IGF signaling through either IGF-1R or IR. Breast cancer cells can escape tamoxifen-induced apoptosis by treatment with IGF-1 most likely through the IGF-mediated activation of AKT and subsequent activation of ER (Lee et al. 1997; Campbell et al. 2001). Targeting IGF-1R with AG-1024 resulted in growth inhibition of tamoxifen-resistant MCF7 breast cells (Knowlden et al. 2005). A recent study showed that BMS-754807 enhanced the antitumor activity of tamoxifen and letrozole in hormone-resistant MCF-7/AC-1 breast cancer models. Interestingly, this activity was not observed with an IGF-1R monoclonal antibody, mAb391, which induced upregulation of IR-A, suggesting a greater susceptibility to

IR-mediated resistance with antibody against IGF-1R (Hillerman et al. 2010). These data suggest that completely blocking the activity of IGF-1R and IR with agents, such as BMS-754807 may have greater promise in extending the benefits of hormonal therapy in breast cancer than the agents targeting IGF-1R alone.

Mechanisms of Sensitivity/Resistance to IGF-1R Inhibitors

A key aspect of successfully developing targeted agents is to identify appropriate biomarkers to select patient populations dependent on the targeted pathway. Use of biomarkers has been postulated to accelerate the drug development process by providing a better understanding of patients who receive benefit from therapy (Carden et al. 2009a). Additionally, understanding of the potential molecular mechanisms of resistance to IGF-1R-targeted compounds could provide the rationale for combining IGF-1R blockade with other therapies to overcome resistance. Several mechanisms of resistance to inhibitors of the IGF signaling pathway have been proposed (Hendrickson and Haluska 2009). This section highlights some of the preclinical findings for the factors involved in both intrinsic and acquired sensitivity/resistance to IGF-1R blockade in human cancer cells, and provides the rationale for possible combination therapies.

IGF-1R/IR Pathway

Preclinical studies have reported that the components of the IGF signaling pathway and its downstream effectors are important determinants for the sensitivity to IGF-targeted treatment (Byron et al. 2006; Cao et al. 2008; Huang et al. 2009; Mukohara et al. 2009; Zha et al. 2009). RNA expression levels of either IGF-1R, IGF-1, IGF-2, IRS1, IRS2, or activated Akt have been shown to significantly correlate with the responsiveness to BMS-536924 in sarcoma cell lines (Huang et al. 2009), to NVP AEW-541, and h10H5 (an antihuman IGF-1R monoclonal antibody) in breast cancer cell lines (Mukohara et al. 2009; Zha et al. 2009), or to R1507 in NSCLC cell lines (Gong et al. 2009). Higher expression of these biomarkers may be indicative of IGF-1R pathway activation and might have clinical utility for identifying patients with tumors displaying the hallmarks of IGF-1R pathway addiction.

The overexpression of IGFBP-3 and IGFBP-6 was found in a panel of sarcoma cell lines with intrinsic resistance to BMS-536924 (Huang et al. 2009). Moreover, higher expression of IGFBP-5 and IGFBP-6 was observed in BMS-536924 acquired-resistant breast cancer cells (Haluska et al. 2007). These results suggest that overexpression of IGFBPs may serve as a resistance mechanism for both intrinsic and acquired resistance to IGF-1R inhibitors by downregulating IGF signaling, diminishing the role of IGF in proliferative and prosurvival pathways.

IR-A was upregulated following in vivo treatment with mAb391, but not with BMS-754807, suggesting that when IGF-1R alone was blocked, IGF signaling can still occur through the IR-A pathway (Haluska et al. 2009). In addition, IR pathway hypersensitivity to insulin was observed in IGF-1R null MEF cells resulting in greater AKT activation; BMS-754807 is able to effectively attenuate the hyperactivity of the IR pathway in IGF-1R null MEF cells (Dinchuk et al. 2010). These results indicate that the upregulation of IR-A, the increase of the IR-A/IR-B ratios, the formation of hybrid receptors, and the hyperactivity of IR pathway may represent an escape mechanism to anti-IGF-1R therapies. Therefore, TKIs that target both IGF-1R and IR may have a therapeutic advantage especially in tumors that have a high IR-A/IGF-1R ratio. A recent study showed that BMS-754807 is able to overcome resistance in Rh41-mAb391R cells, a cell line with acquired resistance to an IGF-1R neutralizing antibody mAb391 (Huang et al. 2010). This suggests that BMS-754807 may have advantage over anti-IGF-1R antibody therapies and be effective in patients who have failed treatment with IGF-1R antibody therapy due to its effective inhibition of both IGF-1R and IR.

Cross Talk Pathways

IGF-1R and other signaling pathways share common downstream effectors, such as PI3K/Akt and RAS/RAF/ERK. Many factors in these pathways that cross talk with the IGF signaling may contribute to resistance to IGF-1R inhibitors. For example, overexpression and activation of EGFR confers resistance to IGF-1R TKIs (Haluska et al. 2008; Haluska ct al. 2009; Huang et al. 2009), which provides a rationale for targeting both IGF-1R and EGFR. Indeed, evidence is accumulating which shows that inhibition of EGFR can increase the sensitivity to IGF-1R inhibition and lead to synergistic activity (Haluska et al. 2008; Carboni et al. 2009; Desbois-Mouthon et al. 2009; Huang et al. 2009; van der Veeken et al. 2009). Furthermore, MET overexpression, as well as PDGFRα amplification and constitutive activation have been shown to be involved in resistance to IGF-1R TKIs (Huang et al. 2009; 2010). These results suggest that resistant cells utilize alternative pathways to escape growth inhibition through compensatory mechanisms. Inhibition of these pathways may prevent or reverse resistance to IGF-1R inhibitors offering a promising strategy for clinical studies.

Others

Other factors have been implicated in sensitivity/resistance to IGF-1R therapies. Predictive gene expression signatures or microRNAs correlate with the responsiveness to IGF-1R targeted agents in different tumor types in in vitro studies (Huang et al. 2009; Pitts et al. 2009; Tan et al. 2009; Zha et al. 2009). Sensitivity to IGF-1R inhibition may also depend on whether the tumor cell has undergone EMT.

Indeed, a better clinical outcome with figitumumab was reported to be associated with expression of E-cadherin, an epithelial biomarker (Karp et al. 2009).

Drug sensitivity depends on several molecular mechanisms, including response to stress. Heat shock proteins (HSPs) are key molecules involved in response to stress. Targeting HSP90 by 17-AAG or siRNA sensitizes the resistant Ewing Sarcoma cell lines to NVP-ADW-742 (Martins et al. 2008), suggesting that HSP90 could be a predictive factor of response to IGF-1R treatment.

Given that clinical data for IGF-1R targeting therapies are only beginning to emerge, the clinical relevance of these factors in resistance to IGF-1R therapies will need to be further tested and validated in clinical studies.

Summary

The IGF axis has emerged as one of the critical components responsible for cellular transformation, survival, and resistance to anticancer therapies. Numerous clinical studies are underway to evaluate the potential of IGF-1R targeted agents. Early clinical results for the IGF-1R antibodies have been encouraging and several small molecule IGF-1R inhibitors are being evaluated in the clinic. It is important to follow the clinical development of TKIs, such as AXL-1717, BMS-754807, INSM-18, OSI-906, and XL-228 with respect to efficacy and the ability to enhance the clinical benefit of cytotoxic and other targeted therapies; an understanding of biomarkers in response/resistance is also critical. The hope remains that TKIs will provide a complementary approach to mAb therapeutics in terms of efficacy and dosing flexibility, particularly in combination studies with cytotoxics and EGFR antagonists, and may well provide a potential advantage over mAb therapeutics due to dual targeting of IGF-1R and IR.

References

Andrews DW, et al. (2001). J Clin Oncol 19(8): 2189–200.
Arteaga CL and Osborne CK (1989). Cancer Res 49(22): 6237–41.
Beech DJ, et al. (2001). Oncol Rep 8(2): 325–9.
Belfiore A (2007). Curr Pharm Des 13(7): 671–86.
Byron SA, et al. (2006). Br J Cancer 95(9): 1220–8.
Camirand A, et al. (2005). Breast Cancer Res 7(4): R570–9.
Campbell RA, et al. (2001). J Biol Chem 276(13): 9817–24.
Cao L, et al. (2008). Cancer Res 68(19): 8039–48.
Carboni JM, et al. (2005). Cancer Res 65(9): 3781–7.
Carboni JM, et al. (2009). Mol Cancer Ther 8(12): 3341–9.
Carden CP, et al. (2009a). Clin Pharmacol Ther 85(2): 131–3.
Carden CP, et al. (2009b). J Clin Oncol (Meeting Abstracts) 27(15S): Abstract 3544.
Casa AJ, et al. (2008). Frontiers in Bioscience 13: 3273–87.
Chakraborty AK, et al. (2008). Cancer Res 68(5): 1538–45.

Chan JM, et al. (1998). Science 279(5350): 563–6.
Chu KC, et al. (2001). Cancer 92(1): 37–45.
Clemens PL, et al. (2009). Molecular Cancer Therapeutics 8(12): Abstract A101.
Cortes J, et al. (2008). ASH Annual Meeting Abstracts 112(11): Abstract 3232.
Cosaceanu D, et al. (2007). Oncogene 26(17): 2423–34.
Cunningham MP, et al. (2006). Int J Oncol 28(2): 329–35.
D'Ambrosio C, et al. (1996). Cancer Res 56(17): 4013–20.
D'cunja J, et al. (2007). Eur J Cancer 43(10): 1581–9.
Desai J, et al. (2010). J Clin Oncol (Meeting Abstracts) 28(7S): Abstract 3104.
Desbois-Mouthon C, et al. (2009). Clin Cancer Res 15(17): 5445–56.
Dinchuk JE, et al. (2010). Endocrinology: manuscript submitted.
Dunn SE, et al. (1997). Cancer Res 57(13): 2687–93.
Engelman JA, et al. (2005). Proc Natl Acad Sci USA. 102(10): 3788–93.
Frasca F, et al. (1999). Mol Cell Biol 19(5): 3278–88.
Garcia-Echeverria C, et al. (2004). Cancer Cell 5(3): 231–9.
Girnita A, et al. (2004). Cancer Res 64(1): 236–42.
Gong Y, et al. (2009). J Clin Oncol (Meeting Abstracts) 27(15S): Abstract 8095.
Gooch JL, et al. (1999). Breast Cancer Res Treat 56(1): 1–10.
Gualberto A and Pollak M (2009). Oncogene 28(34): 3009–21.
Haluska P, et al. (2006). Cancer Res 66(1): 362–71.
Haluska P, et al. (2007). Proceedings from the 15th SPORE Investigators' Workshop.
Haluska P, et al. (2008). Mol Cancer Ther 7(9): 2589–98.
Haluska P, et al. (2009). 32nd San Antonio Breast Cancer Symposium.
Harmenberg J, et al. (2009). Molecular Cancer Therapeutics 8(12): Abstract B256.
Harris LN, et al. (2007). Clin Cancer Res. 13(4): 1198–207.
Harzstark AL, et al. (2007). J Clin Oncol 25(18S).
Hendrickson AW and Haluska P (2009). Curr Opin Investig Drugs 10(10): 1032–40.
Hewish M, et al. (2009). Recent Pat Anticancer Drug Discov 4(1): 54–72.
Hillerman SM, et al. (2010). Proceedings of the 101st Annual Meeting of the AACR; Abstract 363.
Huang F, et al. (2009). Cancer Res 69(1): 161–70.
Huang F, et al. (2010). Cancer Res 70(18): 7221–31.
Hubbard RD and Wilsbacher JL (2007). ChemMedChem 2(1): 41–6.
Ji QS, et al. (2007). Mol Cancer Ther 6(8): 2158–67.
Jones HE, et al. (2004). Endocr Relat Cancer 11(4): 793–814.
Jones HE, et al. (2006). Br J Cancer 95(2): 172–80.
Kalli KR, et al. (2002). Endocrinology 143(9): 3259–67.
Karp DD, et al. (2009). J Clin Oncol 27(15): 2516–22.
Kim HJ, et al. (2007). Mol Cell Biol 27(8): 3165–75.
Knowlden JM, et al. (2005). Endocrinology 146(11): 4609–18.
Kobayashi S, et al. (2005). N Engl J Med. 352(8): 786–92.
Kostler WJ, et al. (2006). J Cancer Res Clin Oncol 132(1): 9–18.
Lee AV, et al. (1997). J Endocrinol 152(1): 39–47.
Lee J, et al. (2007). Mol Pharmacol. 72(4): 1082–93.
LeRoith D, et al. (1995). Ann Intern Med 122(1): 54–9.
Li R, et al. (2009). J Med Chem 52(16): 4981–5004.
Lindsay CR, et al. (2009). J Clin Oncol (Meeting Abstracts) 27(15S): Abstract 2559.
Litzenburger BC, et al. (2009). 32nd San Antonio Breast Cancer Symposium.
Long L, et al. (1995). Cancer Res 55(5): 1006–9.
Lu Y, et al. (2001). J Natl Cancer Inst 93(24): 1852–7.
Macaulay VM, et al. (2001). Oncogene 20(30): 4029–40.
Maiso P, et al. (2008). Br J Haematol 141(4): 470–82.
Martins AS, et al. (2008). Cancer Res 68(15): 6260–70.
Min Y, et al. (2005). Gut 54(5): 591–600.

Mitsiades CS, et al. (2004). Cancer Cell 5(3): 221–30.

Moller DE, et al. (1989). Mol Endocrinol 3(8): 1263–9.

Morgillo F, et al. (2006). Cancer Res 66(20): 10100–11.

Morgillo F, et al. (2007). Clin Cancer Res 13(9): 2795–803.

Mukohara T, et al. (2009). Cancer Lett 282(1): 14–24.

Mulvihill M, et al. (2008). Proceedings of the 101st Annual Meeting of the AACR; Abstract 4893.

Nahta R, et al. (2005). Cancer Res 65(23): 11118–28.

Nahta R, et al. (2007). Mol Cancer Ther 6(2): 667–4.

Nakamura S, et al. (1997). Exp Cell Res. 235(1): 287–94.

Pandini G, et al. (1999). Clin Cancer Res 5(7): 1935–44.

Pandini G, et al. (2002). J Biol Chem 277(42): 39684–95.

Pao W, et al. (2005). PLoS Med. 2(3): e73.

Perer ES, et al. (2000). J Surg Res 94(1): 1–5.

Peretz S, et al. (2001). Proc Natl Acad Sci U S A. 98(4): 1676–81.

Peruzzi F, et al. (1999). Mol Cell Biol 19(10): 7203–15.

Pietrzkowski Z, et al. (1993). Cancer Res 53(5): 1102–6.

Pitts TM, et al. (2009). Molecular Cancer Therapeutics 8(12): Abstract A39.

Pollak M (2008). Curr Opin Pharmacol 8(4): 384–92.

Sciacca L, et al. (1999). Oncogene 18(15): 2471–9.

Sciacca L, et al. (2002). Oncogene 21(54): 8240–50.

Scotlandi K, et al. (2005). Cancer Res 65(9): 3868–76.

Smith DC, et al. (2010). J Clin Oncol (Meeting Abstracts) 28(7S): Abstract 3105.

Tan AC, et al. (2009). Molecular Cancer Therapeutics 8(12): Abstract C22.

Turner BC, et al. (1997). Cancer Res 57(15): 3079–83.

Ulanet DB, et al. (2010). Proc Natl Acad Sci USA.

Valentinis B and Baserga R (2001). Mol Pathol 54(3): 133–7.

van der Veeken J, et al. (2009). Curr Cancer Drug Targets 9(6): 748–60.

Velaparthi U, et al. (2008). J Med Chem 51(19): 5897–900.

Vella V, et al. (2002). J Clin Endocrinol Metab 87(1): 245–54.

Warshamana-Greene GS, et al. (2004). Mol Cancer Ther 3(5): 527–35.

Warshamana-Greene GS, et al. (2005). Clin Cancer Res 11(4): 1563–71.

Wen B, et al. (2001). Br J Cancer 85(12): 2017–21.

Weroha SJ and Haluska P (2008). J Mammary Gland Biol Neoplasia 13(4): 471–83.

Wittman MD, et al. (2009a). J Med Chem 52(23): 7360–3.

Wittman MD, et al. (2009b). Annual Reports in Medicinal Chemistry 44: 281–299.

Zha J, et al. (2009). Mol Cancer Ther 8(8): 2110–21.

Zhang H, et al. (2007). J Clin Invest. 117(8): 2051–8.

Zhang H, et al. (2010). Oncogene in press.

Zhou DJ, et al. (1990). Cancer Res 50(21): 6949–54.

Zimmermann K, et al. (2008). Bioorg Med Chem Lett 18(14): 4075–80.

Zimmermann K, et al. (2010). Bioorg Med Chem Lett 20(5): 1744–8.

Chapter 12
Calories and Cancer: The Role of Insulin-Like Growth Factor-1

Stephen D. Hursting, Sarah D. Smith, Alison E. Harvey, and Laura M. Lashinger

Introduction

The poem "On the Nature of Things," written around 55 BC by Titus Lucretius Carus, is considered to be the first published statement about the potential impact of the overconsumption of food on risk of chronic diseases such as cancer (Lucretius 2008). This apparent connection between excess calorie intake and cancer began to develop into a working hypothesis in the mid-to-late 1800s, following the writings of John Hughes Bennett (1849) and William Lambe (1850). The first tests of the hypothesis that a calorie restriction (CR) dietary regimen can suppress tumors in animal models were reported in 1909 by Moreschi (1909) and extended by Sweet et al. in (1913) and Peyton Rous in (1914). These investigators showed that a low-calorie diet, relative to ad libitum (AL)-fed controls, inhibited the growth of transplanted tumors in mice. Intense interest in the comparison of CR versus AL-fed animals developed in the 1930s, when McCay and Crowell showed that reduced energy intake also increased lifespan in rodents (1934). CR research was further catalyzed by Tannenbaum et al., who consistently showed that the incidence of tumors in mice decreased when food intake was reduced (1944).

As we have previously reviewed, CR has become the most widely studied and effective experimental strategy for increasing median and maximal lifespan in rodents (Hursting et al. 2003). CR is also the most potent, broadly acting dietary intervention for suppressing cancer development or progression in experimental models (Hursting et al. 2003, 2010). A recent report of extended lifespan and delayed

---

S.D. Hursting (✉)
Department of Nutritional Sciences, The University of Texas at Austin,
Austin, TX, USA

Department of Carcinogenesis, The University of Texas MD Anderson Cancer Center,
Smithville, TX, USA
e-mail: shursting@austin.utexas.edu

D. LeRoith (ed.), *Insulin-like Growth Factors and Cancer: From Basic Biology to Therapeutics*, Cancer Drug Discovery and Development,
DOI 10.1007/978-1-4614-0598-6_12, © Springer Science+Business Media, LLC 2012

tumor development in response to CR in rhesus monkeys (Colman et al. 2009) suggests the anticancer effects of CR reported in rodent models extend to primates. The rhesus monkey study involved 46 male and 30 female rhesus macaques (aged 7–14 years at the start of the study), randomized to receive a control diet regimen or a 30% CR regimen and followed for 20 years. Each CR animal's baseline energy intake was reduced by 10% each month over a 3-month period, and then maintained for the duration of the study to achieve the desired 30% CR. The CR regimen reduced the incidence of cancer, cardiovascular disease, and brain atrophy, and 80% of the CR animals were still alive compared to 50% of the controls at the time of the report. These are important and encouraging findings that suggest the mechanisms characterized in animal model studies, and their translation into intervention targets and strategies will have relevance to the prevention and treatment of cancers (particularly those related to obesity) in humans. Unfortunately, the mechanisms underlying this calorie–cancer connection remain unclear.

Given the rising prevalence of obesity in the USA and throughout the world and the emergence of excess weight as a key modulatable risk factor for many cancers, such translation of lessons learned about the energy balance–cancer link from CR studies is urgently needed. The prevalence of obesity has increased dramatically in the last 30 years in the USA (Flegal et al. 2010). As defined by the body mass index (BMI), among adults aged $\geq$20 years in 1999–2002, 65.7% are currently overweight (BMI = 25.0–29.9), 30.6% are obese (BMI $\geq$ 30), and 5.1% are extremely obese (BMI > 40). Between the early 1960s and 2002, mean BMI increased approximately 3 BMI units in both men and women, and similar trends have occurred in children (Ogden et al. 2004). Obesity in adult men and women was associated with increased mortality from cancers of the colon, endometrium, breast (in postmenopausal women), pancreas, esophagus (adenocarcinoma), gallbladder, gastric cardia, liver, kidney (renal cell), and prostate in a large American Cancer Society-funded prospective study (Calle et al. 2003). Findings from this cohort study indicate that approximately 14% of all cancer deaths in men and 20% of all cancer deaths in women are attributable to overweight and obesity (Calle et al. 2003).

This chapter summarizes key findings on the biological mechanisms underlying many of the anticancer effects of CR, with a particular focus on the role of insulin-like growth factor (IGF)-1, its related downstream signaling pathways, and its interactions with other energy balance-related hormones. It also describes some of the epidemiological and experimental evidence linking IGF-1, energy balance, and cancer and the emerging opportunities for investigation that will facilitate the translation of CR research into effective strategies to prevent human cancer.

IGF-1 as a Plausible Mediator of the Anticancer Effects of CR

Several hormones and growth factors serve as intermediate and long-term communicators of nutritional state throughout the body and have been implicated in both energy balance and carcinogenesis (Hursting et al. 2008). These hormones include

IGF-1, insulin, adiponectin, and leptin, as well as several factors associated with inflammation and oxidative stress. In our view, IGF-1 plays a central role in the calorie–cancer connection.

IGF-1 (a 70-amino-acid polypeptide growth factor that shares ~50% homology with insulin) and pituitary-derived growth hormone are key regulators of an endocrine, paracrine, and autocrine signaling network that controls long bone growth and energy metabolism (Yakar et al. 2005). The circulating level of IGF-1 is mainly determined by hepatic synthesis, which is regulated by growth hormone and influenced by nutrient intake, particularly intake of energy and protein (Sara and Hall 1990). Regulation of IGF-1 in extrahepatic tissues is more complex, involving growth hormone, other hormones, and growth factors, and six IGF binding proteins (BPs), which determine the systemic half-life and local availability of IGF-1 (Sara and Hall 1990).

IGF-1 has been identified as a cell cycle progression factor based on its ability in many normal and cancer cell types to stimulate progression through the cell cycle from G1 to S phase (Ma et al. 2009). IGF-1 can also suppress apoptosis in a variety of cell types, and cells overexpressing IGF-1R show decreased apoptosis (LeRoith et al. 1995; Resnicoff et al. 1995). There is mounting evidence that IGF-1 mediates at least some of the antiproliferative, proapoptotic, and anticancer effects of CR through its role in an evolutionarily conserved regulatory pathway that is responsive to energy availability (Pollak 2008). This conclusion does not exclude other mediators, which may be regulated by IGF-1 or function independently of IGF-1. The role of IGF-1 in the anticancer effects of exercise is less clear, with the findings to date consistent with little or no long-term effects of exercise on circulating IGF-1 levels (Rogers et al. 2008; McTiernan et al. 2005). However, IGFBP activity may increase with strenuous physical activity, and thus, overall IGF-1 bioavailability and activity may decrease with exercise (Koistinen et al. 1996).

IGF-1 and insulin interactions: Chronic hyperinsulinemia and insulin resistance increase risk for cancer at several sites (Renehan et al. 2006). However, insulin is generally thought to be mitogenic only under supraphysiologic conditions, so the tumor-enhancing effects of insulin are likely due to indirect effects via IGF-1 receptors, stimulation of IGF-1 production, or interactions with estrogens and other hormones. There is certainly important cross talk between insulin, IGF-1 and their receptors in numerous cancers that are only now beginning to be fully understood, and it is clear that high circulating levels of insulin promote the hepatic synthesis of IGF-1 and decrease the production of IGFBP-1, thus increasing the biologic activity of IGF-1 (Sandhu et al. 2002).

Downstream targets of IGF-1 receptor/insulin receptor signaling: The phosphatidylinositol-3 kinase (PI3K)/Akt pathway is frequently altered in human tumors and is a critical signaling component of the IGF-1 and/or insulin responses that regulate cellular growth and metabolism (Luo et al. 2003). Engagement of the PI3K/Akt pathway allows both intracellular and environmental cues, such as energy availability and growth factor supply, to affect cell growth, proliferation, survival, and metabolism (Engelman et al. 2006).

Activation of receptor tyrosine kinases (RTKs) and/or the Ras protooncogene stimulates PI3K to produce the lipid second messenger, phosphatidyl-inositol-3,4,

5-trisphosphate (PIP3). PIP3 recruits and anchors Akt to the cell membrane where it can be further phosphorylated and activated (Shaw et al. 2006). Akt is a cAMP-dependent, cGMP-dependent protein kinase C protein kinase that when constitutively active is sufficient for cellular transformation by stimulating cell cycle progression and cell survival as well as inhibiting apoptosis (Brazil et al. 2004; Dillon and Muller 2010). Frequently associated with the aberrant Akt signaling commonly seen in human cancers is an elevation in mTOR (mammalian target of rapamycin) signaling (Hay et al. 2005). mTOR is a highly conserved serine/threonine protein kinase, which is activated by Akt and also inhibited by an opposing signal from AMP-activated kinase (AMPK). At the interface of the Akt and AMPK pathways, mTOR dictates translational control of new proteins in response to both growth factor signals and nutrient availability through phosphorylation of its downstream mediators, including S6K and 4EBP-1 (Sarbassov and Sabatini 2005; Guertin and Sabatini 2005). Ultimately, activation of mTOR results in cell growth, cell proliferation, and a resistance to apoptosis.

An important convergent point for these signaling cascades is the tumor suppressor, tuberous sclerosis complex (TSC), reviewed in Kwiatkowki and Manning (2005). Briefly, the TSC binds to and sequesters Rheb, a G-protein required for mTOR activation, thus inhibiting mTOR and downstream targets. However, phosphorylation of the TSC elicits inactivation and Rheb is released, allowing for direct interaction with ATP and subsequent activation of mTOR. Alternatively, when the TSC is inhibited, Rheb is able to phosphorylate and activate mTOR.

Energy balance can influence both the Akt and AMPK pathways of mTOR activation. For example, overweight and obese states are positively associated, as previously mentioned, with high serum levels of IGF-1. We have shown that obesity is associated with enhanced induction of the PI3K/Akt pathway (Moore et al. 2008a). However, nutrient deprivation, by way of calorie restriction, reduced PI3K/Akt and mTOR signaling (Moore et al. 2008a; Jiang et al. 2008), at least in part as a result of decreased circulating levels of IGF-1. Furthermore, genetic reduction of circulating IGF-1 mimics the effects of CR on tumor development and PI3K/Akt/mTOR signaling (Moore et al. 2008b).

Epidemiological Evidence of a Role for IGF-1 in Human Cancer

Abundant epidemiological evidence supports the hypothesis that IGF-1 is involved in human cancer. A pooling project involving analyses of the combined individual data from 17 prospective studies showed that circulating IGF-1 is positively associated with breast cancer risk, independent of menopausal status (The Endogenous Hormones and Breast Cancer Collaborative Group 2010). A report from the Physicians Health Study (Chan et al. 1998) found that plasma IGF-1 levels were linked with a higher risk of developing a prostate malignancy (RR: 4.3; CI: 1.8–10.6). A population-based case–control study also found that increased IGF-1 levels were associated with an increased risk of prostate cancer (Wolk et al. 1998).

Another case–control study demonstrated that levels of IGF-1, but not of IGF-2 or IGFBP-3, were linked with lung cancer (Yu et al. 1999). The first prospective study to investigate whether IGF-1 and/or IGFBP-3 levels are associated with colon cancer risk showed that both elevated levels of IGF-1 and decreased levels of IGFBP-3 were associated with an increased risk of developing colon cancer in men in the Physicians Health Study (Ma et al. 1999). A study nested within the Nurses Health Study subsequently found similar results in women (Giovannucci et al. 2000). A decreased risk of childhood leukemia in association with higher IGFBP3 levels has also been reported (Petridou et al. 1999). Finally, a higher molar ratio of IGF-1/BP3 was associated with increased risk of pancreatic cancer in PLCO screening trial participants (Douglas et al. 2010). The epidemiological association between levels of IGF-1 and IGFBP and the risk of various cancers certainly requires more investigation, particularly additional prospective studies to better establish the temporal nature of any associations. However, when considered together, the multiple human studies reported to date suggest that components of the IGF-1 system are important risk factors in the development of several human cancers.

Experimental Evidence of the Role of IGF-1 in Cancer

The involvement of IGF-1 in cancer was first demonstrated by in vitro studies consistently showing that IGF-1 enhances the growth of a variety of cancer cell lines. These include bladder, brain, breast, cervical, endometrial, esophagus, kidney, liver, lung, ovarian, pancreas, prostate, stomach, and thyroid cancer cell lines, as well as several leukemia and lymphoma cell lines (reviewed in Macaulay 1992).

A markedly increased average and maximal lifespan, at least in part due to a decrease in tumor development, has also been reported in several strains of mutant or genetically modified mice that suffer defects in the production of growth hormone or IGF-1 or in responsiveness to growth hormone (and hence express significantly lower levels of circulating IGF-1). For example, the "little" mouse, with its defective response to hypothalamic-growth-hormone-releasing hormone, lives 20–25% longer than wild-type mice (Flurkey et al. 2001). Laron mice, with a disruption in the growth hormone receptor/binding protein gene, have higher circulating levels of growth hormone than wild-type mice but much lower serum IGF-1 levels, and they live 38–55% longer than wild-type mice (Bartke and Brown-Borg 2004). Mice with primary deficiencies in growth hormone, prolactin, and thyrotropin, caused by failure of the pituitary to differentiate during fetal development, live still longer, 40–64% longer than wild-type mice. These latter examples include the Snell and Jackson dwarf mice, which have a point mutation in the homeotic transcription factor, *Pit1*; and the Ames dwarf mouse, which fails to express Pit1 because of an inactivating point mutation in the *Prop1* transcription factor (Anisimov 2001). As seen with CR, these mutations appear to reduce the onset and/or rate of aging and age-associated cancers, resulting in an extended lifespan (Bartke and Brown-Borg 2004; Anisimov 2001).

In terms of targeted genetic alterations of IGF-1 and their impact on cancer in murine models, tissue-specific overexpression of IGF-1 via the keratin 5 promoter increases spontaneous tumor development (DiGiovanni et al. 2000) and susceptibility to carcinogens (Hursting et al. 2009) and thus decreases lifespan. Liver-specific IGF-1-deficient (LID) mice, which have a deletion in hepatic IGF-1 and consequently have reduced circulating IGF-1 levels, have also been very useful in demonstrating that IGF-1 is an important tumor growth factor in the response to energy balance interventions. Like CR, genetic reduction of IGF-1 in LID mice is associated with decreased mammary (Yiping et al. 2003), colon (Olivo-Marston et al. 2009) skin (Moore et al. 2008b), and pancreatic tumor development and/or growth (Lashinger et al. 2010). Also similar to CR, the reduction in skin (Polunovsky and Houghton 2010) and pancreatic tumors (Lashinger et al. 2010) was associated with reduced steady-state signaling through the Akt/mTOR pathway. Furthermore, restoration of serum IGF-1 levels in LID mice by infusion of recombinant IGF-1 restored pancreatic tumor growth and pancreatic mTOR signaling, providing further support that IGF-1 is an important mediator of the energy balance and cancer link (Lashinger et al. 2010). However, a recent report from Wu et al. suggests differences in chronic versus acute reductions in systemic IGF-1 on obesity-associated hepatic inflammation and tumor metastases, possibly due to differences in the liver microenvironment in response to long-term versus short-term reduction in circulating IGF-1 (2010). Thus, the role of IGF-1 in the energy balance–cancer connection is likely to be complex.

Interactions Between IGF-1 and Other CR-Responsive Fa\tors

A better understanding of the interactions between IGF-1 and other energy balance-related hormones involved in processes associated with carcinogenesis, such as mitogenesis and inflammation, will be very important in understanding and translating the anticancer effects of CR to human disease prevention. Although this chapter focuses on the potential mediating role of IGF-1 in the effects CR, on cancer, we and others have shown that other hormones and growth factors known to interact with IGF-1 and its signaling are also modulated by CR, such as estrogen, leptin, adiponectin, and corticosterone, as well as several cytokines.

Important cross talk has been established between IGF-1 and estrogen signaling (Fagan and Yee 2008). Not only does estrogen receptor (ER) and IGF1R expression typically correlate with each other in cancer tissue, but estradiol (E2), the ligand for ER, and IGF-1 also can synergistically enhance breast cancer cell proliferation in vitro (Mawson et al. 2005). The synergistic relationship between these two pathways occurs as a biological consequence of an interrelated network governed at multiple levels. For example, exposure of breast cancer cells to IGF-1 results in an increased expression of $ER\alpha$ as well as enhancement of its transcriptional activity (reviewed in Sachdev and Yee 2001). Additionally, E2 causes a complementary augmentation of IGF-1 signaling by increasing expression of IGF-1, IGF1R, IGFBPs, and IRS-1 (Fagan and Yee 2008).

Individually, IGF-1 and leptin can promote growth of many cancer cell lines in vitro and have been associated with increased tumor growth in vivo (Hursting et al. 2008). Recent studies have also shown that these molecules and their signaling networks act in concert to synergistically enhance proliferation of some types of cancer cells (Saxena 2008), an effect that is facilitated by a physical interaction between IGF1R and the leptin receptor (ObR) (Ozbay and Nahta 2008). For example, exposure of several breast cancer cell lines to IGF-1 caused activation of the ObR and resultant phosphorylation of leptin-associated signaling components such as STAT3 and Jak2 as well as Akt and Erk (Saxena 2008; Ozbay and Nahta 2008). Moreover, the synergistic activity of IGF-1 and leptin was found to be dependent upon transactivation of the epidermal growth factor receptor (EGFR), signifying yet another layer of complexity (Balana 2001). EGFR is a crucial mediator of survival signaling in many cancers, activation of which occurs from many stimuli, including leptin and IGF-1 (Balana 2001). In fact, some evidence suggests that IGF1R-mediated signaling is augmented through IGF-1's ability to activate EGFR, and leptin-induced activation of the JAK2 and ERK1/2 cascade is also facilitated by EGFR transactivation (Shida 2005).

Metabolic hormones such as leptin, insulin, and IGF-1 have also been shown to interact with inflammation-related pathways, such as NF-κB signaling, at levels observed in obese individuals (Hursting et al. 2008). Our studies with A-Zip/F1 mice, which lack white adipose tissue (and hence have very low adipokine levels) but are diabetic, display high levels of insulin, IGF-1, and inflammatory cytokines, and are highly susceptible to cancer development, support the hypothesis that components of the insulin/IGF-1 and inflammatory pathways may be interrelated targets for breaking the obesity–cancer link (Hursting 2007). Further support for this IGF-1/inflammation interaction comes from our work with LID mice, which demonstrate reductions in both IGF-1 and a broad pane lof cytokine levels (Olivo-Marston et al. 2009; Lashinger et al. 2010). Restoration of IGF-1 levels in LID mice also restored cytokines and inflammation-related signaling (including NF-κB) to control levels (Lashinger et al. 2010). Once bound to their cognate receptor, IGF-1, insulin, and leptin activate Akt, which is an established upstream kinase of the IKK complex (Mitsiades 2002). Subsequently, the activated IKK complex targets IκB-α for degradation and allows the p50/p65 subunits to translocate the nucleus and initiate transcription (Mitsiades 2002). Leptin-stimulated activation of NF-κB has been demonstrated in vitro in human preneoplastic and neoplastic colonic epithelial cells and other cell lines (Fenton et al. 2008; Garafalo and Surmacz 2005). Mitsiades (2002) showed that IGF-1 increased NF-κB DNA binding activity comparable to that of TNF-α. In addition, IGF-1 induced expression of FLIP, XIAP, cIAP-2, and Al/Bfl-1, and survivin, which are downstream genes mediated by NF-κB (Mitsiades 2002).

Together, these findings suggest that energy balance-related hormones, such as IGF-1, insulin, leptin, and other factors, should not be viewed as solitary participants involved in cancer development and progression but as members of an interrelated network collectively orchestrating growth and survival signaling. Additionally, evidence is mounting that factors not traditionally seen as energy-responsive (EGF-R, NF-κB) should also be considered as potential coregulators of energy balance signals.

Calorie Restriction Mimetics

Given how difficult it is for many people to adopt a low calorie diet for an extended period, the identification of pharmacologic agents or natural products that complement or even reproduce the anticancer effects of CR without drastic changes in diet and lifestyle has emerged as a drug development goal. As described above, components of the IGF-1 and Akt/mTOR pathways have emerged as potential key mediators of CR's anticancer effects, and are priority targets for possible CR mimetics. Small-molecule inhibitors of IGF-1 or its receptor, as well as antisense inhibitor approaches and anti-IGF-1 (or its receptor) antibody therapies, are under active development and clinical testing (Sachdev and Yee 2007). In addition, a wide variety of agents with demonstrated cancer chemopreventive or chemotherapeutic activity have been reported to inhibit one or more components of the IGF-1/Akt/mTOR pathway, including selective estrogen receptor modulators, retinoids/rexinoids, and several bioactive food components (Eng-Wong et al. 2003; Lubet et al. 2005; DeAngel et al. 2010; Fang 2006; Anand et al. 2008). mTOR inhibitors have also emerged as potential CR mimetics. In particular, a recent report that rapamycin treatment, even when started late in life, extends life span and delays cancer in mice suggests mTOR is indeed a target for mimicking the effects of CR (Harrison et al. 2009). mTOR inhibitors, including sirolimus (rapamycin), temsirolimus (Torisel), everolimus (Afinitor), and others, are under wide-spread clinical development (Polunovsky and Houghton 2010).

Metformin, an established mTOR inhibitor and promising CR mimetic, is one of the most commonly prescribed drugs for the treatment of type-2 diabetes as well as conditions frequently associated with obesity and insulin resistance such as gestational diabetes and polycystic ovary disease (PCOS) (Sahra et al. 2008). Metformin lowers blood glucose levels by inhibiting gluconeogenesis and improves insulin sensitivity by increasing peripheral glucose uptake. While metformin was first described more than 50 years ago, the exact molecular mechanism of action for this drug has only recently been determined. Metformin activates AMP-activated protein kinase (AMPK) via phosphorylation by the LKB1 tumor suppressor, as recently has been reviewed (Hardie 2008). In brief, AMPK is typically activated in response to metabolic stress, and results in inhibition of ATP-consuming pathways, such as cholesterol synthesis, fatty acid synthesis, and protein translation. Importantly, AMPK inhibits mTOR via activation of the tuberous sclerosis complex 2 (TSC2) tumor suppressor. The TSC1/TSC2 heterodimer forms the TSC complex that negatively regulates mTOR signaling: phosphorylation of TSC2 by AMPK activates this tumor suppressor to repress mTOR and protein synthesis.

Recent preclinical and clinical studies suggest that metformin may be associated with a decreased risk of cancer. Memmott et al. showed that metformin inhibited mTOR signaling and the development of carcinogen-induced lung tumors in mice (2010). In an observational cohort study of diabetics performed by Libby et al, incident cancer was diagnosed among 7.3% of 4,085 metformin users compared with 11.6% of 4,085 comparators ($p < 0.001$) (Libby et al. 2009). Li et al. reported that diabetic patients who had taken metformin had a significantly lower risk of pancreatic cancer compared to those who had not taken metformin (2009). Jiralerspong et al. (2009) reported that among diabetic women with breast cancer undergoing neoadjuvant chemotherapy, those individuals who were on metformin had a higher pathologic complete response rate than those who were on other antidiabetic medication. Finally, Hosono et al. (2010) showed in a short-term clinical trial that metformin decreased colonic epithelial proliferation and the formation of aberrant crypt foci, a precursor of colon cancer development. The results of these studies are provocative and have prompted calls for additional studies to better characterize the role of metformin in both the prevention and treatment of multiple cancers (Pollak 2010).

Genetic or pharmacologic induction of the Sir2/Sirtuin (SIRT)1 family of NAD-dependent deacetylases has also been shown to mimic some of the effects of CR (Firestein et al. 2008). Sirtuin modulators, including resveratrol and its analogues (Signorelli and Ghidoni 2005), as well as other pharmacologic modulators of SIRT1 (Liu et al. 2009), have also shown some anticancer activity, although much of this work has been largely limited to in vitro systems and awaits further verification in vivo.

Conclusions

Based on lessons learned from CR research, this chapter discusses promising molecular targets for breaking the obesity–cancer link, particularly components of the IGF-1/Akt/mTOR pathway. Clearly, no single pathway accounts for all of the anticancer effects of CR. As with most chronic disease intervention strategies, combination approaches that target multiple pathways (and that maximize efficacy and minimize adverse effects) will likely be most successful for preventing cancer. An emerging issue in this area is the relative effects of nature versus nurture, i.e., the contributions of systemic factors (which have been the focus of this review) in the context of cell autonomous effects. The observation by Kalaany and Sabatini that cancer cells with constitutively activated PI3K mutations are proliferative in vitro in the absence of insulin or IGF-1 and form CR-resistant tumors in vivo illustrates this issue (2009). These findings suggest that cell autonomous alterations, such as activating PI3K mutations, may influence the response of cells to CR or CR mimetics. Future studies aimed at further elucidating the mechanisms underlying the anticancer effects of CR, and that exploit this mechanistic information to target CR-responsive pathways through combinations of dietary and pharmacologic approaches, will facilitate the translation of CR research into more effective cancer prevention and control strategies in humans.

References

Lucretius Carus, Titus. On the Nature of Things (Translated by A.E. Stallings). Penguin Press, NY, 2008.

Bennett JH. On Cancerous and Canroid Growths. Sutherland and Knox, Edinburgh, 1849.

Lambe W (with notes and additions by Shew, J.) Water and Vegetable Diet in Consumption, Scrofula, Cancer, Asthma and Other Chronic Diseases. Fowlers and Wells, NY, 1850.

Moreschi C (1909) Beziehungen zwischen Ernahrung und Tumorwachstum. *Zeitschrift fur Immunitatsforsch* 2:661–675.

Sweet JE, Carson-White EP, Saxon GJ. The relation of diets and of castration to the transmissible tumors of rats and mice. J Biol Chem 1913; 15:181–91.

Rous P. The influence of diet on transplanted and spontaneous mouse tumors. J Exp Med 1914; 20:433–51.

McCay CM, Crowell MF. 1934. Prolonging the life span. *Sci. Mon.* 39:405–14.

Tannenbaum A. 1944. The dependence of the genesis of induced skin tumors on the caloric intake during different stages of carcinogenesis. *Cancer Res.* 4:673–79.

Hursting, S.D., Lavigne, J.A., Berrigan, D., Perkins, S.N. and Barrett, J.C. (2003) Calorie restriction, aging, and cancer prevention: mechanisms of action and applicability to humans. *Annu Rev Med*, 54:131–52.

Hursting SD, Smith SM, Lashinger LM, Harvey AE, Perkins SN. Calorie restriction and *Carcinogenesis*: Lessons learned from 30 years of research. *Carcinogenesis* 2010; 31:83–9.

Colman, R.J., Anderson, R.M., Johnson, S.C., Kastman, E.K., Kosmatka, K.J., Beasley, T.M., Allison, D.B., Cruzen, C., Simmons, H.A., Kemnitz, J.W. and Weindruch, R. (2009) Caloric restriction delays disease onset and mortality in rhesus monkeys. *Science*, 325, 201–4.

Flegal KM, Carroll MD, Ogden CL, Curtin LR. Prevalence and trends in obesity among US adults, 1999–2008. JAMA 2010 303:235–41.

Ogden CL, Fryar CD, Carroll MD, Flegal KM. Mean body weight, height, and body mass index, United States 1960–2002. Advance data from vital and health statistics; no 347. Hyattsville, Maryland: National Center for Health Statistics. 2004.

Calle, E.E., Rodriguez, C., Walker-Thurmond, K. and Thun, M.J. (2003) Overweight, obesity, and mortality from cancer in a prospectively studied cohort of U.S. adults. *N Engl J Med*, 348, 1625–38.

Hursting SD, Lashinger LM, Wheatley KW, Rogers CJ, Colbert LH, Nunez, NP, Perkins SN. Reducing the weight of cancer: Mechanistic targets for breaking the obesity-carcinogenesis link. *Best Pract Res Clin Endocrinol Metab*, 2008, 22:659–669.

Yakar, S., Leroith, D. and Brodt, P. (2005) The role of the growth hormone/insulin-like growth factor axis in tumor growth and progression: Lessons from animal models. *Cytokine Growth Factor Rev*, 16, 407–20.

Sara, V.R. and Hall, K. (1990) Insulin-like growth factors and their binding proteins. *Physiol Rev*, 70, 591–614.

Ma QL, Tang TL, Yin JY, Peng ZY, Yu M, Liu ZQ, Chen FP. Role of insulin-like growth factor-1 in regulating cell cycle progression. Biochem Biophys Res Comm 2009; 389:150–5.

LeRoith, D., Baserga, R., Helman, L. and Roberts, C.T., Jr. (1995) Insulin-like growth factors and cancer. *Ann Intern Med*, 122, 54–9.

Resnicoff, M., Abraham, D., Yutanawiboonchai, W., Rotman, H.L., Kajstura, J., Rubin, R., Zoltick, P. and Baserga, R. (1995) The insulin-like growth factor I receptor protects tumor cells from apoptosis in vivo. *Cancer Res*, 55, 2463–9.

Pollak, M. (2008) Insulin and insulin-like growth factor signalling in neoplasia. *Nat Rev Cancer*, 8, 915–28.

Rogers CJ, Colbert LH, Berrigan D, Greiner JW, Perkins SN, Hursting SD. Physical activity and cancer prevention: Pathways and targets for intervention. *Sports Medicine 2008*; 38(4): 221–57.

McTiernan A, Sorensen B, Yasui Y, Tworoger SS, Ulrich CM, Irwin ML, Rudolph RE, Stanczyk FZ, Schwartz RS, Potter JD. No effect of exercise on insulin-like growth factor-1 and insulin-like binding protein 3 in postmenopausal women: a 12-month randomized clinical trial. Cancer Epidemiol Biomarkers Prev 14:1020, 2005.

Koistinen H, Koistinen R, et al. Effect of marathon run on serum IGF-1 and IGF-binding protein 1 and 3 levels. J Appl Physiol 1996; 80(3): 760–4.

Renehan AG, Frystyk J, Flyvbjerg A. Obesity and cancer risk: the role of the insulin-IGF axis. Trends Endocrinol Metab 2006; 17:328–36.

Sandhu MS, Dunger DB, Giovannucci EL. Insulin, insulin-like growth factor, IGF binding proteins, their biologic interactions, and colorectal cancer. JNCI 2002; 94:972–80.

Luo, J., Manning, B. D., and Cantley, L. C. Targeting the PI3K-Akt pathway in human cancer: rationale and promise. *Cancer Cell, 4:* 257–62, 2003.

Engelman, J. A., Luo, J., and Cantley, L. C. The evolution of phosphatidylinositol 3-kinases as regulators of growth and metabolism. *Nat Rev Genet, 7:* 606–19, 2006.

Shaw, R. J., and Cantley, L. C. Ras, PI(3)K and mTOR signaling controls tumor cell growth. *Nature*, 441: 424–30, 2006.

Brazil, D. P., Yang, Z. Z., and Hemmings, B. A. Advances in protein kinase B signalling: AKTion on multiple fronts. *Trends Biochem Sci, 29:* 233–42, 2004.

Dillon RL, Muller WJ. Distinct biological roles for the AKt family in mammary tumor progression. Cancer Res 2010; 70:426064.

Hay, N. The Akt-mTOR tango and its relevance to cancer. *Cancer Cell, 8:* 179–83, 2005.

Sarbassov DD, Sabatini DM. Redox regulation of the nutrient-sensitive raptor-mTOR pathway and complex. J Biol Chem 2005; 280: 39505–39509.

Guertin, D.A. and D.M. Sabatini, An expanding role for mTOR in cancer. Trends Mol Med, 2005. 11(8): p. 353–61.

Kwiatkowki DJ, Manning BD. Tuberous sclerosis: a GAP at the crossroads of multiple signaling pathways. Hum Mol Genetics 2005; 14:R251-8.

Moore T, Beltran L, Carbijal S, Strom S, Traag J, Hursting SD, DiGiovanni J, Dietary energy balance modulates signaling through the Akt/mTOR pathway in multiple tissues. Cancer Prev Res 2008; 1:65–76.

Jiang, W., Z. Zhu, Thompson H. Dietary energy restriction modulates the activity of amp-activated protein kinase, akt, and mammalian target of rapamycin in mammary carcinomas, mammary gland, and liver. cancer research, 2008. 68: p. 5492–5499.

Moore T, Carbijal S., Beltran L, Perkins SN, Hursting SD, DiGiovanni J, Reduced susceptibility to two-stage skin carcinogenesis in mice with low circulating IGF-1 levels. Cancer Res, 2008. 68: p. 3680–8.

The Endogenous Hormones and Breast Cancer Collaborative Group. Insulin-like growth factor-q (IGF1), IGF binding protein 3 (IGFBP3) and breast cancer risk: pooled individual data analysis of 17 prospective studies. Lancet Oncology 11:530–42, 2010.

Chan JM, Stampfer MJ, Giovannucci E, et al. 1998. Plasma insulin-like growth factor-I and prostate cancer risk: a prospective study. *Science* 279:563–66.

Wolk A, Mantzoros CS, Andersson SO, et al. 1998. Insulin-like growth factor 1 and prostate cancer risk: a population-based, case-control study. *J. Natl. Cancer Inst.* 90:911–15.

Yu H, Spitz MR, Mistry J, et al. 1999. Plasma levels of insulin-like growth factor--I and lung cancer risk: a case-control analysis. *J. Natl. Cancer Inst.* 91:151–56.

Ma J, Pollak MN, Giovannucci E, et al. 1999. Prospective study of colorectal cancer risk in men and plasma levels of insulin-like growth factor (IGF)-I and IGF-binding protein-3. *J. Natl. Cancer Inst.* 91:620–25.

Giovannucci E, Pollak MN, Platz EA, et al. 2000. A prospective study of plasma insulin-like growth factor-1 and binding protein-3 and risk of colorectal neoplasia in women. *Cancer Epidemiol. Biomarkers Prev.* 9:345–49.

Petridou E, Dessypris N, Spanos E, et al. 1999. Insulin-like growth factor-I and binding protein-3 in relation to childhood leukaemia. *Int. J. Cancer* 80:494–96.

Douglas JB, Silverman DT, Pollak MN, Tao Y, Soliman AS, Stolzenberg-Solomon R. Serum IGF-1, IGF-II, IGFBP-3 and IGF-1/BP-3 molar ratio and risk of pancreatic cnacer in the PLCO cancer screening trial. Cancer Epidemiol Biomarkers Prev 2010; 19:2298–306.

Macaulay, V.M. (1992) Insulin-like growth factors and cancer. *Br J Cancer*, 65, 311–20.

Flurkey K, Papaconstantinou J, Miller RA, Harrison DE. 2001. Lifespan extension and delayed immune and collagen aging in mutant mice with defects in growth hormone production. *Proc. Natl. Acad. Sci. USA* 98:6736–41.

Bartke A, Brown-Borg HM. Life extension in the dwarf mouse. Curr Topics Dev Biol 2004; 63:189–225.

Anisimov VN. 2001. Mutant and genetically modified mice as models for studying the relationship between aging and carcinogenesis. *Mech. Ageing Dev. 122*:1221–55.

DiGiovanni J, Bol DK, Wilker E, et al. 2000. Constitutive expression of insulin-like growth factor-1 in epidermal basal cells of transgenic mice leads to spontaneous tumor promotion. *Cancer Res.* 60:1561–70.

Hursting SD, Perkins SN, Lavigne JA, Beltran L, Haines DC, Hill HL, Alvord WG, Barrett JC, DiGiovanni J. Urothelial overexpression of insulin-like growth factor-1 increases susceptibility to *p*-Cresidine-induced bladder carcinogenesis in transgenic mice. *Mol Carcinogenesis* 2009; 48:671–7.

Yiping Wu, Karen Cui, Keiko Miyoshi, Lothar Hennighausen, Jeffrey E. Green, Jennifer Setser, Derek LeRoith, Shoshana Yakar. Reduced Circulating Insulin-like Growth Factor I Levels Delay the Onset of Chemically and Genetically Induced Mammary Tumors. Cancer Res 2003; 63:4384–88.

Olivo-Marston S, Hursting SD, Lavigne J, Perkins SN, Marouf R, Yakar S, Harris CC. Genetic reduction of insulin-like growth factor-1 inhibits azoxymethane-induced colon tumorigenesis in mice. *Mol Carcinogenesis* 2009, 48:1071–6.

Lashinger LM, Malone LM, McArthur MJ, Goldberg JA, Daniels EA, Pavone A, Colby JK, Perkins SN, Fischer SM, Hursting SD. Genetic reduction of insulin-like growth factor-1 mimics the anticancer effects of calorie restriction on cyclooxygenase-2-drive pancreatic cancer. Cancer Prev Res 2010; in press.

Polunovsky V and Houghton PJ (2010). mTOR pathway and mTOR inhibitors in cancer therapy. New York, NY: Humana Press.

Wu Y, Brodt P, Sun H, Mejia W, Novosyadlyy R, Nunez N, Chen X, Mendoza A, Hong SH, Khanna C, Yakar S. Insulin-like growth factor-I regulates the liver microenvironment in obese mice and promotes liver metastasis Cancer Res 70: 57–67, 2010.

Fagan DH, Yee D. Crosstalk between IGF1R and estrogen receptor signaling in breast cancer. J Mammary Gland Biol Neoplasia. 2008; 13: 423–9.

Mawson A, Lai A, Carroll JS, Sergio CM, Mitchell CJ, and Sarcevic B. Estrogen and insulin/IGF-1 cooperatively stimulate cell cycle progression in MCF-7 breast cancer cells through differential regulation of c-Myc and cyclin D1. *Mol Cell Endocrinol* 2005; 229(1–2): 161–73.

Sachdev D and Yee D. The IGF system and breast cancer. Endocr Relat Cancer 2001; 8(3): 197–209.

Saxena NK, Taliaferro-Smith L, Knight BB, Merlin D, Anania FA, O'Regan RM, and Sharma D. Bidirectional crosstalk between leptin and insulin-like growth factor-I signaling promotes invasion and migration of breast cancer cells via transactivation of epidermal growth factor receptor. *Cancer Res* 2008; 68(23): 9712–22.

Ozbay T and Nahta R. A novel unidirectional cross-talk from the insulin-like growth factor-I receptor to leptin receptor in human breast cancer cells. *Mol Cancer Res* 2008; 6(6): 1052–8.

Balañá ME, Labriola L, Salatino M, Movsichoff F, Peters G, Charreau EH, and Elizalde PV. Activation of ErbB-2 via a hierarchical interaction between ErbB-2 and type I insulin-like growth factor receptor in mammary tumor cells. *Oncogene* 2001; 20(1): 34–47.

Shida D, Kitayama J, Mori K, Watanabe T and Nagawa H. Transactivation of epidermal growth factor receptor is involved in leptin-induced activation of janus-activated kinase 2 and extracellular signal-regulated kinase 1/2 in human gastric cancer cells. *Cancer Res* 2005; 65(20): 9159–63.

Hursting SD, Lashinger LM, Colbert LH, Rogers CJ, Wheatley KW, Nunez NP, Mahabir S, Barrett JC, Forman MR, and Perkins SN. Energy balance and carcinogenesis: underlying pathways and targets for intervention. *Curr Cancer Drug Targets* 2007; 7(5): 484–91.

Mitsiades CS, Mitsiades N, Poulaki V, Schlossman R, Akiyama M, Chauhan D, Hideshima T, Treon SP, Munshi NC, Richardson PG, and Anderson KC. Activation of NF-kappaB and upregulation of intracellular anti-apoptotic proteins via the IGF-1/Akt signaling in human multiple myeloma cells: therapeutic implications. *Oncogene* 2002; 21(37): 5673–83.

Fenton JI, Birmingham JM, Hursting SD, and Hord NG. Adiponectin blocks multiple signaling cascades associated with leptin-induced cell proliferation in Apc Min/+ colon epithelial cells. *Int J Cancer* 2008; 122(11): 2437–45.

Fang J, Zhou Q, Shi XL, Jiang BH. Luteolin inhibits insulin-like growth factor 1 receptor signaling in prostate cancer cells. *Carcinogenesis* 2007; 28(3): 713–23.

Garafalo C and Surmacz E. Leptin and cancer. Cell Phys 2005; 207:12–22.

Sachdev D and Yee D. Disrupting insulin-like growth factor signaling as a potential cancer therapy. Mol Cancer Therap 2007; 6:1–12.

Eng-Wong J, Hursting SD, Perkins SN, Zujewski J. Effects of raloxifene on insulin-like growth factor (IGF)-1, IGF-binding protein-3 and leptin in premenopausal women at high risk for breast cancer. *Cancer Epidemiol Biomarkers Prev* 2003; 12:1468–73.

Lubet RA, Christov K, Nunez N, Hursting SD, Steele VE, Juliana MM, Eto I, Grubbs CJ. Effects of the RXR agonist targretin in the methylnitrosourea-induced mammary cancer model: Dose response curves, cancer cell proliferation and apoptosis, and serum IGF-1 levels. *Carcinogenesis* 2005; 26:441–8.

DeAngel RD, Smith SD, Perkins SN, Glickman R, Hursting SD. Anti-tumor effects of ursolic acid in a mouse model of postmenopausal breast cancer. *Nutr Cancer* 2010; in press.

Fang J. Luteolin inhibits insulin-like growth factor 1 receptor signaling in prostate cancer cells. Carcinogenesis 2006; 28:713–23.

Anand P, Sundaram C, et al. Curcumin and Cancer: an "old-age" disease with an "age-old" solution. Cancer Letters 2008; 267(1): 133–64.

Harrison, D.E., Strong, R., Sharp, Z.D., Nelson, J.F., Astle, C.M., Flurkey, K., Nadon, N.L., Wilkinson, J.E., Frenkel, K., Carter, C.S., Pahor, M., Javors, M.A., Fernandez, E. and Miller, R.A. (2009) Rapamycin fed late in life extends lifespan in genetically heterogeneous mice. *Nature*, 460, 392–5.

Sahra IB, et al. The antidiabetic drug metformin exerts an antitumoral effect in vitro and in vivo through a decrease in cyclin D1 levels. Oncogene 2008; 27:3576–3586.

Hardie DG. AMPK: A regulator of energy balance in the single cell and the whole organism. Int J Obes 2008; 32:S7–12.

Memmott RM, et al. Metformin prevents tobacco carcinogen-induced lung tumorigenesis. Cancer Prevention Res 2010; 3:1066–76.

Libby G, Donnelly LA, Donnan PT, Alessi DR, Morris AD, Evans JM. New users of metformin are at low risk of incident cancer: a cohort study among people with type 2 diabetes. Diabetes Care. 2009;32(9):1620–5. PMCID: 2732153.

Li D, Yeung SC, Hassan MM, Konopleva M, Abbruzzese JL. Antidiabetic therapies affect risk of pancreatic cancer. Gastroenterology. 2009;137(2):482–8.

Jiralerspong S, Palla SL, Giordano SH, Meric-Bernstam F, Liedtke C, Barnett CM, et al. Metformin and pathologic complete responses to neoadjuvant chemotherapy in diabetic patients with breast cancer. J Clin Oncol. 2009;27(20):3297–302.

Hosono et al. Metformin suppresses colorectal aberrant crypt foci in a short-term clinical trial. Cancer Prevention Res 2010; 3:1077–83.

Pollak M. Metformin and other biguanides in oncology: advancing the research agenda. Cancer Prev Res 2010; 3:1060–65.

Firestein, R., Blander, G., Michan, S., Oberdoerffer, P., Ogino, S., Campbell, J., Bhimavarapu, A., Luikenhuis, S., de Cabo, R., Fuchs, C., Hahn, W.C., Guarente, L.P. and Sinclair, D.A. (2008) The SIRT1 deacetylase suppresses intestinal tumorigenesis and colon cancer growth. *PLoS One*, 3, e2020.S.

Signorelli, P. and Ghidoni, R. (2005) Resveratrol as an anticancer nutrient: molecular basis, open questions and promises. *J Nutr Biochem*, 16, 449–66.

Liu, T., Liu, P.Y. and Marshall, G.M. (2009) The critical role of the class III histone deacetylase SIRT1 in cancer. *Cancer Res*, 69, 1702–5.

Kalaany NY, Sabatini DM. Tumours with PI3K activation are resistant to dietary restriction. Nature 2009; 458:725–31.

Chapter 13
Cancer Cell Metabolism

Akash Patnaik, Jason W. Locasale, and Lewis C. Cantley

"Insulin-Resistant" States and Cancer

There is mounting clinical and epidemiologic evidence for a relationship between insulin-resistant states, such as obesity, type II diabetes, or metabolic syndrome and several cancers (Table 13.1). One large prospective study reported that for men with a BMI > 35 kg/m^2, the relative risk of mortality from any cancer was 1.23 that of the normal weight reference population (BMI, 18.5–24.9 kg/m^2). Similar findings were observed in women with a BMI of 30–34.9 kg/m^2, increasing to 1.62 in those with a BMI >40 kg/m^2 (Calle et al. 2003).

The intriguing relationship between obesity and cancer may have its mechanistic underpinnings in an altered adipokine milieu found in obese relative to normal weight-individuals, which results in a generalized proinflammatory state that predisposes an individual to cancer. Recent evidence suggests that low-adiponectin states, such as obesity, are associated with increased prostate cancer (PCa) risk (Michalakis et al. 2007). Adiponectin activates adenosine monophosphate-dependent protein kinase (AMPK), an evolutionarily conserved regulator of cellular energy homeostasis that protects cells from energy stress (Zakikhani et al. 2008). A mechanistic model for obesity-induced cancers is illustrated in Fig. 13.1.

L.C. Cantley (✉)
Division of Signal Transduction, Department of Medicine, Beth Israel Deaconess Medical Center, Boston, MA, USA

Department of Systems Biology, Harvard Medical School, Boston, MA, USA
e-mail: lewis_cantley@hms.harvard.edu

D. LeRoith (ed.), *Insulin-like Growth Factors and Cancer: From Basic Biology to Therapeutics*, Cancer Drug Discovery and Development,
DOI 10.1007/978-1-4614-0598-6_13, © Springer Science+Business Media, LLC 2012

Table 13.1 Cancers associated with obesity, type II diabetes, and hyperinsulinemia

Hematologic cancers
Non-Hodgkin's lymphoma
Multiple myeloma
Gastrointestinal cancers
Colorectal cancer
Pancreatic cancer
Gastric cardia cancer
Extrahepatic biliary cancer
Esophageal adenocarcinoma
Hepatocellular carcinoma
Cholangiocarcinoma
Gynecologic cancers
Breast cancer
Endometrial cancer
Cervical adenocarcinoma

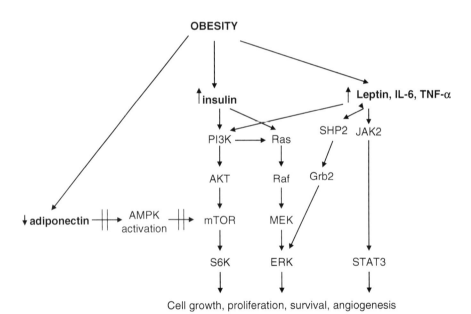

Fig. 13.1 Mechanistic model for obesity-induced cancers. The obesogenic phenotype results in an organismal metabolic dysfunction characterized by an alteration in hormonal and/or inflammatory cytokine levels: increased insulin, IGF-1, leptin, and tumor necrosis factor-α, and decreased adiponectin, respectively. These alterations can directly impact signaling pathways within the tumor to increase cell growth, proliferation, survival, and angiogenesis. *AMPK* AMP-activated protein kinase, *PI3K* PI-3 kinase, *mTOR* mammalian target of rapamycin

AMPK and Cancer

AMPK is an evolutionarily conserved energy-sensing serine/threonine protein kinase, consisting of a catalytic subunit (α) and two regulatory subunits (β and γ). At the cellular level, AMPK is activated by metabolic stresses that deplete ATP and increase AMP (e.g., exercise, hypoxia, glucose deprivation). At the level of the organism, enzyme activity is also under the control of hormones and cytokines, such as adiponectin and leptin (Hardie 2008). Activation of AMPK reduces plasma insulin levels, suppresses ATP-consuming metabolic functions (such as synthesis of fatty acids (FAs), sterols, glycogen, and proteins), and increases ATP-producing activities (glucose uptake, FA oxidation, and mitochondrial biogenesis) to restore energy homeostasis. Thus, AMPK functions as a central metabolic sensor that governs glucose and lipid metabolism.

A critical kinase involved in AMPK activation is the well-known tumor suppressor LKB1 (Woods et al. 2003). LKB1 germ-line mutations are responsible for Peutz–Jegher syndrome, predisposing carriers to hamartomas and a variety of malignant epithelial tumors (Jenne et al. 1998). Additionally, homozygous deletions in the LKB1-binding partner STRADA, that is essential for its full activity, are found in patients with abnormal brain development characterized in part by megalencephaly (Orlova et al. 2010). Interestingly, over 80% of LKB-1 knockout mice develop prostatic intraepithelial neoplasia (PIN) which is a precursor to prostate cancer (PCa) (Pearson et al. 2008; Shackelford and Shaw 2009). This suggests that the LKB1–AMPK pathway may regulate growth as a link between cancer and energy homeostasis. Indeed, when physiologically or pharmacologically activated, AMPK acts in a tumor suppressor-like fashion. It inhibits key lipogenic enzymes by direct phosphorylation [Acetyl-CoA carboxylase (ACC), 3-hydroxy-3-methyl-glutaryl-CoA (HMG-CoA reductase)] and by transcriptional regulation [ATP citrate lyase (ACLY), fatty acid synthase (FAS)] through the suppression of the transcriptional factor sterol regulatory element-binding protein 1 (SREBP-1). In addition, AMPK inhibits the mTOR pathway through direct phosphorylation of tuberous sclerosis complex 2 protein (TSC2) and the mTOR-associated factor raptor that comprises part of the mTORC1 signaling complex (Fig. 13.2). Finally, it induces cell cycle arrest or apoptosis through phosphorylation of p53 and FOXO3a (Shackelford and Shaw 2009). Thus, activated AMPK can simultaneously regulate multiple oncogenic pathways. In particular, it may simultaneously inhibit two of the major pathways (lipogenic and PI3K/mTOR pathways) that drive carcinogenesis by antagonizing the activity of Akt at multiple downstream effectors, including SREBP-1, TSC-2, and mTORC1.

Decreased AMPK activity has been found to contribute to the metabolic abnormalities involved in metabolic syndrome (Luo et al. 2005; Ruderman and Prentki 2004), a constellation of metabolic manifestations that include insulin resistance, blood glucose abnormalities, elevated triglycerides, and low HDL. Moreover, a recent study revealed an association between polymorphisms in the PRKAA2 gene (encoding the $\alpha2$ subunit of AMPK) and susceptibility to insulin resistance and diabetes in the Japanese population (Horikoshi et al. 2006). This result is consistent

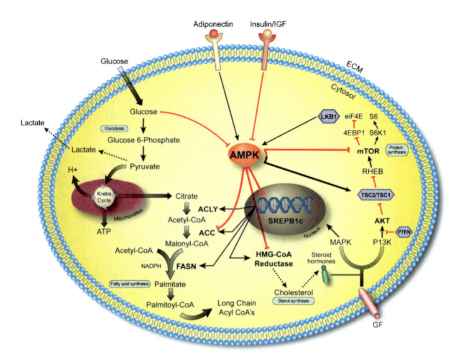

Fig. 13.2 AMPK regulates multiple metabolic and signaling pathways deregulated in cancer. Activation of AMPK can inhibit these pathways by direct phosphorylation of key lipogenic enzymes [ACC, in particular isoform 1, HMG-CoA reductase] and key kinases (the complex TSC1/TSC2 and the mTOR-associated factor raptor) or by regulating transcription through SREBP1c. *Red and black arrows* indicate activation and inhibition, respectively. Tumor suppressor genes are represented in *violet hexagonal boxes. AMPK* AMP-activated protein kinase, *SREBP1c* sterol regulatory element-binding protein-1c, *ACLY* ATP citrate lyase, *ACC* acetyl-CoA carboxylase, *FASN* fatty acid synthase, *HMG-CoA reductase* 3-hydroxy-3-methyl-glutaryl-CoA reductase, *MAPK* mitogen-activated protein kinase, *PI3K* phosphatidylinositol-3-kinase, *PTEN* phosphatase and tensin homolog, *TSC2/TSC1* tuberous sclerosis complex 1/2, *RHEB* Ras homolog enriched in brain, *mTOR* mammalian target of rapamycin, *4EBP1* 4E-binding protein 1, *S6K1* S6 kinase 1, *eiF4E* eukaryotic translation initiation factor 4, *GF* growth factors. *Adapted from Zadra et al. (2010)*

with gene deletion studies that had previously shown a role for the α2 subunit of AMPK in controlling insulin sensitivity in mice (Viollet et al. 2003). Interestingly, the same locus correlates with PCa risk (Matsui et al. 2004), suggesting that AMPK dysregulation may provide a mechanistic link between obesity/metabolic syndrome and PCa. Consequently, drugs that ameliorate MS conditions through AMPK activation (Table 13.2) may be beneficial for cancer prevention and treatment.

The antidiabetic drug metformin inhibits complex I of the mitochondrial respiratory chain (Takane et al. 2008), resulting in increased AMP/ATP ratio and secondary activation of the AMPK pathway. This results in decreased hepatic gluconeogenesis, and secondary reduction in serum insulin and glucose levels, respectively. At supraphysiologic millimolar concentrations, metformin also activates AMPK in cancer cell lines in vitro. While its precise antitumor mechanism is currently unclear (see section "AMPK Activators" for detailed discussion of metformin's proposed

13 Cancer Cell Metabolism

Table 13.2 Current direct and indirect AMPK activators

Activator	Effect on AMPK	Mechanism
Metformin	Indirect	Increase AMP/ATP by inhibition of complex 1 of mitochondrial respiratory chain
TZDs	Indirect	Increase PPARγ-mediated release of adiponectin, which consequently activates AMPK
Deguelin	Indirect	Not fully clarified. Decrease of ATP
Epigallocatechin-3-gallate	Indirect	Activation of the AMPK activator CaMKK
Barberin	Indirect	Increase AMP/ATP by inhibition of mitochondrial function
α-Lipoic acid	Indirect	n.d.
Resveratrol	Indirect	Not fully clarified. Possible activation of SIRT1 and consequent deacetylation of the AMPK activator LKB1
AICAR	Direct	AMP mimetic
A-769662	Direct	Allosteric binding of β1 AMPK subunit
PT1	Direct	Allosteric binding of α1 AMPK subunit

Adapted from Zadra et al. (2010)

n.d. not determined yet, *TZDs* thiazolidinediones, *CAMKK* calmodulin-dependent protein kinase kinase, *SIRT1* sirtuin 1, *AICAR* 5-aminoimidazole-4-carboxamide-1-b-riboside

antitumor mechanisms), a recent study examined the potential role of metformin in a diet-induced colon cancer xenograft model (Algire et al. 2008). Tumors from mice on the high-energy diet were approximately twice the volume of those of mice on the control diet, 17 days following the subcutaneous injection of MC38 colon carcinoma cells. These findings were correlated with the observation that the high-energy diet led to elevated serum insulin levels, as well as increased phosphorylated AKT, and increased expression of FAS in the tumor cells. Metformin blocked the effect of the high-energy diet on tumor growth, reduced insulin levels, and attenuated the effect of diet on phosphorylation of AKT and expression of FAS. Furthermore, the administration of metformin led to the activation of AMPK, the inhibitory phosphorylation of ACC, the upregulation of BNIP3 and increased apoptosis in the tumor, as estimated by poly (ADP-ribose) polymerase (PARP) cleavage. These findings could be explained by both an *indirect* effect of metformin on tumor growth and survival via inhibition of hepatic gluconeogenesis and reduction in serum insulin levels, and a *direct* effect on signaling pathways within the tumor. The study suggests a potential role for this agent in the management of a metabolically defined subset of cancers (see section "AMPK Activators").

Fatty Acid Metabolism and Cancer

Cancer cells display elevated rates of de novo free fatty acid (FFA) synthesis, largely due to increased expression of FAS. Newly synthesized FFAs are converted to neutral lipid stores, including mono-, di-, or triacylglycerols. FAS is a multifunctional enzyme that catalyzes the terminal steps in the synthesis of the 16-carbon fatty acid palmitate in cells (Wakil 1989). In normal cells, FAS expression levels are relatively low because fatty acid is generally supplied by dietary fatty acid. In contrast, FAS is expressed at significantly higher levels in a variety of human epithelial cancers, including breast, thyroid, colon, ovary, lung, and prostate (Menendez and Lupu 2007). Overexpression of FAS has also been reported in hematological malignancies, including leukemia, multiple myeloma, and diffuse large B-cell lymphoma (Pizer et al. 1996; Wang et al. 2008). Moreover, several reports have shown that FAS expression levels correlate with tumor progression, aggressiveness, and metastasis (Kuhajda 2006). For example, FAS expression levels are predictive of poor prognosis in breast and prostate cancer (Kuhajda 2006). As FAS has been strongly linked to tumor cell proliferation and is preferentially expressed in cancer cells, it represents an attractive target for novel anticancer therapy (Menendez and Lupu 2007; Kuhajda 2006).

Recent studies have suggested that there is a functional interaction between FAS enzymatic activity and different receptor tyrosine kinases (RTK), such as HER2 (Menendez et al. 2004) and c-Met (Coleman et al. 2009). RTKs and their specific ligands are essential components of intracellular signaling pathways used for the control of growth, differentiation, and survival. Both HER2 and c-Met have been implicated in tumor growth, invasion, and metastasis in a variety of human cancers via the PI3-kinase/AKT and MAPK signaling pathways, respectively (Engelman et al. 2006).

In the context of prostate cancer, exacerbation of de-novo FA and sterol synthesis due to overexpression of key enzymes (ATP citrate lyase, Acetyl-CoA carboxylase, FAS, HMG-CoA-reductase) and increased protein synthesis due to hyperactivation of mTOR are common features of both primary and advanced PCa (Swinnen et al. 2000; Rossi et al. 2003; Ettinger et al. 2004). These alterations are induced both by androgen and by the activated PTEN/PI3K/Akt/mTOR signaling pathways, respectively, the latter being deregulated in a large fraction of human prostate cancers. Indeed, deletions/mutations in the tumor suppressor PTEN are found in 30% of primary PCa and in over 60% of metastatic PCa (Sansal and Sellers 2004).

While acquisition of the lipogenic phenotype appears to be a critical event in the metabolic transformation of cancer cells, recent data suggests that cancer cells can subvert a lipolytic enzyme, monoacylglycerol lipase (MAGL), to remodel their lipogenic state into the genesis of protumorigenic signals (Nomura et al. 2010). MAGL was found to be highly expressed in melanoma, ovarian, and breast cancer cell lines and primary tumors, respectively, where it appears to regulate a fatty acid network enriched in oncogenic bioactive lipids (phosphatidic acid, lysophosphatidic acid, and PGE_2) that promote tumor invasion, migration, and survival. Interestingly, impairments in MAGL-dependent tumor growth are rescued by a high-fat diet, suggesting that exogenous sources of fatty acids can contribute to malignancy in cancers lacking MAGL activity (Nomura et al. 2010).

Amino Acid Metabolism and Cancer

A recent study utilized a high-throughput metabolomics approach to distinguish normal (benign) prostate, localized and metastatic prostate cancer (Sreekumar et al. 2009). Among the 1,126 metabolites they isolated from samples of prostate tissue, serum and urine, they found 87 that distinguish prostate cancer from benign prostate tissue. Of this group, six metabolites were of particular interest because their levels were even higher in metastatic cancer. The authors pursued one of these metabolites as a possible biomarker for cancer progression: sarcosine – a derivative of the amino acid glycine because of its elevation in metastatic disease and link to potential disease mechanisms.

Sarcosine (N-methylglycine) is generated by the enzymatic transfer of a methyl group from S-adenosylmethionine to glycine in vivo. This reaction is catalyzed by the enzyme glycine-N-methyltransferase (GNMT), which is expressed at high levels in the mammalian liver, exocrine pancreas, and prostate. GNMT plays a central part in modulating the cellular pool of S-adenosylmethionine, which is the main methyl donor for several essential reactions that regulate gene expression and protein activity; these include cytosine methylation of DNA, lysine methylation of histone proteins and arginine methylation of histones and other proteins. In an earlier study, this group found that the levels of the methyltransferase enzyme EZH2, which transfers methyl groups to lysine 27 of histone H3, are higher during the progression of prostate cancer and other tumors. Their latest data are suggestive of a transcriptional link between cancer progression and GNMT activity, through the binding of both the androgen receptor and the oncogene *ERG* to the promoter sequence of the *GNMT* gene in cancer cells. This study also found that the addition of sarcosine to benign prostate epithelial cells promotes invasive properties in these cells, whereas lowering GNMT levels in a prostate-cancer cell line reduces its invasiveness (Sreekumar et al. 2009). Taken together, these findings suggest a potential role for sarcosine as a biomarker for prostate-cancer progression, and provide evidence for a functional role of this metabolite in enhancing the malignant phenotype, at least in the context of prostate cancer.

Enhanced Rates of Glucose Uptake and the Warburg Effect

Prior to the discovery of oncogenes and tumor suppressor genes in the 1970s, cancer was considered a metabolic disease (Warburg 1956). Altered metabolism in tumors compared to normal tissues was first described by Otto Warburg who found that many tumors metabolize glucose through a fermentative metabolism resulting in lactate production (Warburg et al. 1924). Now referred to as the Warburg Effect, this form of glucose metabolism occurs even in the presence of oxygen and has also been termed aerobic glycolysis. Warburg accounted for this observation by postulating that tumor cells maintained defective mitochondrial respiration. However, it is now believed that tumor cells in large part have fully functioning respiratory chains and intact mitochondrial physiology (Deberardinis et al. 2008a).

The more plausible explanation for decreased oxidative phosphorylation in tumors is that aerobic glycolysis allows for tumor cells to adapt their metabolism for more efficient anabolic metabolism and cell-autonomous survival and proliferation in an environment absent of contact of extracellular matrix (Vander Heiden

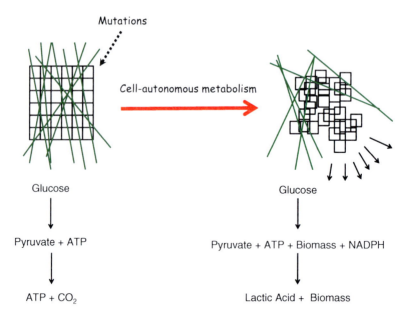

Fig. 13.3 Altered metabolism in tumor cells. Upon cell transformation, cancer cells acquire a cell-autonomous metabolism that allows for proliferation outside the context of interaction with the extracellular matrix. The transformed cells switch their glucose metabolism from that of primarily energy production to anabolic metabolism involving the production of biomass and NADPH, respectively

et al. 2009) (Fig. 13.3). Lactate also likely has multiple non cell-autonomous effects for tumor cells by lowering local pH to enhance invasiveness by disrupting the extracellular matrix as well as to keep tumor-attacking immune cells away.

Furthermore, aerobic glycolysis, when coupled to what is often observed to be enhanced rates of glucose uptake may allow for more efficient anabolic metabolism. The likely consequences of enhanced anabolic metabolism come from requirements imposed by balancing the stoichiometry of the overall chemical equation for glycolysis. Considering the overall chemical equation for glycolysis, it is apparent that glycolysis consumes NAD+ and ADP to generate NADH and ATP. For high rates of glycolysis to be maintained in tumors, NAD+ and ADP must be regenerated. NAD+ can be generated by lactate production via lactate dehydrogenase, whereas how sufficient ADP is generated is poorly understood and a subject of future study. By maintaining high rates of glucose uptake and relatively low rates of oxidative phosphorylation, the carbon atoms from glucose can be diverted into anabolic processes rather than oxidized to CO_2. These anabolic pathways include amino acid synthesis, glycerol synthesis used for the synthesis of lipids, and de novo nucleotide synthesis originating from the pentose phosphate pathway and the folate pool.

Large relative rates of glucose uptake are observed in most (but not all) tumors as evidenced by the use of positron emission tomography (PET) imaging for analyzing tumor status (Vander Heiden et al. 2009). PET positive tumors account for nearly 80% of solid tumors and PET imaging using radioactive fluorodeoxyglucose (FDG-PET) remains one of the most powerful imaging diagnostics for monitoring cancer status and disease progression. FDG-PET measures the glucose that is taken up and captured by cells.

Cellular Metabolic Reprogramming in Cancer by Oncogenes and Tumor Suppressor Genes

Accumulating evidence indicates that most oncogenes and tumor suppressor genes play critical roles in regulating metabolism (Locasale et al. 2009). The PI3K pathway is known to regulate glucose uptake by acutely stimulating the translocation of glucose transporters to the plasma membrane, in the case of muscle and fat cells, and by enhancing expression of genes involved in glucose uptake and metabolism in all cells. A recent study also implicates KRAS mutations as having an effect on increasing glucose uptake (Yun et al. 2009). Glut1 was one of the most upregulated genes expressed in a KRAS-mutated HCT116 colon cancer cell line when compared to an isogenic wild-type KRAS expressing cell line. Interestingly, the study also demonstrated that wild-type KRAS expressing cells spontaneously acquire KRAS gain-of-function mutations when subjected to growth conditions in low glucose. Provocatively, this finding suggested that KRAS mutations manifest their transformative potential by virtue of enhancing glucose metabolism and may have evolved through a selective pressure to achieve a hyperactive glucose metabolism.

Additionally, growth factor signaling pathways can also regulate metabolism through posttranslational modifications. AKT can phosphorylate glycolytic enzymes hexokinase (HK) and phosphofructokinase2 (PFK2) (Manning and Cantley 2007). HK phosphorylates glucose to initiate the first step in glycolysis involving glucose capture. AKT phosphorylation of HK is believed to be an activating modification. PFK2 regulates the levels of fructose 2,6-bisphosphate which in turn allosterically regulates the activity of PFK and all points downstream in glycolysis beyond the fructose 1,6-bisphosphate generating step (Bensaad et al. 2006).

Furthermore, hyperactivation of growth factor signaling often leads to increased mTOR signaling. Accumulating evidence points to mTOR as having direct control of metabolism-related transcription factors, including HIF and SREBP-1 (Laplante and Sabatini 2010; Kaelin et al. 2008). HIF induces the expression of glycolysis related genes. SREBP-1induces genes involved in cholesterol and fatty acid synthesis.

Enhanced expression of MYC is one of the most common events in human cancers (Meyer and Penn 2008). KRAS mutations lead to hyperactivation of MYC via MAPK phosphorylation. Developmental pathways, often mutated in cancer, such as the Wnt and Hedgehog signaling pathways also activate MYC. MYC is also the most commonly amplified gene in all of human cancer (Beroukhim et al. 2010). MYC is now known to regulate the expression of diverse sets of metabolic genes. Glutamine uptake and metabolism is directly regulated by MYC through expression of glutaminase enzymes (Wise et al. 2008).

Glutamine has numerous cellular functions (DeBerardinis et al. 2008b). Glutamine is involved in the synthesis of glutathione, which is present in millimolar quantities in cells and regulates the removal of reactive oxygen species. Glutamine is also involved in de novo nucleotide and amino acid metabolism and, when converted to glutamate by transamination, provides a nitrogen source for numerous anabolic reactions in cells. Glutamine has also been observed to have, in some contexts, a catabolic function in which it has been shown to flux into the Krebs cycle via alpha-ketoglutarate.

MYC has also been shown to regulate the expression of PKM2, a splice variant of pyruvate kinase that is expressed in all cancer and proliferating cells and is believed to confer a growth advantage to cells (David et al. 2010). MYC likely has a number of other metabolic functions as a candidate list of MYC-regulated genes included many genes involved in metabolism (Dang et al. 2008).

Tumor suppressor genes also have metabolic functions. p53, the most commonly mutated gene in human cancers, has several appreciated metabolic functions. p53 regulates the expression of TIGAR and SCO2 (Vousden and Ryan 2009). TIGAR regulates the levels of fructose-2,6-phosphate and is believed to control flux in the pentose phosphate pathway. SCO2 regulates the activity of the cytochrome c oxidase (COX) complex that provides a link from p53 to mitochondrial physiology. p53 has also recently been shown to regulate glutamine metabolism by inducing the expression of glutaminase (Hu et al. 2010; Suzuki et al. 2010). Other tumor suppressors also may have effects on metabolism.

Pharmaceuticals Targeting the Cancer Cell Metabolome

As a result of our increased understanding of the metabolic circuitry that drives the malignant phenotype, there are a number of pharmaceuticals that target the cancer metabolome already in clinical use or currently under investigation (Tennant et al. 2010).

Antimetabolite Chemotherapy

The advent of modern chemotherapy originated after World War II from Sydney Farber's observation that soldiers in the tropics with anemia could be treated with B vitamins and folic acid. B vitamins were known to be enzyme cofactors contributing to enhanced folate metabolism. In these patients, it was observed that enhancing metabolism induced blood cell growth. Conversely, this observation led to the molecular concept that targeting folate metabolism might reduce growth in neoplastic settings. Folate antagonists were found to induce partial remission in certain leukemias providing the basis for antineoplastic chemical therapy (Farber et al. 1948). Methotrexate, aminopterin, and other folate antagonists remain some of the

13 Cancer Cell Metabolism

most common chemotherapeutic frontline drugs for treating hematologic cancers as well as solid tumors, often leading to complete remission in some disease settings (Jolivet et al. 1983).

Directly downstream of folate metabolism is nucleotide metabolism and the antineoplastic properties of folate antagonists are believed to be a result of inhibiting nucleotide synthesis. Additional chemotherapies have been developed that target nucleotide synthesis and these have proven to be very effective. These agents include 5-fluorouracil and gemcitabine, among others (Chabner and Roberts 2005).

AMPK Activators

Aminoimidazole-4-carboxamide-1-β-D-ribofuranoside (AICAR), an AMP mimetic and intermediate in the AMP biosynthetic pathway, has been shown to inhibit ex vivo proliferation of prostate cancer cell lines and inhibit tumor growth in PCa xenograft models (Ben Sahra et al. 2008). However, AICAR is not specific for AMPK, it has limited oral bioavailability and frequently induces an increase in blood levels of lactic acid and uric acid. The possibility of novel small molecules able to allosterically activate AMPK has been greatly fostered by the recent publication of the crystal structure of AMPK (Xiao et al. 2007). Abbott laboratories has pioneered this area and identified A-769662, a thinopyridone AMPK activator that activates the enzyme by binding the β1 subunit (Cool et al. 2006). A-769662 has been shown to delay tumor development and decrease tumor incidence in PTEN+/– mice with a hypomorphic LKB1 allele (Huang et al. 2008). A second small-molecule activator (PT1), not yet well characterized, has also been recently reported (Pang et al. 2008).

Several observations made in population studies point toward the use of metformin for cancer treatment and/or prevention. First, diabetic patients treated with metformin have a dramatic decrease in cancer risk and cancer-specific mortality compared to diabetic patients treated with insulin (Currie et al. 2009). Second, metformin use was associated with a 44% risk reduction in prostate cancer among Caucasian men (Wright and Stanford 2009). Third, a retrospective study of >2,500 breast cancer patients treated with neoadjuvant chemotherapy showed that patients taking metformin had significantly higher pathologic complete responses than patients not taking metformin (Jiralerspong et al. 2009).

As described in section "AMPK and Cancer," the mechanism of action for metformin's putative antitumor effect is not completely understood and has been ascribed to both *direct* and *indirect* effects. Metformin's *direct* effects on tumor have been partly attributed to AMPK activation. This results in inhibition of mTOR and p70S6K activity and decreased translational efficiency in prostate (Ben Sahra et al. 2008) and breast cancer cell lines (Dowling et al. 2007), respectively. However, inhibition of AMPK using siRNA did not prevent the antiproliferative effect of metformin in PCa cell lines, even though S6K1 phosphorylation was inhibited, suggesting that its effects can be independent of AMPK. Since metformin decreases ATP levels and elevates

AMP levels, it could potentially affect many cellular functions that are sensitive to changes in these nucleotides. In fact, it has been argued that agents that decrease ATP levels are more likely to kill tumors that lack the ability to activate AMPK (Shaw et al. 2004). In vitro studies have also shown that metformin treatment has an inhibitory effect on nuclear factor-kappa B (NF-κB) and Erk 2/5 activation by an AMPK-independent mechanism (16, personal communication). Recent work has demonstrated that metformin treatment inhibited transformation and selectively killed *cancer stem cells* from four genetically distinct breast cancer lines. In xenograft breast cancer models, combination therapy using metformin and doxorubicin or tamoxifen reduced tumor size and resulted in prolonged remissions (Hirsch et al. 2009).

Metformin's *indirect* effect on tumor proliferation can be explained via inhibition of hepatic gluconeogenesis and increased glucose uptake in skeletal muscle (Kim et al. 2008) thereby decreasing circulating glucose, insulin, and IGF-1 levels, and thereby blocking stimulation of the insulin/IGF-1 pathway in tumor cells.

The retrospective clinical studies have generated a great deal of enthusiasm for incorporating metformin into clinical trials (Goodwin et al. 2009). Understanding how biguanides mediate their anticancer effect is critical before launching clinical trials for human cancer. For example, pAMPK levels in breast cancer tumors are extremely variable (Hadad et al. 2009). If this pathway mediates antitumor effects, a specific group of PCa patients with the AMPK activation signature could be targeted for clinical trials with biguanides (actually, metformin might work better in tumors that lack functional AMPK). Alternatively, if the antitumor effects of biguanides are predominant by an indirect mechanism, then PCa patients most likely to benefit might be those with concomitant insulin resistance. Therefore, although metformin is very safe and remarkably inexpensive, it is critical to lay the groundwork before embarking on trials in metastatic disease.

Inhibitors of Lipogenesis

ACC, FASN, and HMG-CoA reductase are responsible for the synthesis of malonyl-CoA, the saturated FA palmitate, and mevalonate (the precursor of cholesterol), respectively, and their roles in the pathogenesis and progression of prostate cancer is well established (Menendez and Lupu 2007; Migita et al. 2009). Small-molecule FASN inhibitors (cerulein, C75, C93, Orlistat), HMG-CoA reductase inhibitors (statins), and ACC inhibitors (such as soraphen A) have shown promising preclinical results both in vitro and in vivo (Flavin et al. 2010; Murtola 2010; Beckers et al. 2007). So far, the use of FAS inhibitors as systemic drugs has been hampered by pharmacologic limitations and side effects of weight loss (Flavin et al. 2010). However, recent reports have described new potent FAS inhibitors identified through high-throughput screening as a testimony of the continuous interest in FAS as a therapeutic target (Flavin et al. 2010). Moreover, recent data showed a reduced incidence of PCa among statin users in the Finnish Prostate Cancer Screening Trial, associated with lower PSA levels (Murtola 2010). This evidence suggests that interfering with lipid metabolism represents an important direction to pursue. At present, two clinical trials are ongoing to investigate the effect of statin therapy prior to prostatectomy (NCT00572468) or during external beam radiation therapy (NCT00580970). A more accurate stratification of patients eligible for lipogenic pathway-inhibiting therapies is plausible due to the increasing development of new PET-based metabolic imaging techniques. In fact, lipid metabolism is being investigated by [11][C]- and [18][F]-labeled acetate or choline. Both of these tracers have shown increased sensitivity in the detection of primary, recurrent, and metastatic PCa (Picchio et al. 2009).

Targets in Central Carbon Metabolism

Exploiting the altered glucose metabolism that is seen in many tumors offers multiple avenues to target cancer cell metabolism. The unique isoform of pyruvate kinase, PKM2, provides an attractive cancer target as its expression occurs only in proliferating tissues and tumors (Christofk et al. 2008). Since PKM2 is intrinsically a less active enzyme than its counterparts that are expressed in differentiated tissue, one strategy is to allosterically activate PKM2 and a class of these compounds is currently being pursued in preclinical settings (Boxer et al. 2010).

Other means of intervening in central carbon metabolism may be promising as well. Azaserine, a glutamate antagonist has antineoplastic properties and was at one point subjected to clinical trials (Stock et al. 1954). Bromopyruvate (BrPyr), an alkylating agent with reported antiglycolytic activity has been shown to selectively inhibit tumor growth in xenograft models of KRAS-mutated cell lines (Yun et al. 2009; da Silva et al. 2009). Dichloroacetate, a pyruvate dehydrogenase kinase inhibitor appears to have some clinical response in patients with advanced stage glioblastoma and can be given in doses that affect mitochondrial physiology in patients (Michelakis et al. 2010). Inhibiting pyruvate dehydrogenase is predicted to enhance the rate of glycolytic carbon entering the Krebs cycle. Inhibiting lactate dehydrogenase has also shown to be effective in some preclinical settings (Fantin et al. 2006).

Conclusion

The transformation of cells from a normal to malignant state is accompanied by reprogramming of metabolic pathways, which include those that participate in energy stress, lipid, amino acid, and glucose metabolism. While we have gained appreciation that deregulated metabolism is a defining feature of cancer, the precise relative contribution of these biochemical changes to pathogenesis remains unclear. An insight into the interplay between these metabolic pathways provides a deeper understanding of disease mechanisms and contributes to the development of novel, personalized cancer therapies.

References

Calle, E.E., et al., *Overweight, obesity, and mortality from cancer in a prospectively studied cohort of US adults.* New England Journal of Medicine, 2003. **348**(17): p. 1625–1638.

Michalakis, K., et al., *Serum adiponectin concentrations and tissue expression of adiponectin receptors are reduced in patients with prostate cancer: A case control study.* Cancer Epidemiology Biomarkers & Prevention, 2007. **16**(2): p. 308–313.

Zakikhani, M., et al., *The Effects of Adiponectin and Metformin on Prostate and Colon Neoplasia Involve Activation of AMP-Activated Protein Kinase.* Cancer Prevention Research, 2008. **1**(5): p. 369–375.

Hardie, D.G., *AMPK: a key regulator of energy balance in the single cell and the whole organism.* International Journal of Obesity, 2008. **32**: p. S7–S12.

Woods, A., et al., *LKB1 is the upstream kinase in the AMP-activated protein kinase cascade.* Curr Biol, 2003. **13**(22): p. 2004–8.

Jenne, D.E., et al., *Peutz-Jeghers syndrome is caused by mutations in a novel serine threonine kinase.* Nature Genetics, 1998. **18**(1): p. 38–44.

Orlova, K.A., et al., *STRAD alpha deficiency results in aberrant mTORC1 signaling during corticogenesis in humans and mice.* Journal of Clinical Investigation, 2010. **120**(5): p. 1591–1602.

Pearson, H.B., et al., *Lkb1 deficiency causes prostate neoplasia in the mouse.* Cancer Research, 2008. **68**(7): p. 2223–2232.

Shackelford, D.B. and R.J. Shaw, *The LKB1-AMPK pathway: metabolism and growth control in tumour suppression.* Nature Reviews Cancer, 2009. **9**(8): p. 563–575.

Luo, Z.J., et al., *AMPK, the metabolic syndrome and cancer.* Trends in Pharmacological Sciences, 2005. **26**(2): p. 69–76.

Ruderman, N. and M. Prentki, *AMP kinase and malonyl-CoA: Targets for therapy of the metabolic syndrome.* Nature Reviews Drug Discovery, 2004. **3**(4): p. 340–351.

Horikoshi, M., et al., *A polymorphism in the AMPK alpha 2 subunit gene is associated with insulin resistance and type 2 diabetes in the Japanese population.* Diabetes, 2006. **55**(4): p. 919–923.

Viollet, B., et al., *Physiological role of AMP-activated protein kinase (AMPK): insights from knockout mouse models.* Biochemical Society Transactions, 2003. **31**: p. 216–219.

Matsui, H., et al., *Genomewide linkage analysis of familial prostate cancer in the Japanese population.* Journal of Human Genetics, 2004. **49**(1): p. 9–15.

Takane, H., et al., *Polymorphism in human organic cation transporters and metformin action.* Pharmacogenomics, 2008. **9**(4): p. 415–422.

Algire, C., et al., *Metformin attenuates the stimulatory effect of a high-energy diet on in vivo LLC1 carcinoma growth.* Endocrine-Related Cancer, 2008. **15**(3): p. 833–839.

Wakil, S.J., *FATTY-ACID SYNTHASE, A PROFICIENT MULTIFUNCTIONAL ENZYME.* Biochemistry, 1989. **28**(11): p. 4523–4530.

Menendez, J.A. and R. Lupu, *Fatty acid synthase and the lipogenic phenotype in cancer pathogenesis.* Nature Reviews Cancer, 2007. **7**(10): p. 763–777.

Pizer, E.S., et al., *Fatty acid synthase (FAS): A target for cytotoxic antimetabolites in HL60 promyelocytic leukemia cells.* Cancer Research, 1996. **56**(4): p. 745–751.

Wang, W.Q., et al., *Increased fatty acid synthase as a potential therapeutic target in multiple myeloma.* Journal of Zhejiang University-Science B, 2008. **9**(6): p. 441–447.

Kuhajda, F.P., *Fatty acid synthase and cancer: New application of an old pathway.* Cancer Research, 2006. **66**(12): p. 5977–5980.

Menendez, J.A., et al., *Pharmacological inhibition of fatty acid synthase (FAS): A novel therapeutic approach for breast cancer chemoprevention through its ability to suppress Her-2/neu (erbB-2) oncogene-induced malignant transformation.* Molecular Carcinogenesis, 2004. **41**(3): p. 164–178.

Coleman, D.T., R. Bigelow, and J.A. Cardelli, *Inhibition of fatty acid synthase by luteolin posttranscriptionally down-regulates c-Met expression independent of proteosomal/lysosomal degradation.* Molecular Cancer Therapeutics, 2009. **8**(1): p. 214–224.

Engelman, J.A., J. Luo, and L.C. Cantley, *The evolution of phosphatidylinositol 3-kinases as regulators of growth and metabolism.* Nat Rev Genet, 2006. **7**(8): p. 606–19.

Swinnen, J.V., et al., *Selective activation of the fatty acid synthesis pathway in human prostate cancer.* International Journal of Cancer, 2000. **88**(2): p. 176–179.

Rossi, S., et al., *Fatty acid synthase molecular signatures expression defines distinct in prostate cancer.* Molecular Cancer Research, 2003. **1**(10): p. 707–715.

Ettinger, S.L., et al., *Dysregulation of sterol response element-binding proteins and downstream effectors in prostate cancer during progression to androgen independence.* Cancer Research, 2004. **64**(6): p. 2212–2221.

Sansal, I. and W.R. Sellers, *The biology and clinical relevance of the PTEN tumor suppressor pathway.* Journal of Clinical Oncology, 2004. **22**(14): p. 2954–2963.

Nomura, D.K., et al., *Monoacylglycerol Lipase Regulates a Fatty Acid Network that Promotes Cancer Pathogenesis.* Cell, 2010. **140**(1): p. 49–61.

Sreekumar, A., et al., *Metabolomic profiles delineate potential role for sarcosine in prostate cancer progression.* Nature, 2009. **457**(7231): p. 910–914.

Warburg, O., *On the origin of cancer cells.* Science, 1956. **123**(3191): p. 309–14.

Warburg, O., K. Posener, and E. Negelein, *Ueber den Stoffwechsel der Tumoren* Biochemische Zeitschrift, 1924. **152**: p. 319–344.

Deberardinis, R.J., et al., *The biology of cancer: metabolic reprogramming fuels cell growth and proliferation.* Cell Metab, 2008. **7**(1): p. 11–20.

VanderHeiden, M.G., L.C. Cantley, and C.B. Thompson, *Understanding the Warburg effect: the metabolic requirements of cell proliferation.* Science, 2009. **324**(5930): p. 1029–33.

Locasale, J.W., L.C. Cantley, and M.G. Vander Heiden, *Cancer's insatiable appetite.* Nature Biotechnology, 2009. **27**(10): p. 916–917.

Yun, J., et al., *Glucose Deprivation Contributes to the Development of KRAS Pathway Mutations in Tumor Cells.* Science, 2009. 18; **325**(5947): p. 1555–9.

Manning, B.D. and L.C. Cantley, *AKT/PKB signaling: Navigating downstream.* Cell, 2007. **129**(7): p. 1261–1274.

Bensaad, K., et al., *TIGAR, a p53-inducible regulator of glycolysis and apoptosis.* Cell, 2006. **126**(1): p. 107–20.

Laplante, M. and D.M. Sabatini, *mTORC1 activates SREBP-1c and uncouples lipogenesis from gluconeogenesis.* Proceedings of the National Academy of Sciences of the United States of America, 2010. **107**(8): p. 3281–3282.

Kaelin, W.G., Jr. and P.J. Ratcliffe, *Oxygen sensing by metazoans: the central role of the HIF hydroxylase pathway.* Mol Cell, 2008. **30**(4): p. 393–402.

Meyer, N. and L.Z. Penn, *MYC - TIMELINE Reflecting on 25 years with MYC.* Nature Reviews Cancer, 2008. **8**(12): p. 976–990.

Beroukhim, R., et al., *The landscape of somatic copy-number alteration across human cancers.* Nature, 2010. **463**(7283): p. 899–905.

Wise, D.R., et al., *Myc regulates a transcriptional program that stimulates mitochondrial glutaminolysis and leads to glutamine addiction.* Proc Natl Acad Sci U S A, 2008. **105**(48): p. 18782–7.

DeBerardinis, R.J., et al., *Brick by brick: metabolism and tumor cell growth.* Current Opinion in Genetics & Development, 2008. **18**(1): p. 54–61.

David, C.J., et al., *HnRNP proteins controlled by c-Myc deregulate pyruvate kinase mRNA splicing in cancer.* Nature, 2010. **463**(7279): p. 364–U114.

Dang, C.V., et al., *The interplay between MYC and HIF in cancer.* Nat Rev Cancer, 2008. **8**(1): p. 51–6.

Vousden, K.H. and K.M. Ryan, *p53 and metabolism.* Nature Reviews Cancer, 2009. **9**(10): p. 691–700.

Hu, W.W., et al., *Glutaminase 2, a novel p53 target gene regulating energy metabolism and antioxidant function.* Proceedings of the National Academy of Sciences of the United States of America, 2010. **107**(16): p. 7455–7460.

Suzuki, S., et al., *Phosphate-activated glutaminase (GLS2), a p53-inducible regulator of glutamine metabolism and reactive oxygen species.* Proceedings of the National Academy of Sciences of the United States of America, 2010. **107**(16): p. 7461–7466.

Tennant, D.A., R.V. Duran, and E. Gottlieb, *Targeting metabolic transformation for cancer therapy.* Nature Reviews Cancer, 2010. **10**(4): p. 267–277.

Farber, S., et al., *TEMPORARY REMISSIONS IN ACUTE LEUKEMIA IN CHILDREN PRODUCED BY FOLIC ACID ANTAGONIST, 4-AMINOPTEROYL-GLUTAMIC ACID (AMINOPTERIN).* New England Journal of Medicine, 1948. **238**(23): p. 787–793.

Jolivet, J., et al., *THE PHARMACOLOGY AND CLINICAL USE OF METHOTREXATE.* New England Journal of Medicine, 1983. **309**(18): p. 1094–1104.

Chabner, B.A. and T.G. Roberts, *Timeline - Chemotherapy and the war on cancer.* Nature Reviews Cancer, 2005. **5**(1): p. 65–72.

Ben Sahra, I., et al., *The antidiabetic drug metformin exerts an antitumoral effect in vitro and in vivo through a decrease of cyclin D1 level.* Oncogene, 2008. **27**(25): p. 3576–3586.

Xiao, B., et al., *Structural basis for AMP binding to mammalian AMP-activated protein kinase.* Nature, 2007. **449**(7161): p. 496-U14.

Cool, B., et al., *Identification and characterization of a small molecule AMPK activator that treats key components of type 2 diabetes and the metabolic syndrome.* Cell Metabolism, 2006. **3**(6): p. 403–416.

Huang, X., et al., *Important role of the LKB1-AMPK pathway in suppressing tumorigenesis in PTEN-deficient mice.* Biochem J, 2008. **412**(2): p. 211–21.

Pang, T., et al., *Small molecule antagonizes autoinhibition and activates AMP-activated protein kinase in cells.* Journal of Biological Chemistry, 2008. **283**(23): p. 16051–16060.

Currie, C.J., C.D. Poole, and E.A.M. Gale, *The influence of glucose-lowering therapies on cancer risk in type 2 diabetes.* Diabetologia, 2009. **52**(9): p. 1766–1777.

Wright, J.L. and J.L. Stanford, *Metformin use and prostate cancer in Caucasian men: results from a population-based case-control study.* Cancer Causes & Control, 2009. **20**(9): p. 1617–1622.

Jiralerspong, S., et al., *Metformin and pathologic complete responses to neoadjuvant chemotherapy in diabetic patients with breast cancer.* J Clin Oncol, 2009. **27**(20): p. 3297–302.

Dowling, R.J.O., et al., *Metformin inhibits mammalian target of rapamycin-dependent translation initiation in breast cancer cells.* Cancer Research, 2007. **67**(22): p. 10804–10812.

Shaw, R.J., et al., *The tumor suppressor LKB1 kinase directly activates AMP-activated kinase and regulates apoptosis in response to energy stress.* Proc Natl Acad Sci U S A, 2004. **101**(10): p. 3329–35.

Hirsch, H.A., et al., *Metformin Selectively Targets Cancer Stem Cells, and Acts Together with Chemotherapy to Block Tumor Growth and Prolong Remission (vol 69, pg 7507, 2009).* Cancer Research, 2009. **69**(22): p. 8832–8833.

Kim, Y.D., et al., *Metformin inhibits hepatic gluconeogenesis through AMP-activated protein kinase-dependent regulation of the orphan nuclear receptor SHP.* Diabetes, 2008. **57**(2): p. 306–314.

Goodwin, P.J., J.A. Ligibel, and V. Stambolic, *Metformin in Breast Cancer: Time for Action.* Journal of Clinical Oncology, 2009. **27**(20): p. 3271–3273.

Hadad, S.M., et al., *Histological evaluation of AMPK signalling in primary breast cancer.* Bmc Cancer, 2009. **9**.

Migita, T., et al., *Fatty Acid Synthase: A Metabolic Enzyme and Candidate Oncogene in Prostate Cancer.* Journal of the National Cancer Institute, 2009. **101**(7): p. 519–532.

Flavin, R., et al., *Fatty acid synthase as a potential therapeutic target in cancer.* Future Oncology, 2010. **6**(4): p. 551–562.

Murtola, T.J., *Men Presenting for Radical Prostatectomy on Preoperative Statin Therapy Have Reduced Serum Prostate Specific Antigen EDITORIAL COMMENT.* Journal of Urology, 2010. **183**(1): p. 124–124.

Beckers, A., et al., *Chemical inhibition of Acetyl-CoA carboxylase induces growth arrest and cytotoxicity selectively in cancer cells.* Cancer Research, 2007. **67**(17): p. 8180–8187.

Picchio, M., et al., *PET-CT for treatment planning in prostate cancer.* Quarterly Journal of Nuclear Medicine and Molecular Imaging, 2009. **53**(2): p. 245–268.

Christofk, H.R., et al., *The M2 splice isoform of pyruvate kinase is important for cancer metabolism and tumour growth.* Nature, 2008. **452**(7184): p. 230–3.

Boxer, M.B., et al., *Evaluation of Substituted N,N'-Diarylsulfonamides as Activators of the Tumor Cell Specific M2 Isoform of Pyruvate Kinase.* Journal of Medicinal Chemistry, 2010. **53**(3): p. 1048–1055.

Stock, C.C., et al., *AZASERINE, A NEW TUMOUR-INHIBITORY SUBSTANCE - STUDIES WITH CROCKER MOUSE SARCOMA-180.* Nature, 1954. **173**(4393): p. 71–72.

da Silva, A.P.P., et al., *Inhibition of energy-producing pathways of HepG2 cells by 3-bromopyruvate.* Biochemical Journal, 2009. **417**: p. 717–726.

Michelakis, E.D., et al., *Metabolic modulation of glioblastoma with dichloroacetate.* Sci Transl Med, 2010. **2**(31): p. 31ra34.

Fantin, V.R., J. St-Pierre, and P. Leder, *Attenuation of LDH-A expression uncovers a link between glycolysis, mitochondrial physiology, and tumor maintenance.* Cancer Cell, 2006. **9**(6): p. 425–34.

Chapter 14
Overlaps Between the Insulin and IGF-I Receptor and Cancer

Antonino Belfiore and Roberta Malaguarnera

Abbreviations

IGF	Insulin growth factor
IR	Insulin receptor
IGF-IR	IGF-I receptor
IGFBP	IGF-binding protein
IRS-1 and -2	Insulin receptor substrates 1 and -2
HR	Hybrid receptor
GH	Growth hormone
MAPK	Mitogen-activated protein kinase
PI3K	Phosphatidylinositol 3-kinase
NEFA	Nonesterified fatty acids
PKC	Protein kinase C
T2DM	Type 2 diabetes mellitus
M6P/IGF-IIR	Mannose-6-phosphate/IGF-II receptor

Introduction

The Insulin Growth Factor (IGF) system consists of two related peptides, namely, IGF-I and IGF-II, three membrane-bound receptors (the insulin receptor (IR), the IGF-I receptor (IGF-IR), and the mannose-6-phosphate receptor/IGF-II receptor (M6P/IGF-IIR), and six high-affinity IGF-binding proteins (IGFBP-1 to -6).

A. Belfiore (✉)
Endocrinology, Department of Clinical and Experimental Medicine,
University of Catanzaro, Catanzaro, Italy
e-mail: belfiore@unicz.it

D. LeRoith (ed.), *Insulin-like Growth Factors and Cancer: From Basic Biology to Therapeutics*, Cancer Drug Discovery and Development,
DOI 10.1007/978-1-4614-0598-6_14, © Springer Science+Business Media, LLC 2012

This complex network is involved in various cellular processes, which basically include the regulation of somatic growth and cell metabolism in relation to nutrient availability.

Despite a high homology between insulin and IGFs and between IR and IGF-IR, it is commonly held that insulin mainly mediates metabolic effects through IR, whereas IGFs mainly regulate growth processes through IGF-IR (Nakae et al. 2001). However, the IR and the IGF-IR have some degree of functional connection and overlap, which are significant during prenatal life, but are limited in adult life by various molecular mechanisms that include the following: tissue-specific receptor expression, different regulation of ligand bioavailability, differential expression and function of IR isoforms and IR/IGF-IR hybrids.

This signaling specificity is often disrupted in cancer. In fact, a role for both IGF-IR and IR in cancer is supported by several studies (LeRoith and Roberts 2003; Pollak et al. 2004; Belfiore 2007). Moreover, insulin resistance and compensatory hyperinsulinemia, newly recognized risk factors for cancer (Fair et al. 2007), are also associated with reduced insulin signaling specificity. We briefly review the molecular bases responsible for insulin and IGFs signaling specificity in physiology as well as the mechanisms causing disruption of signal specificity in cancer.

Molecular Bases of Insulin and IGFs Signaling Specificity

Although the intracellular signaling pathways of the two receptors are similar, IR and IGF-IR clearly have a different biological role (Nakae et al. 2001). The IR pathway has a central role in glucose homeostasis, while the IGF-IR pathway is crucial in mediating body growth in response to pituitary growth hormone (GH). These functional differences are especially evident in postnatal life, while IR and IGF-IR closely cooperate in regulating cell proliferation in prenatal life. Genetic data obtained from knockout mice indicate that both IR and IGF-IR are required for optimal embryonic development and glucose metabolism (Liu et al. 1993; Accili et al. 1996). In fact, IR knockout mice show unimpaired glucose metabolism in prenatal life (Accili et al. 1996; Louvi et al. 1997) and die by diabetic ketoacidosis only after birth.

Factors accounting for insulin and IGFs specificity in adult life are briefly described.

Tissue-Specific IR and IGF-IR Distribution

The different tissue distribution of IR and IGF-IR is a major mechanism to prevent signaling overlap between insulin and IGFs. The major insulin target tissues are liver, adipose tissue, and skeletal muscle. These tissues possess the highest IR content and the appropriate intracellular enzymatic machinery to regulate glucose and lipid metabolism. In humans, liver may contain up to fourfold IR than muscle and more than tenfold IR than adipose tissue (Pezzino et al. 1989). Other studies have found smaller differences between these tissues (Kotzke et al. 1995). The IR is also expressed at high levels in the brain, and at lower levels in pancreas, monocytes, granulocytes, erythrocytes, and fibroblasts (Kaplan 1984). The effect of insulin is typically not metabolic in these tissues.

Regarding IGF-IR, IGF-IR mRNA is widespread during embryonic mouse development being most abundant in developing nervous system, muscle, and kidney (Bondy et al. 1990), consistent with the role of IGFs in mediating growth and differentiation at this stage. After birth, IGF-IR mRNA falls dramatically, whereas IGF-I mRNA increases. In humans, IGF-IR is expressed ubiquitously being more abundant in placenta and in skeletal muscle (Murphy 2006). However, in muscle, IGF-IR is four- to fivefold less abundant than IR (Spampinato et al. 2000). In the rabbit, IGF-IR expression is higher in fat (100%) and brain tissues (50%) as compared with heart, kidney, lung, and spleen ($\approx$30%). Liver and muscle show the lowest content (less than 10% in fat) as compared to other tissues (Bailyes et al. 1997).

However, exhaustive data regarding a comparative measurement of IR and IGF-IR content in human tissues are lacking.

Generation of IR Isoforms and Their Tissue-Specific Distribution

In mammals, the *Ir* gene has acquired a small additional exon (exon 11), which encodes a stretch of 12 amino-acid residues at the carboxyl terminus of the IR α-subunit. Mammals have also acquired the ability to differentially skip this exon in a developmental and tissue-specific manner (Hernandez-Sanchez et al. 2008). Accordingly, two IR isoforms can be generated, isoform A (IR-A), lacking exon 11, and isoform B (IR-B), which includes exon 11 (Seino and Bell 1989; Yamaguchi et al. 1993). IR isoform measurement has shown that IR-B accounts for more than 75–95% of total IR expression in liver, 45–78% in skeletal muscle, 60–70% in adipose tissue, 45% in placenta, and 0% in lymphocytes (Benecke et al. 1992).

Unlike IR-B, which is a highly specific receptor for insulin, IR-A exhibits high affinity for insulin, intermediate affinity for IGF-II, and low affinity for IGF-I (Frasca et al. 1999). Because of these characteristics, IR isoform differential expression has emerged as an important mechanism for regulating developmental and tissue-specific cross talk between insulin and IGFs.

Given that IR-A binds IGF-II with similar affinity to IGF-IR (Frasca et al. 1999), in cells expressing these two receptors, the biological effects of IGF-II maybe mediated by both receptors according to their molar ratio. Accordingly, the IGF-II/IR-A loop is important for growth in the fetus, where the IR-A:IGF-IR is relatively high (Louvi et al. 1997). In liver, the low IR-A and IGF-IR expression is protective against excessive proliferation stimulation by high levels of locally produced IGFs.

By contrast, IGF-I binds to IR-A with a much lower affinity than to IGF-IR (Frasca et al. 1999). Therefore, IGF-I may signal through IR-A only in cells with very high IR-A:IGF-IR ratios (Sacco et al. 2009).

Differential Activation of Intracellular Substrates and Biological Effects Following IR and IGF-IR Activation

Subtle differences in the recruitment/activation of intracellular mediators by IR and IGF-IR are believed to contribute to the biological response specificity of insulin and IGFs (Urso et al. 1999). Some substrates appear to be preferentially interacting with IR, such as the adapter protein Grb10 (Laviola et al. 1997) and the membrane protein CEACAM-2, both involved in receptor downregulation (Soni et al. 2000). By contrast, Crk-II adaptor protein (Beitner-Johnson and LeRoith 1995), and 14-3-3 proteins preferentially interact with the IGF-IR (Furlanetto et al. 1997). IGF-IR, but not IR stimulation, induces the expression of *twist*, a gene with antiapoptotic role (Dupont et al. 2001a). Conversely, IR, but not IGF-IR stimulation, causes PKCδ activation in keratinocytes (Shen et al. 2001). The two receptors may even cause opposite effects: IGF-IR induces α-5 integrin upregulation and Fak phosphorylation, whereas IR induces α-5 integrin downregulation (Palmade et al. 1994) and Fak dephosphorylation (Pillay et al. 1995).

Global gene expression studies, performed in cells transfected with either IR or IGF-IR and in cells expressing TrkC/IR or TrkC/IGF-IR chimeric receptors (Dupont et al. 2001b; Mulligan et al. 2002) have shown that most genes are similarly regulated by the two receptors. However, a subset of genes especially involved in the regulation of proliferation, adhesion, and differentiation were selectively responsive to IGF-I, while other genes were selectively regulated by insulin.

As far as biological effects are concerned, Rat1 fibroblasts were found more sensitive to mitogenesis when overexpressing IGF-IR and stimulated with IGF-I than when overexpressing similar numbers of IRs and stimulated with insulin (Sasaoka et al. 1996). These data could not be reproduced in NIH-3T3 fibroblasts where both receptors stimulated DNA synthesis to a similar extent (Mastick et al. 1994).

IGF-IR has a unique permissive effect on cell transformation, as assessed in mouse fibroblasts lacking the endogenous IGF-IR (R⁻ cells). This effect could not be reproduced by IR overexpression (Sell et al. 1994; Valentinis et al. 1994) and was attributed to the function of IGF-IR C-terminus, which lacks homology with the IR (O'Connor et al. 1997). However, in NIH3T3 fibroblasts, expressing endogenous IGF-IR, IR overexpression is sufficient to induce a ligand-dependent transformed phenotype (Giorgino et al. 1991).

Ligand Bioavailability

Regulation of IGFs bioavailability by specific binding proteins (IGFBPs) is a major mechanism of signaling specificity between insulin and IGFs. More than 90% of IGFs circulates bound to IGFBPs, whereas insulin circulates free. IGFBP-1 and IGFBP-3 are the best characterized of the six circulating IGFBPs (Rajaram et al. 1997). IGFBP-3 binds approximately 75% of both IGFs and, by forming a ternary complex with an acid-labile subunit (ALS), it increasing IGFs half-life (Rajaram et al. 1997). Other IGFBPs form binary complexes with IGFs allowing selective transport to various tissues. Only approximately 1% of IGFs circulates free. IGFBPs generally inhibit IGFs actions by reducing their bioavailability and IGFBPs proteolysis and phosphorylation regulate site-specific availability of free IGFs.

Tissue-specific IGF-II availability is also regulated by IGF-II binding to M6P/IGF-IIR (Kornfeld 1992). M6P/IGF-IIR is a multifunctional transmembrane glycoprotein with no enzymatic activity that targets IGF-II to endocytosis and to lysosomal degradation, thus reducing IGF-II signaling.

Disruption of Insulin and IGFs Signaling Specificity in Cancer Patients

Signaling specificity between insulin and IGFs that exist at the level of normal adult organs and tissues is usually disrupted in malignant tumors by a variety of mechanisms, which increase the level of cross talk between the IR and IGF-IR.

Most of these changes involving ligands and receptors of the IGF system occur in malignant cells because of genetic and/or epigenetic changes that are only partially understood. Moreover, insulin resistance and compensatory hyperinsulinemia, which are common findings in cancer patients, may also enhance cross talk between insulin and IGFs signals. Insulin resistance may occur in cancer patients because of a variety of reasons. Type 2 diabetes mellitus (T2DM) and obesity are common disorders, and both are characterized by insulin resistance. Obesity is present in approximately 30% of the population in the western countries and T2DM in 5–7%. A variety of anticancer therapies including hormonal therapies are also associated with insulin resistance and (Redig and Munshi 2010).

We briefly discuss the mechanisms (Table 14.1) as well as the possibility that some of these mechanisms may lead to the activation of unbalanced intracellular signaling that elicit unique biological effects in cancer cells.

Deregulated Autocrine and Paracrine Production of IGFs in Cancer

It is well established that both IGF-I and IGF-II may be expressed at high levels in cancer and function in an autocrine and/or paracrine manner (Samani et al. 2007). In breast and prostate cancer IGF-II is expressed both by the malignant cells and by stromal cells adjacent to epithelial malignant cells (Tennant et al. 1996; Rasmussen and Cullen 1998). In thyroid cancer, autocrine IGF-II increases along with cancer dedifferentiation (Vella et al. 2002). Overexpression of IGF-II in the primary tumor has been shown to be predictive of metastases in colorectal (Hakam et al. 1999) and adrenal cortical carcinomas (Gicquel et al. 2001).

Table 14.1 Major factors implicated in insulin and IGFs signaling specificity in adult differentiated tissues and frequent alterations leading to extensive cross talk between IR and IGF-IR in cancer

	Adult differentiated tissues		Cancer cells	
Receptor/ligand	Expression	Effect	Expression	Effect
IR-B	High only in liver, muscle, fat	Binds only insulin	May increase	Response to high insulin levels
IR-A	Low/ubiquitous	Limited IGF-II signaling via IR-A	Mostly high	Enhanced IGF-II and IGF-I signaling via IR-A
		No IGF-I signaling via IR-A		Favors dedifferentiation?
IGF-IR	Low/ubiquitous	IGF-I effects > IGF-II effects	High	Enhanced IGF-I and IGF-II signaling via IGF-IR
IR-A:IGF-IR ratio	Low	IGF-I effects > IGF-II effects	May increase	IGF-II effects ≥ IGF-I effects
		Favors differentiation?		Favors dedifferentiation?
HR (especially HR-A)	Low	Limited IGF-I and IGF-II signaling via HR	High	IGF-I and IGF-II activate both IR and IGF-IR substrates
Atypical IR and IGF-IR	Not reported	–	May occur	Bind insulin and IGFs
M6P/IGF-IIR	Widespread	Reduces IGF-II signaling	May be reduced	Enhanced IGF-II signaling
IGF-I	Regulated by GH	Signals via IGF-IR	Frequently autocrine	Enhanced IGF-I signaling
IGF-II	Partially regulated by GH	Signals according to IR-A:IGF-IR ratio	Frequently autocrine	Enhanced IGF-II signaling via IGF-IR, IR-A, HR

14 Overlaps Between IGF-IR and IR and Cancer

Autocrine IGF-I expression plays a role in colon (Michell et al. 1997) and prostate cancer (DiGiovanni et al. 2000) and in Ewing's sarcoma (Strammiello et al. 2003).

Deregulated IGFs production provides high growth factor concentrations that act not only through the IGF-IR but also through IR-A and IR/IGF-IR hybrids, with the consequence of activating receptor-specific intracellular substrates.

Reduced M6P/IGF-IIR Expression

Reduced M6P/IGF-IIR expression may occur in a variety of malignancies owing to loss of heterozygosity involving the related gene with or without concomitant point mutations in the remaining allele (Yamada et al. 1997). By acting in concert with IGF-II autocrine production this contributes to increased IGF-II availability in cancer.

Amplification of IGF-IR Signaling by IR Overexpression and Enhanced IR/IGF-IR Hybrids Formation

Both IR and IGF-IR are often overexpressed in cancer cells. The first direct evidence that IR may be overexpressed in malignant cells was obtained by Papa et al. (1990) in human breast cancer. By analyzing a large casistic, they found that IR content was approximately sevenfold higher in cancer than in the normal breast tissue. IR expressed by breast cancer cells is fully functional and is responsible of insulin mediated growth in these cells (Milazzo et al. 1992a). Subsequent studies demonstrated that IR is also overexpressed in a variety of malignancies, including cancer of the thyroid, colon, lung, and ovary, and sarcomas (Beck et al. 1994; Frasca et al. 1999; Vella et al. 2002).

These malignancies often overexpress the IGF-IR (Papa et al. 1993; Pandini et al. 1999; Samani et al. 2007) (Strammiello et al. 2003). IGF-IR may be overexpressed not only in primary cancers but also in nodal metastases (Koda et al. 2003).

Both for IR and IGF-IR, dimerization of two α–β hemireceptors occurs as an early posttranslational process in the endoplasmic reticulum. Because of the high homology between the IR and the IGF-IR (Ullrich et al. 1986), an IR hemireceptor may assemble with an IGF-IR hemireceptor, forming hybrid IR/IGF-IR receptors (HRs). The in vivo presence of HRs in various organs has been demonstrated by various studies (Moxham and Jacobs 1992; Soos et al. 1993; Bailyes et al. 1997). We showed that HRs are usually overexpressed in cancer cells and, in the majority of cases, exceed the IR or the IGF-IR content (Pandini et al. 1999).

Functionally, HRs are considered high-affinity IGF-I binding sites (Soos et al. 1993). Accordingly, when cells with a high HR:IGF-IR ratio are exposed to IGF-I, HRs autophosphorylation exceeds IGF-IR autophosphorylation, suggesting that most of the IGF-I effect is mediated by HRs. Both in vitro and in mouse xenografts cancer cell growth could be more efficiently inhibited by antibodies blocking both IGF-IR and HRs, as compared with antibodies targeting only IGF-IR (Pandini et al. 2007). One conclusion is, therefore, that IR overexpression amplifies cancer cell response not only to insulin but also to IGF-I through HRs. The implications of HR formation may even be more complex, as further discussed in section "IR-A/IGF-IR Hybrids."

IR-Mediated IGFs Signaling

Unbalanced IR-A Overexpression

Both IR isoforms may be overexpressed in cancer, but usually IR-A predominates, representing 60–100% of total IR. IR-A:IR-B ratio in favor of IR-A has been demonstrated in both epithelial and nonepithelial malignancies, including cancer of the breast, thyroid, lung, colon and a variety of human sarcomas (Frasca et al. 1999; Vella et al. 2002). This is particularly intriguing, as IR-A is predominantly expressed and sustains growth in fetal life while IR-B predominates in most adult tissues (Frasca et al. 1999; Belfiore 2007).

Unlike IR-B, which is a highly specific receptor for insulin, IR-A exhibits high affinity for insulin, intermediate affinity for IGF-II and low affinity for IGF-I (Frasca et al. 1999). Several studies have now firmly established that IGF-II elicits significant biological effects via IR-A. In mouse fibroblasts expressing only IR-A and not IGF-IR (R$^-$/IR-A cells), IGF-II was a more potent mitogen than insulin itself (Frasca et al. 1999), while in human rabdomyosarcoma cells lacking functional IGF-IR and expressing almost only IR-A, IGF-II was more potent than insulin in inducing cell migration (Sciacca et al. 2002). IR-A overexpression and enhanced IGF-II autocrine production often coexist in some malignancies, such as breast and thyroid cancer or sarcomas (Sciacca et al. 2002; Vella et al. 2002). IGF-II binds both to IR-A and IGF-IR with similar affinity, therefore, IR-A overexpression amplifies IGF-II effects in cancer cells and serves as a signaling diversification factor, as IR-A and IGF-IR elicit different downstream signals (see section "Activation of Unbalanced Intracellular Signaling by Insulin and IGFs in Cancer").

In spite of the homology with IGF-II, IGF-I binds with high affinity only to the IGF-IR and its affinity for the IR-A is approximately tenfold lower than that of IGF-II (Frasca et al. 1999). However, IGF-I binding affinity for the IR-A is higher than its affinity for the IR-B. Until very recently, the biological activity of IGF-I through IR was considered negligible. However, IGF-I can induce significant downstream signaling through overexpressed IR-A in cells lacking IGF-IR (Sacco et al. 2009). These findings are in partial agreement with a recent study reporting that IGF-I may elicit biological effects through both IR-A and IR-B (Denley et al. 2007). Taken together, these data strongly suggest that IGF-I may activate intracellular signaling and biological effects in cancer cells with high IR-A:IGF-IR ratio.

Atypical IRs

Atypical IRs with high affinity binding for both insulin and IGFs have been described in human placenta and in human lymphoblastoid cells (Jonas and Cox 1991). No studies have been performed on atypical IRs using recent technologies, therefore, is not clear whether they overlap with the IR-A or are a distinct entity. No studies on atypical IRs are available in cancer.

Activation of IGF-IR Signaling by Insulin

IR-A/IGF-IR Hybrids

As previously discussed, HRs are generally considered fully functional IGF-I binding sites (Soos et al. 1993). However, IR hemireceptors involved in HR may exclude or include exon 11, leading to the formation of HR-A (containing IR-A hemireceptors) or HR-B (containing IR-B hemireceptors). Therefore, cancer cells predominantly express HR-A. The question arises whether HR-A have different functional activities than HR-B. Data on this issue are inconclusive. We found that HR-A are activated by IGFs and insulin according to the following hierarchy: IGF-I > IGF-II >> insulin while HR-B behave more similarly to homodimeric IGF-IR, which are fairly specific for IGF-I but also bind IGF-II with lower affinity (Pandini et al. 2002). In our hands insulin was able to transphosphorylate IGF-IR beta chain and recruit IGF-IR-specific intracellular substrates, such as Crk-II, in cells expressing HR-A but not in cell expressing HR-B (Pandini et al. 2002). However, two other studies were unable to confirm HR-A activation by insulin and reported either high or low affinity of IGF-II for both HRs (Slaaby et al. 2006; Benyoucef et al. 2007). By binding to HR, IGF-I may transphosphorylate IR beta chain (Slaaby et al. 2006). Therefore, while the high affinity of HRs for IGF-I is well established, more studies are required to assess HRs affinity for IGF-II and insulin.

Atypical IGF-IR

Atypical IGF-IRs with high affinity for both IGF-I and insulin have been described in human breast cancer cells MCF-7 cells, where they exceed typical IGF-IRs (Milazzo et al. 1992b; Soos et al. 1993). These atypical IGF-IRs are reminiscent of atypical IGF-IRs found in fetal muscle (Alexandrides and Smith 1989) and in a subclone of mouse myoblasts, where they derive from differential posttranslational processing of the product of the IGF-IR gene (Navarro et al. 2008). Additional studies are required to understand the presence and the possible impact of atypical IGF-IRs in human cancer.

Increase of IGFs Synthesis and/or Bioavailability Mediated by Hyperinsulinemia

Insulin resistance, often present in cancer patients, may represent an additional factor enhancing the cross talk between the insulin and the IGFs pathways. At least 80% of circulating IGF-I is produced in the liver under the control of GH, which also regulates liver production of IGFBP-3. However, insulin also regulates liver IGF-I production, both directly and also indirectly, by upregulating GH receptors. Insulin also increases IGF-I bioavailability through the downregulation of IGFBP-1 and IGFBP-2, both of which inhibit IGF-I actions (Frystyk 2004). Insulin decreases IGFBP-1 gene transcription and decreases IGFBP-2 synthesis at translational level.

Elevated serum IGFBP-1 levels and low free IGF-I are observed in presence of low-insulin levels, while low serum IGFBP-1 levels and high free IGF-I are associated with chronic or short-term hyperinsulinemia (Frystyk 2004). IGFBP-2 does not respond to acute changes in insulin but increases during chronic low insulin concentrations (Sandhu et al. 2002). Accordingly, low levels of IGFBP-2 and high free IGF-I concentrations occur in conditions characterized by insulin resistance and compensatory hyperinsulinemia. Under these conditions, elevated free IGF-I may suppress GH with consequent reduction of IGF-I and IGFBP-3 production by the liver.

Few data are available on the regulation of IGFBP-4, -5, and -6 and their effect on free and total IGF levels. In vitro studies indicate that IGF-I-mediated actions are inhibited by IGFBP-4 and -6 and stimulated by IGFBP-5 (Frystyk 2004).

Activation of Unbalanced Intracellular Signaling by Insulin and IGFs in Cancer

In cancer cells, disruption of the physiological balance between receptors of the insulin/IGF system and altered ligand production may lead to the activation of unbalanced intracellular signaling, which favor the recruitment/activation of substrates more effectively associated with the regulation of proliferation, apoptosis, and migration rather than with glucose metabolism. In cancer patients affected by insulin resistance, unbalanced intracellular signaling through IRs may also be generated by chronic hyperinsulinemia.

IGFs Signaling Through the IR-A and Preferential Activation of Mitogenesis and Migration

Studies carried out in cells null for the IGF-IR and overexpressing the IR isoform A (R⁻/IR-A cells) have shown that both IGF-I and IGF-II elicit a peculiar signaling pattern as compared to insulin. Although binding with a lower affinity than insulin, both IGFs activate p70S6K and ERK1/2 at levels similar to those elicited by insulin, while Akt activation was somehow parallel to receptor autophosphorylation. As a consequence, IGFs favor the activation balance toward p70S6K and ERK, rather than toward Akt. The mechanisms, through which IGFs cause such unique signaling, are incompletely understood and appear to involve preferential activation of IRS-2 rather than IRS-1 and less efficient activation of intracellular feed-back mechanisms involved in signal termination through protein kinases C (Sacco et al. 2009).

These mechanisms may account for the more potent mitogenic and migratory effect of IGF-II in respect to insulin (Morrione et al. 1997; Frasca et al. 1999; Sciacca et al. 2002) and for the partially different gene expression of the two ligands in cells expressing only IR-A (Pandini et al. 2003).

IR Isoform Balance and Cell Differentiation

In various cell systems, IR isoform switching to predominant IR-B expression is associated with cell differentiation. Differentiation of brown preadipocytes into mature adipocytes is concomitant with a marked increase in total IR content and with IR isoform switch from IR-A to IR-B (Entingh et al. 2003). A similar IR isoform switching also occurs in 3T3-L1 cells (Kosaki and Webster 1993), in murine 32D hemopoietic cells (Sciacca et al. 2003) and in human hepatoblastoma cells (HepG2 cells) (Kosaki and Webster 1993; Pandini et al. 2002) when induced to differentiate. Data obtained in 32D cells also indicated that IR-A transfection preferentially induces mitogenic and antiapoptotic signals, whereas IR-B predominantly induces cell differentiation (Sciacca et al. 2003).

The molecular mechanisms for the opposite effects of IR-A and IR-B on cell differentiation are unclear. Besides having a different affinity for IGFs, the two IR isoforms may also elicit subtly different intracellular signaling in response to insulin (Leibiger et al. 2001).

Together, these results suggest that the high IR-A:IR-B ratio, often found in cancer, may adversely affect cell differentiation.

Unbalanced Signaling in Insulin Resistant Patients

Insulin resistance and compensatory hyperinsulinemia are associated with a defect in the proximal part of the insulin signaling network. In particular, studies conducted in obese Zucker (fa/fa) rats as well as in insulin-resistant patients have revealed that the PI3K pathway is selectively blunted as compared with the MAPK pathway (Jiang et al. 1999; Cusi et al. 2000). Mechanisms accounting for this selective impairment of PI3K-Akt activation mainly involve serine and threonine phosphorylation of the IR β-chain and/or IRS-1 phosphorylation at serine residues caused by increased circulating levels of NEFA and inflammatory cytokines with consequent activation of intracellular kinases, such as PKCs (Gual et al. 2005). Under these conditions, the attenuation of the PI3K pathway contrasts with the effectiveness of insulin in activating the MAPK pathway, which may even increase (Jiang et al. 1999; Cusi et al. 2000).

Therefore, insulin resistance may cause impaired glucose homeostasis in insulin target tissues while stimulating cell proliferation in other tissues (e.g., cancer).

Concluding Remarks

Insulin and IGFs exert multiple and nonoverlapping roles in physiology. Signaling and functional specificity between insulin and IGFs, however, are frequently disrupted in cancer by a variety of mechanisms. As a consequence, the level of overlap between insulin and IGFs, which is relatively low in normal differentiated adult cells, is often elevated in cancer cells. Insulin resistance and hyperinsulinemia are common in cancer patients because of concomitant obesity and/or T2DM and/or anticancer therapies and may contribute to deranged signaling in cancer cells. Hyperinsulinemia and promiscuous receptors, which bind IGFs and insulin, represent remarkable barriers to IGF-IR targeting therapies in cancer. The next challenge will be to discover therapies that are able to block IR-A-related signaling pathways while not inducing insulin resistance and T2DM.

Conflict of Interest The authors declare that they have no conflict of interest.

Acknowledgments This work was partially supported by grants from the AIRC (Associazione Italiana per la Ricerca sul Cancro) and PRIN-MIUR 2008 (Ministero Italiano Università e Ricerca) to A.B.

References

Accili D, Drago J, Lee EJ, et al (1996) Early neonatal death in mice homozygous for a null allele of the insulin receptor gene. Nat Genet 12:106–109

Alexandrides TK, Smith RJ (1989) A novel fetal insulin-like growth factor (IGF) I receptor. Mechanism for increased IGF I- and insulin-stimulated tyrosine kinase activity in fetal muscle. J Biol Chem 264:12922–12930

Bailyes EM, Nave BT, Soos MA, et al (1997) Insulin receptor/IGF-I receptor hybrids are widely distributed in mammalian tissues: quantification of individual receptor species by selective immunoprecipitation and immunoblotting. Biochem J 327 (Pt 1):209–215

Beck EP, Russo P, Gliozzo B, et al (1994) Identification of insulin and insulin-like growth factor I (IGF I) receptors in ovarian cancer tissue. Gynecol Oncol 53:196–201

Beitner-Johnson D, LeRoith D (1995) Insulin-like growth factor-I stimulates tyrosine phosphorylation of endogenous c-Crk. J Biol Chem 270:5187–5190

Belfiore A (2007) The role of insulin receptor isoforms and hybrid insulin/IGF-I receptors in human cancer. Curr Pharm Des 13:671–686

Benecke H, Flier JS, Moller DE (1992) Alternatively spliced variants of the insulin receptor protein. Expression in normal and diabetic human tissues. J Clin Invest 89:2066–2070

14 Overlaps Between IGF-IR and IR and Cancer 275

Benyoucef S, Surinya KH, Hadaschik D, et al (2007) Characterization of insulin/IGF hybrid receptors: contributions of the insulin receptor L2 and Fn1 domains and the alternatively spliced exon 11 sequence to ligand binding and receptor activation. Biochem J 403:603–613

Bondy CA, Werner H, Roberts CT, Jr., et al (1990) Cellular pattern of insulin-like growth factor-I (IGF-I) and type I IGF receptor gene expression in early organogenesis: comparison with IGF-II gene expression. Mol Endocrinol 4:1386–1398

Cusi K, Maezono K, Osman A, et al (2000) Insulin resistance differentially affects the PI 3-kinase- and MAP kinase-mediated signaling in human muscle. J Clin Invest 105:311–320

Denley A, Carroll JM, Brierley GV, et al (2007) Differential activation of insulin receptor substrates 1 and 2 by insulin-like growth factor-activated insulin receptors. Mol Cell Biol 27:3569–3577

DiGiovanni J, Kiguchi K, Frijhoff A, et al (2000) Deregulated expression of insulin-like growth factor 1 in prostate epithelium leads to neoplasia in transgenic mice. Proc Natl Acad Sci U S A 97:3455–3460

Dupont J, Fernandez AM, Glackin CA, et al (2001a) Insulin-like growth factor 1 (IGF-1)-induced twist expression is involved in the anti-apoptotic effects of the IGF-1 receptor. J Biol Chem 276:26699–26707

Dupont J, Khan J, Qu BH, et al (2001b) Insulin and IGF-1 induce different patterns of gene expression in mouse fibroblast NIH-3T3 cells: identification by cDNA microarray analysis. Endocrinology 142:4969–4975

Entingh AJ, Taniguchi CM, Kahn CR (2003) Bi-directional regulation of brown fat adipogenesis by the insulin receptor. J Biol Chem 278:33377–33383

Fair AM, Dai Q, Shu XO, et al (2007) Energy balance, insulin resistance biomarkers, and breast cancer risk. Cancer Detect Prev 31:214–219

Frasca F, Pandini G, Scalia P, et al (1999) Insulin receptor isoform A, a newly recognized, high-affinity insulin-like growth factor II receptor in fetal and cancer cells. Mol Cell Biol 19:3278–3288

Frystyk J (2004) Free insulin-like growth factors -- measurements and relationships to growth hormone secretion and glucose homeostasis. Growth Horm IGF Res 14:337–375

Furlanetto RW, Dey BR, Lopaczynski W, et al (1997) 14-3-3 proteins interact with the insulin-like growth factor receptor but not the insulin receptor. Biochem J 327 (Pt 3):765–771

Gicquel C, Bertagna X, Gaston V, et al (2001) Molecular markers and long-term recurrences in a large cohort of patients with sporadic adrenocortical tumors. Cancer Res 61:6762–6767

Giorgino F, Belfiore A, Milazzo G, et al (1991) Overexpression of insulin receptors in fibroblast and ovary cells induces a ligand-mediated transformed phenotype. Mol Endocrinol 5:452–459

Gual P, Le Marchand-Brustel Y, Tanti JF (2005) Positive and negative regulation of insulin signaling through IRS-1 phosphorylation. Biochimie 87:99–109

Hakam A, Yeatman TJ, Lu L, et al (1999) Expression of insulin-like growth factor-1 receptor in human colorectal cancer. Hum Pathol 30:1128–1133

Hernandez-Sanchez C, Mansilla A, de Pablo F, et al (2008) Evolution of the insulin receptor family and receptor isoform expression in vertebrates. Mol Biol Evol 25:1043–1053

Jiang ZY, Lin YW, Clemont A, et al (1999) Characterization of selective resistance to insulin signaling in the vasculature of obese Zucker (fa/fa) rats. J Clin Invest 104:447–457

Jonas HA, Cox AJ (1991) Insulin receptor sub-types in a human lymphoid-derived cell line (IM-9): differential regulation by insulin, dexamethasone and monensin. J Recept Res 11:813–829

Kaplan SA (1984) The insulin receptor. J Pediatr 104:327–336

Koda M, Sulkowski S, Garofalo C, et al (2003) Expression of the insulin-like growth factor-I receptor in primary breast cancer and lymph node metastases: correlations with estrogen receptors alpha and beta. Horm Metab Res 35:794–801

Kornfeld S (1992) Structure and function of the mannose 6-phosphate/insulinlike growth factor II receptors. Annu Rev Biochem 61:307–330

Kosaki A, Webster NJ (1993) Effect of dexamethasone on the alternative splicing of the insulin receptor mRNA and insulin action in HepG2 hepatoma cells. J Biol Chem 268:21990–21996

Kotzke G, Schutt M, Missler U, et al (1995) Binding of human, porcine and bovine insulin to insulin receptors from human brain, muscle and adipocytes and to expressed recombinant alternatively spliced insulin receptor isoforms. Diabetologia 38:757–763

Laviola L GF, Chow JC, Baquero JA, Hansen H, Ooi J, Zhu J, Riedel, H SR (1997) The adapter protein Grb10 associates preferentially with the insulin receptor as compared with the IGF-1 receptor in mouse fibroblasts. J Clin Invest 99:830–837

Leibiger B, Leibiger IB, Moede T, et al (2001) Selective insulin signaling through A and B insulin receptors regulates transcription of insulin and glucokinase genes in pancreatic beta cells. Mol Cell 7:559–570

LeRoith D, Roberts CT, Jr. (2003) The insulin-like growth factor system and cancer. Cancer Lett 195:127–137

Liu JP, Baker J, Perkins AS, et al (1993) Mice carrying null mutations of the genes encoding insulin-like growth factor I (Igf-1) and type 1 IGF receptor (Igf1r). Cell 75:59–72

Louvi A, Accili D, Efstratiadis A (1997) Growth-promoting interaction of IGF-II with the insulin receptor during mouse embryonic development. Dev Biol 189:33–48

Mastick CC, Kato H, Roberts CT, Jr., et al (1994) Insulin and insulin-like growth factor-I receptors similarly stimulate deoxyribonucleic acid synthesis despite differences in cellular protein tyrosine phosphorylation. Endocrinology 135:214–222

Michell NP, Langman MJ, Eggo MC (1997) Insulin-like growth factors and their binding proteins in human colonocytes: preferential degradation of insulin-like growth factor binding protein 2 in colonic cancers. Br J Cancer 76:60–66

Milazzo G, Giorgino F, Damante G, et al (1992a) Insulin receptor expression and function in human breast cancer cell lines. Cancer Res 52:3924–3930

Milazzo G, Yip CC, Maddux BA, et al (1992b) High-affinity insulin binding to an atypical insulin-like growth factor-I receptor in human breast cancer cells. J Clin Invest 89:899–908

Morrione A, Valentinis B, Xu SQ, et al (1997) Insulin-like growth factor II stimulates cell proliferation through the insulin receptor. Proc Natl Acad Sci U S A 94:3777–3782

Moxham CP, Jacobs S (1992) Insulin/IGF-I receptor hybrids: a mechanism for increasing receptor diversity. J Cell Biochem 48:136–140

Mulligan C, Rochford J, Denyer G, et al (2002) Microarray analysis of insulin and insulin-like growth factor-1 (IGF-1) receptor signaling reveals the selective up-regulation of the mitogen heparin-binding EGF-like growth factor by IGF-1. J Biol Chem 277:42480–42487

Murphy LJ (2006) Insulin-like growth factor-I: a treatment for type 2 diabetes revisited. Endocrinology 147:2616–2618

Nakae J, Kido Y, Accili D (2001) Distinct and overlapping functions of insulin and IGF-I receptors. Endocr Rev 22:818–835

Navarro M, Joulia D, Fedon Y, et al (2008) The atypical alpha2beta2 IGF receptor expressed in inducible c2.7 myoblasts is derived from post-translational modifications of the mouse IGF-I receptor. Growth Horm IGF Res 18:412–423

O'Connor R, Kauffmann-Zeh A, Liu Y, et al (1997) Identification of domains of the insulin-like growth factor I receptor that are required for protection from apoptosis. Mol Cell Biol 17:427–435

Palmade F S-CO, Coquelet C, Bonne C (1994) Insulin-like growth factor-1 (IGF-1) specifically binds to bovine lens epithelial cells and increases the number of fibronectin receptor sites. Curr Eye Res 13:531–537

Pandini G, Vigneri R, Costantino A, et al (1999) Insulin and insulin-like growth factor-I (IGF-I) receptor overexpression in breast cancers leads to insulin/IGF-I hybrid receptor overexpression: evidence for a second mechanism of IGF-I signaling. Clin Cancer Res 5:1935–1944

Pandini G, Frasca F, Mineo R, et al (2002) Insulin/insulin-like growth factor I hybrid receptors have different biological characteristics depending on the insulin receptor isoform involved. J Biol Chem 277:39684–39695

Pandini G, Medico E, Conte E, et al (2003) Differential gene expression induced by insulin and insulin-like growth factor-II through the insulin receptor isoform A. J Biol Chem 278:42178–42189

Pandini G, Wurch T, Akla B, et al (2007) Functional responses and in vivo anti-tumour activity of h7C10: a humanised monoclonal antibody with neutralising activity against the insulin-like growth factor-1 (IGF-1) receptor and insulin/IGF-1 hybrid receptors. Eur J Cancer 43:1318–1327

14 Overlaps Between IGF-IR and IR and Cancer

Papa V, Pezzino V, Costantino A, et al (1990) Elevated insulin receptor content in human breast cancer. J Clin Invest 86:1503–1510

Papa V, Gliozzo B, Clark GM, et al (1993) Insulin-like growth factor-I receptors are overexpressed and predict a low risk in human breast cancer. Cancer Res 53:3736–3740

Pezzino V, Papa V, Trischitta V, et al (1989) Human insulin receptor radioimmunoassay: applicability to insulin-resistant states. Am J Physiol 257:E451–457

Pillay TS, Sasaoka T, Olefsky JM (1995) Insulin stimulates the tyrosine dephosphorylation of pp125 focal adhesion kinase. J Biol Chem 270:991–994

Pollak MN, Schernhammer ES, Hankinson SE (2004) Insulin-like growth factors and neoplasia. Nat Rev Cancer 4:505–518

Rajaram S, Baylink DJ, Mohan S (1997) Insulin-like growth factor-binding proteins in serum and other biological fluids: regulation and functions. Endocr Rev 18:801–831

Rasmussen AA, Cullen KJ (1998) Paracrine/autocrine regulation of breast cancer by the insulin-like growth factors. Breast Cancer Res Treat 47:219–233

Redig AJ, Munshi HG (2010) Care of the cancer survivor: metabolic syndrome after hormone-modifying therapy. Am J Med 123:87 e81-86

Sacco A, Morcavallo A, Pandini G, et al (2009) Differential signaling activation by insulin and insulin-like growth factors I and II upon binding to insulin receptor isoform A. Endocrinology 150:3594–3602

Samani AA, Yakar S, LeRoith D, et al (2007) The role of the IGF system in cancer growth and metastasis: overview and recent insights. Endocr Rev 28:20–47

Sandhu MS, Dunger DB, Giovannucci EL (2002) Insulin, insulin-like growth factor-I (IGF-I), IGF binding proteins, their biologic interactions, and colorectal cancer. J Natl Cancer Inst 94:972–980

Sasaoka T, Ishiki M, Sawa T, et al (1996) Comparison of the insulin and insulin-like growth factor 1 mitogenic intracellular signaling pathways. Endocrinology 137:4427–4434

Sciacca L, Mineo R, Pandini G, et al (2002) In IGF-I receptor-deficient leiomyosarcoma cells autocrine IGF-II induces cell invasion and protection from apoptosis via the insulin receptor isoform A. Oncogene 21:8240–8250

Sciacca L, Prisco M, Wu A, et al (2003) Signaling differences from the A and B isoforms of the insulin receptor (IR) in 32D cells in the presence or absence of IR substrate-1. Endocrinology 144:2650–2658

Seino S, Bell GI (1989) Alternative splicing of human insulin receptor messenger RNA. Biochem Biophys Res Commun 159:312–316

Sell C, Dumenil G, Deveaud C, et al (1994) Effect of a null mutation of the insulin-like growth factor I receptor gene on growth and transformation of mouse embryo fibroblasts. Mol Cell Biol 14:3604–3612

Shen S, Alt A, Wertheimer E, et al (2001) PKCdelta activation: a divergence point in the signaling of insulin and IGF-1-induced proliferation of skin keratinocytes. Diabetes 50:255–264

Slaaby R, Schaffer L, Lautrup-Larsen I, et al (2006) Hybrid receptors formed by insulin receptor (IR) and insulin-like growth factor I receptor (IGF-IR) have low insulin and high IGF-1 affinity irrespective of the IR splice variant. J Biol Chem 281:25869–25874

Soni P, Lakkis M, Poy MN, et al (2000) The differential effects of pp120 (Ceacam 1) on the mitogenic action of insulin and insulin-like growth factor 1 are regulated by the nonconserved tyrosine 1316 in the insulin receptor. Mol Cell Biol 20:3896–3905

Soos MA, Field CE, Siddle K (1993) Purified hybrid insulin/insulin-like growth factor-I receptors bind insulin-like growth factor-I, but not insulin, with high affinity. Biochem J 290 (Pt 2):419–426

Spampinato D, Pandini G, Iuppa A, et al (2000) Insulin/insulin-like growth factor I hybrid receptors overexpression is not an early defect in insulin-resistant subjects. J Clin Endocrinol Metab 85:4219–4223

Strammiello R, Benini S, Manara MC, et al (2003) Impact of IGF-I/IGF-IR circuit on the angiogenetic properties of Ewing's sarcoma cells. Horm Metab Res 35:675–684

Tennant MK, Thrasher JB, Twomey PA, et al (1996) Protein and messenger ribonucleic acid (mRNA) for the type 1 insulin-like growth factor (IGF) receptor is decreased and IGF-II mRNA is increased in human prostate carcinoma compared to benign prostate epithelium. J Clin Endocrinol Metab 81:3774–3782

Ullrich A, Gray A, Tam AW, et al (1986) Insulin-like growth factor I receptor primary structure: comparison with insulin receptor suggests structural determinants that define functional specificity. Embo J 5:2503–2512

Urso B, Cope DL, Kalloo-Hosein HE, et al (1999) Differences in signaling properties of the cytoplasmic domains of the insulin receptor and insulin-like growth factor receptor in 3T3-L1 adipocytes. J Biol Chem 274:30864–30873

Valentinis B, Porcu PL, Quinn K, et al (1994) The role of the insulin-like growth factor I receptor in the transformation by simian virus 40 T antigen. Oncogene 9:825–831

Vella V, Pandini G, Sciacca L, et al (2002) A novel autocrine loop involving IGF-II and the insulin receptor isoform-A stimulates growth of thyroid cancer. J Clin Endocrinol Metab 87:245–254

Yamada T, De Souza AT, Finkelstein S, et al (1997) Loss of the gene encoding mannose 6-phosphate/insulin-like growth factor II receptor is an early event in liver carcinogenesis. Proc Natl Acad Sci U S A 94:10351–10355

Yamaguchi Y, Flier JS, Benecke H, et al (1993) Ligand-binding properties of the two isoforms of the human insulin receptor. Endocrinology 132:1132–1138

Index

A

Acetyl-CoA carboxylase (ACC), 247
Acid-labile subunit (ALS), 75, 267
Adiponectin, 47
Aging and cancer
  balancing factors, 33
  carcinogenesis, 27
  dietary restriction, 29
  IGFs, 32–33
  molecular aetiology
    gene mutations, 25
    lung cancer, 26
    PI3k–Akt/PKB pathway, 27
  neoplastic lesions, 28
  occult tumours and clinical cancers
    autopsy, 29
    breast cancer, 31
    genetic risk, 31–32
    neoplastic lesions, 29–30
    prostate cancer, 30
    sporadic cancers, 31
  rats, 28
Alveolar rhabdomyosarcoma (ARMS),
      148–149
AMG479, 202–203
Androgen-independent (AI) disease, 85
Androgen receptors (AR), 85, 160
Ataxia-telangiectasia mutated (ATM), 223
Autopsy, 29
AVE1642, 201–202

B

Benzimidazoles, 219–220
BIIB022, 203

Body mass index (BMI), 37
BRCA1
  breast and ovarian cancer, 164
  immunohistochemical analysis,
      165
  prostate cancer, 166
Breast cancer, 27
  aging, 31
  cytotoxic and hormonal therapy, 73
  diagnosis, 73
  gene signatures, 78–79
  IGF-I and IGFBP–3, 123–125
  IGF ligands and bindings proteins
    angiogenic factor, 76
    postmenopausal women, 75–76
    tumor cell growth, 76–77
  IGF–1R expression and adaptor proteins,
      77–78
  IGF signaling, 74–75
  IGF targeting, 79
  indirect evidence, 15
  meta-analysis, 126
  obesity, 14
  resistance, 78
  risk factor, 123
  serologic evidence
    blood donation, 16
    EPIC study, 16
    estrogen receptor, 17
    IGFBP–3 and risk, 17–18
    insulin/C-peptide, 18
    meta-analyses, 17
    premenopausal and postmenopausal,
      15–16
  targeted therapy, 73–74

D. LeRoith (ed.), *Insulin-like Growth Factors and Cancer: From Basic Biology
to Therapeutics*, Cancer Drug Discovery and Development,
DOI 10.1007/978-1-4614-0598-6, © Springer Science+Business Media, LLC 2012

C

Calorie restriction (CR)
  animal model, 232
  anticancer effects, 232–234
  cancer
    epidemiological evidence of, 234–235
    experimental evidence of, 235–236
  chronic diseases, 231
  cytokines, 237
  energy balance-related hormones, 237–238
  estrogen receptor, 236
  leptin, 237
  metabolic hormones, 237
  mimetics, 238–239
Cancer
  adipocytokines, 53–54
  adipose tissue and insulin resistance
    adiponectin, 47
    interleukin–6, 45–46
    leptin, 47
    resistin, 46
    tumor necrosis factor alpha, 45
  aging (*see* Aging and cancer)
  breast cancer (*see* Breast cancer)
  calorie restriction (*see* Calorie restriction (CR))
  estrogen, 54–55
  hyperglycemia and, 50–51
  and hyperinsulinemia, 48–50
  hyperlipidemia and, 51–53
  insulin analogues, 55–56
  insulin resistance, 44–45
  insulin signaling, 42–44
  metformin, 56–58
  obesity, 39–40, 42, 54–55
  prostate cancer (*see* prostate cancer)
  thiazolidinediones, 58–59
  type 2 diabetes, 40–42
Cancer cell metabolism
  amino acid metabolism and, 250–251
  AMPK and, 247–249
  fatty acid metabolism, 249–250
  glucose uptake rates, 251–253
  hyperinsulinemia, 245, 246
  obesity, 245, 246
  oncogenes and tumor suppressor genes, 253–254
  pharmaceuticals targeting
    AMPK activators, 255–256
    antimetabolite chemotherapy, 254–255
    central carbon metabolism, 257
    lipogenesis inhibitors, 256–257

  type II diabetes, 245, 246
  Warburg effect, 251–253
Castrate-resistant prostate cancer (CRPC), 96
Catechols, 221–222
Chronic myeloid leukemia (CML), 221
Colorectal cancer (CRC), 27, 126–128
  indirect evidence, 5
  serologic evidence
    IGFBP–3 and risk, 8
    IGF–1 concentrations, 6
    insulin/C-peptide, 8–9
    risk factors, 6–7
Cyclin-dependent kinases (CDKs), 109

D

Dihydrotestosteron (DHT), 86

E

Electrophoretic mobility shift assays (EMSA), 164
Embryonal rhabdomyosarcoma (ERMS), 148–149
Endoplasmic reticulum (ER), 111
Epidermal growth factor (EGF), 78
Epidermal growth factor receptor (EGFR), 204
Epithelial ovarian cancer (EOC), 78–79
Epithelial-to-mesenchymal transition (EMT), 182
Estrogen, 54–55
Estrogen receptors (ER), 17, 160, 236
Estrogen receptor-signaling pathway, 205
European Prospective Investigation into Cancer and Nutrition (EPIC), 7, 16, 40, 76, 123, 129
Ewing's sarcoma family of tumors (ESFT), 149–150

F

Fatty acids (FAs), 247
Focal adhesion kinase (FAK), 109
Forkhead transcription factors (FOXO), 106
Free fatty acid (FFA), 44, 249

G

Gastrointestinal stromal tumor (GIST), 151
Glitazones. *See* Thiazolidinediones
Glycine-*N*-methyltransferase (GNMT), 251
Glycogen synthase kinase 3 (GSK3), 106
Growth hormone (GH), 264

Index 281

H
Heat shock proteins (HSPs), 227
Hormonal therapy, 224–225
Human umbilical vein endothelial cells (HUVECs), 109

I
IMC-A12, 202
Imidazopyrazines, 218–219
Inhibitor of apoptosis (IAP), 94
Insulin and IGFs signaling specificity
  cancer patients
    atypical IGF-IR and IRs, 271
    autocrine and paracrine production, 267, 269
    hyperinsulinemia, 272
    IR-A/IGF-IR hybrids, 271
    IR/IGF-IR hybrids formation, 269–270
    reduced M6P/IGF-IIR expression, 269
    unbalanced IR-A, 270
  molecular bases
    intracellular substrates and biological effects, 266
    IR isoforms and tissue-specific distribution, 265
    ligand bioavailability, 266–267
    tissue-specific IR, 264–265
  molecular mechanisms, 264
  unbalanced intracellular signaling
    insulin resistant patients, 273–274
    IR isoform balance and cell differentiation, 273
    mitogenesis and migration, 272–273
Insulin degrading enzyme (IDE), 94–95
Insulin-like growth factor I (IGF–1)
  calorie restriction (*see* Calorie restriction (CR))
  deficiency
    A2058 cells, 114
    Akt, 107
    angiogenesis, 119–120
    anti-IGF-IR antibodies, 130
    breast cancer, 123–126
    calcineurin/NFAT pathway, 108
    calorie-restriction, 122
    cancer cell lines, 114–115
    canonical and noncanonical signaling pathways, 106, 107
    caveoli, 109
    CDKs, 109–110
    cell adhesion, 116–118
    colorectal cancer, 126–128
    cytoskeletal arrangements, 115–116

    folding process, 111–112
    GH/IGF–1 axis, 129, 130
    lung tumors, 121
    MAPK pathway, 107–108
    molecular chaperones, 112–113
    mTORC1, 106–107
    paxillin activation, 116
    p53 gene, 110
    prostate cancer, 128–129
    PTEN, 111
    Rho family, 113–114
    RTK family, 106
    tissue remodeling, 118–119
    TKI, 130
    WT1, 110–111
    XBP–1 protein, 112
  epidemiologic evidence
    breast cancer, 14–18
    colorectal cancer, 5–9
    IGFBP–3 level, 4–5
    prostate cancer, 9–14
  physiology and mechanism
    IGF system, 2
    insulin, 2, 3
    level, determinants of, 4
    receptor signaling, 2–3
Insulin-like growth factor-I receptor (IGF-IR)
  acquired tumor resistance mechanisms, 207
  AKT activation, 206
  AMG479, 202–203
  animal models, 196–198
  animal tumor models, 181, 182
  anti-IGF-IR antibody-targeting strategies, 195–196
  AVE1642, 201–202
  BIIB022, 203
  cancer therapies
    chemotherapy, 222
    ErbB family-targeted therapies, 223–224
    hormonal therapy, 224–225
    radiation therapy, 223
  chemotherapy, 204
  clinical trials, 198, 199
  Cre recombinase, 180
  CT domain, 193–194
  cysteine-rich region, 193
  disruption
    liver, 187
    pancreas, 185–186
    prostate cancer, 186–187
  drug sensitivity, 227
  embryonic stem cells, 179–180

Insulin-like growth factor-I receptor (IGF-IR)
(*cont.*)
  estrogen receptor-signaling pathway, 205
  gene expression
    androgen receptor signaling pathway,
      169–170
    breast and ovarian cancer, 164
    disrupted transcription factors, 168
    estrogen receptor signaling pathways,
      168–169
    immunohistochemical analysis, 165
    KLF, 161, 162
    MCF-7, 163
    MS, 162, 163
    multiple tumor suppressors, 170–171
    p53, 166–167
    potential epigenetic regulation,
      171–172
    prostate cancer, 166
    renal cancer, 167
    role, 159
    tumors, 160–161
  hemizygotes, 180
  human testing, 198
  IGF–1R ATP-competitive inhibitors
    benzimidazoles, 219–220
    imidazopyrazines, 218–219
    pyrrolopyrimidines, 216–218
    pyrrolotriazines, 220–221
    2,4,6-triaminopyrimidine, 221
  IGF–1R/IR pathway, 225–226
  IMC-A12, 202
  LKB/AMP kinase pathway, 206–207
  lung, 184–185
  mammary gland
    CD8-IGFIR transgenic mice, 181, 182
    developmental stage, 184
    kras gene, 183
    MTB-IGFIR transgenic mice, 182–183
    traztuzumab-resistant tumors, 184
  MK0646, 200–201
  NSCLC patients, 200
  R1507, 201
  rtTA, 180–181
  salivary gland, 187–188
  SCH717454, 201
  signaling pathways, 226
  SiRNA, 207
  small-molecule IGF–1R inhibitors, 216
  substrate inhibitors
    catechols, 221–222
    picropodophyllotoxin, 222
  tamoxifen, 205
  toxicity, 204

  tumor xenograft growth, 204–205
  tyrosine kinase activity, 194–195
  VEGF receptor activation, 206
Insulin receptor substrates (IRSs), 106
Interleukin–6, 45–46

K

Krüppel-like factor–6 (KLF6), 162

L

Leimyosarcoma, 147
Leptin, 47
Liver IGF–1 deficient (LID), 121
Loss of heterozygosity (LOH), 149
Loss of imprinting (LOI), 149
Lung cancer, 26

M

Mass spectroscopy (MS), 162
Metformin, 56–58
Mitogen-activated protein kinase (MAPK),
  106, 147
MK0646, 200–201
Monoacylglycerol lipase (MAGL), 250
Mouse mammary tumor virus (MMTV),
  121, 182

N

Nonsmall cell lung carcinoma (NSCLC),
  74, 197
Nordihydroguaiaretic acid (NDGA), 221
Nuclear factor of activated T cells
  (NFAT), 108
Nuclear receptors
  androgen receptor signaling pathway,
    169–170
  estrogen receptor signaling pathways,
    168–169

O

Obesity
  adipocytokines, 53–54
  adipose tissue and insulin resistance
    adiponectin, 47
    interleukin–6, 45–46
    leptin, 47
    resistin, 46
    tumor necrosis factor alpha, 45
  breast cancer, 14

Index

and cancer, 39–40, 54–55
estrogen, 54–55
hyperglycemia and cancer, 50–51
hyperinsulinemia and cancer, 48–50
hyperlipidemia and cancer, 51–53
insulin resistance, 44–45
insulin signaling, 42–44
and type 2 diabetes, 38–39, 42
Osteosarcoma, 150

P

Pediatric preclinical testing program
(PPTP), 152
Pediatric sarcomas
clinical trials, 153–155
ESFT, 149–150
GIST, 151
IGF–1R antibody therapy, 152–153
IGF signaling pathway, 147–148
mTOR inhibitors, 153
osteosarcoma, 150
preclinical models, 152
rhabdomyosarcoma, 148–149
RMS xenograft growth, 152
synovial sarcomas, 151
TKIs, 152
Phosphatase and tensin homolog
(PTEN), 111
Phosphofrucktokinase2 (PFK2), 253
Phosphoinositide-dependent kinase 1
(PDK1), 106
Phosphoinositide–3-kinase (PI3K), 106
Phosphotyrosine-binding (PTB), 43
Picropodophyllin (PPP), 114, 183
Picropodophyllotoxin (PPP), 222
Platelet-derived growth factor receptor alpha
(PDGFRA), 151
Positron emission tomography (PET), 252
Postmenopausal breast cancer, 15–16
Prostate cancer, 128–129
aging, 30
AI disease, 85
carcinogenesis
castration resistant cells, 97
cixutumumab, 98
figitumumab therapy, 98
IGFBP–3 levels, 96
castration, 87–88
dihydrotestosterone, 87
IAP, 94
IGF-IR
androgen modulation, 90
AR phosphorylation, 90–91

AR signaling, 94–95
cell transformation, 89
inhibitor androgen synthesis, 86–87
nuclear translocation, 91–93
indirect evidence, 10
insulin receptor substrate–1 (IRS–1),
93–94
potential interaction, 88–89
serologic evidence
advanced and nonadvanced prostate
cancer, 12
diagnostic marker, 13
IGF–1 and risk, 11
IGFBP–3, 13
insulin and C-peptide levels, 13–14
low/high-grade, 12
Prostate carcinogenesis
castration resistant cells, 97
cixutumumab, 98
figitumumab therapy, 98
IGFBP–3 levels, 96
Prostate-specific antigen (PSA), 29
Prostatic intraepithelial neoplasia (PIN), 247
Pyrrolopyrimidines, 216–218
Pyrrolotriazines, 220–221

R

R1507, 201
Radiation therapy, 223
Receptor tyrosine kinases (RTKs), 106,
233, 250
Resistin, 46
Reverse tetracycline transactivator
(rtTA), 180
Rhabdomyosarcoma (RMS), 148–149

S

Sarcosine, 251
SCH717454, 201
Sex hormone binding globulin (SHBG), 49
Src homology collagen (SHC), 107
Synovial sarcomas, 151

T

Tamoxifen, 205
TATA-binding protein (TBP), 166
Tetracycline response element (TRE), 181
Thiazolidinediones, 58–59
2,4,6-Triaminopyrimidine, 221
Tuberous sclerosis complex (TSC), 234
Tumor necrosis factor-α, 45

Type 2 diabetes
  adipose tissue and insulin resistance
    adiponectin, 47
    interleukin–6, 45–46
    leptin, 47
    resistin, 46
    tumor necrosis factor alpha, 45
  cancer, 40–41
    hyperglycemia, 50–51
    hyperinsulinemia, 48–50
    hyperlipidemia, 51–53
  insulin analogues, 55–56
  insulin resistance, 44–45
  insulin signaling, 42–44
  metformin, 56–58
  obesity, 38–39, 42
  thiazolidinediones, 58–59

Tyrosine kinase inhibitors (TKIs), 130, 152, 216

V
Vascular endothelial growth factor (VEGF), 119, 193, 206
von-Hippel Lindau gene (VHL), 111, 160

W
Wilms tumor protein 1 (WT1), 110, 160
Wiskott–Aldrich syndrome protein (WASP), 114

X
X-box-binding protein–1 (XBP–1), 112